Sourcebook of
Occupational
Rehabilitation

Plenum Series in Rehabilitation and Health

SERIES EDITORS

Michael Feuerstein
Uniformed Services University of the Health Sciences (USUHS)
Bethesda, Maryland

and

Anthony J. Goreczny
University of Indianapolis
Indianapolis, Indiana

ENABLING ENVIRONMENTS: Measuring the Impact of Environment on
Disability and Rehabilitation
Edited by Edward Steinfeld and Gary Scott Danford

HANDBOOK OF HEALTH AND REHABILITATION PSYCHOLOGY
Edited by Anthony J. Goreczny

INTERACTIVE STAFF TRAINING: Rehabilitation Teams that Work
Patrick W. Corrigan and Stanley G. McCracken

SOURCEBOOK OF OCCUPATIONAL REHABILITATION
Edited by Phyllis M. King

A Continuation Order Plan is available for this series. A continuation order will bring delivery of each new volume immediately upon publication. Volumes are billed only upon actual shipment. For further information please contact the publisher.

Sourcebook of
Occupational
Rehabilitation

Edited by

Phyllis M. King
*University of Wisconsin
Milwaukee, Wisconsin*

Plenum Press • New York and London

Library of Congress Cataloging-in-Publication Data

Sourcebook of occupational rehabilitation / edited by Phyllis M. King.
        p.   cm. -- (Plenum series in rehabilitation and health)
    Includes bibliographical references and index.
    ISBN 0-306-45842-X
    1. Occupational diseases--Patients--Rehabilitation. 2. Industrial
accidents--Patients--Rehabiliatation. 3. Medical rehabilitation.
I. King, Phyllis M. II. Series.
RC964.S6665 1998
617.4'703--dc21   98-39286
                                                                     CIP

ISBN 0-306-45842-X

© 1998 Plenum Press, New York
A Division of Plenum Publishing Corporation
233 Spring Street, New York, N.Y. 10013

http://www.plenum.com

Printed in the United States of America

Contributors

Gunnar B. J. Andersson, Department of Orthopedic Surgery, Rush-Presbyterian–St. Luke's Medical Center, 1653 West Congress Parkway, Chicago, Illinois 60612

Donald S. Bloswick, Department of Mechanical Engineering, University of Utah, Salt Lake City, Utah 84112

Paula C. Bohr, Program in Occupational Therapy, Washington University School of Medicine, St. Louis, Missouri 63108

Robert E. Breslin, Center for Occupational Health, University of Cincinnati Medical Center, Cincinnati, Ohio 45267

Daniel M. Doleys, Pain and Rehabilitation Institute, Suite 200, 700 Monteclair Road, Birmingham, Alabama 35209

Thomas M. Domer, Schneidman, Myers, 700 West Michigan Avenue, Milwaukee, Wisconsin 53201-0442

Edward F. Ellingson, Zerrecon Inc., 1549 North 51st Street, Milwaukee, Wisconsin 53208

Robert B. Fillingim, Department of Psychology, University of Alabama at Birmingham, Birmingham, Alabama 35209

Lawrence P. Hanrahan, Wisconsin Division of Health and Departments of Industrial Engineering and Preventive Medicine, University of Wisconsin–Madison, Madison, Wisconsin 53703

Kurt T. Hegmann, Department of Preventive Medicine, Medical College of Wisconsin, Milwaukee, Wisconsin, 53226

Susan J. Isernhagen, Isernhagen & Associates, 1015 E. Superior Street, Duluth, Minnesota 55802

Brad Joseph, Ford Motor Company, 1500 Century Drive, Dearborn, Michigan 48210

Phyllis M. King, Occupational Therapy Program, University of Wisconsin–Milwaukee, Milwaukee, Wisconsin 53201

Joshua C. Klapow, Department of Psychology, University of Alabama at Birmingham, Birmingham, Alabama 35294

Deborah E. Lechner, Division of Physical Therapy, School of Health Related Professions, University of Alabama at Birmingham, Birmingham, Alabama 35294

Sally Maki, NovaCare, 260 East Highland Avenue, Milwaukee, Wisconsin 53151

Leonard N. Matheson, Occupational Therapy Program, Washington University School of Medicine, St. Louis, Missouri 63108

J. Steven Moore, Department of Nuclear Engineering, School of Rural Public Health, Texas A&M University, College Station, Texas 77843

Linda Ogden Niemeyer, Rehabilitation Technology Works, 2195 Club Center Drive, Suite G, San Bernardino, California 92408

Richard Perlman, Research Fellow, University of Birmingham, United Kingdom, and Department of Economics, University of Wisconsin–Milwaukee, Milwaukee, Wisconsin 53201

Lisa L. Perry, Anthem Blue Cross and Blue Shield, Suite 150, 8845 Governor's Hill Drive, Cincinnati, Ohio 45242

Jeffrey Rothman, Director of Physical Therapy Programs, College of Staten Island, City University of New York, Staten Island, New York 10314

Robin L. Saunders, The Saunders Group, 4250 Norex Drive, Chaska, Minnesota 55318

Donald E. Shrey, Department of Physical Medicine and Rehabilitation, University of Cincinnati Medical Center, Cincinnati, Ohio 45267

Roger O. Smith, Occupational Therapy Program, University of Wisconsin–Milwaukee, Milwaukee, Wisconsin 53201

Mark R. Stultz, Medronic Neurological, Advanced Pain Therapies, 800 53rd Avenue N.E., Minneapolis, Minnesota 55421

Anne K. Tramposh, Advantage Health Systems, 8704 Bourgade, Lenexa, Kansas 66216

Tim Villnave, Department of Mechanical Engineering, University of Utah, Salt Lake City, Utah 84112

Preface

The demand for effective occupational rehabilitation practices has never been greater. A multitude of factors are driving the need for more effective work-injury prevention and rehabilitation measures. The costs of treatment and compensation for work-related injuries continue to soar. Accelerated work demands, an aging workforce, and advancements in technology and information management set the stage for development, exacerbation, or maintenance of a variety of work-related health problems. These health problems, in turn, affect productivity, quality of life for the worker, and relations in the workplace.

This book covers concepts and practices related to the field of occupational rehabilitation. It synthesizes the knowledge of academia, clinical practice, and business to further the understanding of mechanisms and management of work-related disorders. It is intended to serve as a source of information and inspiration to those dedicated to work-injury prevention and management. The range of concepts—from prevention to rehabilitation—illustrates the depth, breadth, and impact of the field of occupational rehabilitation. Boundaries are not defined because the field continues to evolve and define best practice.

The book is divided into four parts: (1) "Forces Impacting Practice in Occupational Rehabilitation," (2) "Prevention of Work Injury," (3) "Assessment of Work-Related Disorders," and (4) "Rehabilitation of Work-Related Disorders." It acknowledges the contributions of multiple disciplines to the field of occupational rehabilitation. Each profession brings a unique perspective. However, it is through the combined efforts of these disciplines that strength is gained in acknowledging all aspects of care and an appreciation of the whole is realized.

Part I begins by examining the forces impacting practice in occupational rehabilitation. A consideration of the changing demographics of the workforce, with an aging population and an increase in female participation, addresses who this new work population is and what prevention and rehabilitation programs must be consider. Occupational and employment trends and the associations discovered between certain occupations and work-related disorders provide the context within which occupational rehabilitation practice now positions itself.

Rehabilitation professionals are often faced with decisions related to employee hiring, placement and retention, work restrictions, employee safety and injury prevention, and (for more severely disabled individuals) vocational rehabilitation, and benefits entitlement. Chapter 3 examines the legal context within which the professional must function.

Chapter 4 discusses reimbursement issues in an era of health care reform. Occupational rehabilitation is experiencing the transition from fee-for-service reimbursement to managed care. No longer is the patient the primary customer. Managed care has influenced practice — and will continue to do so. It behooves the occupational rehabilitation professional to be aware of these changing conditions.

Chapter 5 considers the forces active in the design of a continuum of care. This continuum is anchored on one end by the stage of prehire and on the other end by the stage of retire. Along the continuum is the constant matching of workers' functional abilities with ongoing analysis of the requirements of the job.

Part II examines a number of health promotion and injury-prevention strategies. Education and training are aimed at influencing human behavior. Likewise, wellness and fitness programs recognize the importance of lifestyle behavior and its effect on health. Both of these strategies support and encourage self-responsibility.

The application of ergonomics principles in the workplace is a prevention strategy that considers the interaction of a number of variables — the environment, the person, and the job. Preemployment and preplacement screening practices consider these same elements by matching human capabilities with job demands within legal parameters. Surveys and surveillance techniques are used to monitor the conditions of this matching and serve as a system that alerts all parties to potential health problems.

Prevention strategies have recently come under the spotlight as methods with significant potential to reduce costs incurred from work-related injuries and improve and promote health and safety in the workplace. A philosophy of prevention has far-reaching positive effects on individuals' personal and work lives. The full extent of these effects is yet to be realized.

Part III examines methods used to evaluate physical ability and the extent of impairment. Greater reliance on functional capacity evaluations for the determination of a disability and readiness to return to work has precipitated investigative activities aimed at identifying the most important features of a well-designed evaluation system and created a desire to standardize these practices as they are identified.

Fundamental to the practice of occupational rehabilitation is work analysis. Breaking down tasks into discrete performance components provides insight into functional abilities and potential health risks and hazards.

Part IV examines models of care and concepts in service delivery. A common thread that runs through the chapters in this section is the view that the workplace is an integral part of comprehensive intervention. Until recently, rehabilitation of work-related injuries has primarily been practiced outside the workplace. However, a plethora of recent research activities suggests variables inside the workplace play a vital role in the determination of return-to-work outcomes. With this awareness, rehabilitation providers have adapted their practice to include collaboration with employers. This scenario has given rise to on-site therapy programs and job modifications and accommodations performed at the worksite.

Actively involving the employer in a worker's rehabilitation introduces more players to the team. This change, coupled with the arrival of managed health care, has created a greater need for coordination of rehabilitation services. Case management, vocational rehabilitation, and disability management programs have responded to this need by expanding services.

Pain management and work rehabilitation programs have long recognized that rehabilitation is a multidimensional experience. Chapter 19 explicitly addresses the notion of the client being at the center of this perspective, and describes a model of human development that explores the linkages of occupational competence and motivation.

As we move into the twenty-first century, ongoing research efforts and the development of collaborative relationships between business and health care professionals will continue to give way to innovative approaches aimed at promoting health and safety in the workplace. As long as quality of life is a concern, and work holds meaning in people's lives, occupational rehabilitation will have a role to play.

Acknowledgments

This book is the realization of a vision supported by many people. I sincerely acknowledge and thank the contributors for sharing their time and expertise to convey a sense of the past, clarify the present, and offer insight into the future of the field of occupational rehabilitation. A special thank you to Michael Feuerstein for encouraging me to consider the breadth of this field and expand the contents of this book. I appreciate the support of my colleagues in academia at the University of Wisconsin–Milwaukee for providing an infrastructure conducive to the creation of this work. Organizational groups such as the Wisconsin Work Programs Network and the Occupational Injury Prevention and Rehabilitation Society have served as inspirations in modeling leadership and bringing together professionals from various disciplines to collaborate on research, education, and practice in the field of occupational rehabilitation. Consulting opportunities within the state of Wisconsin, particularly at Kohler Company, have fostered insight and provided valuable application experiences to enact best practices.

I thank Plenum Press for accepting the challenge of publishing this work. Their staff provided commendable professional service that made the production process a positive experience.

Finally, a heartfelt thank you to my husband, Ted, and my two sons, Brandon and Ted, who have been pillars of support.

Contents

I

FORCES IMPACTING PRACTICE IN OCCUPATIONAL REHABILITATION

1

The Changing Workplace

Richard Perlman and Phyllis M. King

Work is going global. Worldwide competition has accelerated and so have the demands of work. Coupled with these increased work demands are an aging workforce, advancements in technology, and a work environment characterized by ever-increasing cognitive and interpersonal complexity. Exposure to this interactive set of factors can set the stage for the development, exacerbation, or maintenance of a variety of work-related health problems. These problems in turn can affect productivity, cooperation within the workplace, workers' quality of life, and, ultimately, the extent of work disability (Feuerstein, 1991).

This chapter places the issue of work-related disorders within the broader context of a changing workforce and industrial and occupational employment trends. It prefaces a closer look, in the chapters that follow, at the associations between these factors and work-related disorders.

With a greater appreciation of the dynamics of these issues—particularly their interactions—the field of occupational rehabilitation can better understand the need for services and develop effective intervention strategies to maintain and/or improve health and safety in the changing world of work.

THE CHANGING WORKFORCE

One would probably be more surprised if the workforce composition had remained stable over the years rather than have changed. Nonetheless, the changes have been so dramatic that they warrant a close examination of their magnitude and the underlying forces that precipitated them, and recent trends in the changing workforce composition.

The two designations *workforce* and *composition* should be clarified at the outset.

Richard Perlman • Research Fellow, University of Birmingham, United Kingdom, and Department of Economics, University of Wisconsin–Milwaukee, Milwaukee, Wisconsin 53201.   **Phyllis M. King** • Occupational Therapy Program, University of Wisconsin–Milwaukee, Milwaukee, Wisconsin 53201.

Sourcebook of Occupational Rehabilitation, edited by Phyllis M. King. Plenum Press, New York, 1998.

Workforce, to be precise, refers to the technical labor statistic of the "labor force" (used hereafter interchangeably with workforce), which includes all those individuals 16 years of age and older, not in institutions, who are gainfully employed or unemployed at the time of the U.S. Labor Department's monthly estimates. Composition of the labor force, a much more vague and elusive term, describes the workforce through detailing its two components: who works and what they do.

"Who works" describes the changing pattern of two basic demographic categories—age and sex gender. Regarding age, the formal definition of the labor force eliminates a large group from consideration—children under 16. Everyone else, except those persons who are institutionalized (e.g., in prisons or nursing homes), is in the potential labor force. No explanation of sexual/gender categories is necessary.

In considering "what they do," discussion centers around the changing U.S. pattern of employment by industry and by occupational mix (related in part to the decline of labor unions) and the demographic aspects of workforce distribution.

"Who Works?"—The Labor Force

Before concentrating on the labor force itself, we should study the fundamental factor in its variations in relative size—the changing age composition of the overall population. The facts of the baby-boom bulge and the aging of America are well known, but the details of these phenomena are still impressive. From a study of the overall population change, we move to the labor force, examining changes in the Labor Force Participation Rate (LFPR) (defined when discussed), comparing this rate with that of other advanced economies, and noting the relative changes among demographic groups.

The U.S. Population, 1950–1995

Over a 45-year period, 1950–1995, the U.S. population rose from 152.3 million to 263.0 million (figures rounded to the nearest hundred thousand). Expressed in relative terms, it rose 72.7%, or at an annual rate of about 1.2%, which is not especially noteworthy. But when we look at population changes for specific age groups, we find significant deviation from the overall slightly upward trend; these variations have an important impact on the age composition of the current and future labor force.

As Table 1.1, which includes only those individuals 16 and over, the potential labor

Table 1.1. U.S. Population by Potential Labor Force

Year	Population total	Age group (%)			
		16–24	25–44	45–64	65 and over
1950	109.1*	20.2**	45.7	30.8	12.4
1965	131.6	27.3	46.9	38.9	18.5
1980	172.5	38.8	63.5	44.5	25.7
1995	201.5	32.3	83.5	52.2	33.5
% change	84.7	59.9	82.7	69.5	270.2

*Population totals rounded to the nearest hundred thousand. **Percentage of growth for each age group rounded to the nearest one-tenth.
SOURCE: Economic Report of the President (1996), *Annual Report of the Council of Economic Advisors*, Washington, DC: U.S. Government Printing Office.

force, illustrates the most dramatic change occurs in the oldest group (65 and over), those least likely to participate in the labor force. The explanation of this sharp divergence from the overall growth trend is not difficult to find: It is the steady long-run growth in the average life span, resulting from improvements in health care and the promotion and practice of healthier lifestyles. The dramatic increase among the 65 and over age group has nothing to do with baby boomers, the large group born in the post–World War II period. The oldest of these baby boomers is now about 50 years old. They now are mainly described as the 25–44 age group. The large relative growth in that group since 1965 is also noteworthy, indicating that the aging of the total population will carry through well into the twenty-first century. The significance of the aging population on the workforce relates to the formal definition of the labor force itself, which as mentioned earlier consists of those 16 years of age and over (not in institutions), and the basic statistic of labor force activity, in the Labor Force Participation Rate (LFPR), which equals

$$\frac{\text{Labor Force (LF)}}{\text{Labor Force Potential (LFP)}}$$

The Labor Force Participation Rate (LFPR) and Its Composition by Sex

Because the conventional retirement age remains at 65, although Social Security is gradually raising its full-benefit age to 67, the aging of the population imposes a strong negative influence on the LFPR. An increasing number of older people who do not tend to be active participants in the world of work are included in the labor force potential.

Despite this strong negative effect of the aging of the U.S. population, the overall U.S. LFPR has experienced steady but slow growth over the period from 1950 to the late 1980s and has stabilized since. The source of this stabilizing force, which counteracts the negative effect of the aging of the population, is the strong growth in the female participation rates, at least until about 1990. (See Table 1.2, which presents the overall LFPRs and gender categories.)

The main reason for the decline in the male rate has already been noted: the aging of the population with an expanded group (65 and over) who are voluntarily out of the

Table 1.2. Labor Force Participation
Rates (LFPRs) Overall
and by Gender

Year	LFPRs all civilian workers (%)	LFPRs by gender (%)	
		Male	Female
1950	59.2*	86.4	33.9
1965	58.9	80.7	39.3
1980	63.8	77.4	51.5
1990	66.4	76.1	57.5
1995	66.6	75.0	58.9

*LFPRs rounded to the nearest one-tenth.
Source: Economic Report of the President (1996), p. 321. *Annual Report of the Council of Economic Advisors*, Washington, DC: U.S. Government Printing Office.

labor force. But females are aging, too. Obviously, then, their LFPR must have risen because of a sharp growth in participation by women of conventional working age. Several reasons for this increase can be offered.

1. The slowdown in growth and the actual decline in real wages, giving impetus to the two-worker household.
2. The greatly improved link between the education of women and the world of work. Long gone are the old-fashioned women's colleges that in effect steered women away from work.
3. The change in the industrial and occupational mix (to be discussed in the next section) from jobs that were physically demanding to those requiring white-collar skill development and higher education.

The most dramatic changes in participation among large-scale demographic groups appeared among women. Table 1.3 further breaks down this group's demographic data to include marital status and children's ages. Probably the most significant aspect of this table is the recent extremely high participation rate of women with children. (In comparing data from Tables 1.2 and 1.3, we note that only single women with children under 6 years of age have a lower rate than women as a whole.) The need for income is a driving force behind these statistics, with the burden of child care having somewhat of a negative influence on participation. (Note the higher rate for women with children 6 to 17, which for the year 1995 exceeds the overall male rate, except for the single women subgroup.) Leading to the high 1995 LFPR for women with children was the very strong growth

**Table 1.3. Labor Force Participation
Rates (LFPRs) for Women
with Children by Age
of Child and Marital Status**

Children under 6

	LFPRs by marital status (%)		
Year	Single	Married	Widowed, separated, divorced
1960	n/a	18.6	40.3
1970	n/a	30.3	52.1
1980	44.1	45.1	60.1
1990	48.7	58.9	62.0
1995	53.0	63.5	64.2
Children 6 to 17			
1960	n/a	39.0	65.9
1970	n/a	49.2	66.9
1980	67.6	61.7	74.6
1990	64.7	67.8	79.7
1995	67.0	76.2	79.5

*LFPRs rounded to nearest one-tenth.
SOURCE: U.S. Department of Commerce, Bureaus of the Census, (1996), *Statistical Abstract of the United States*, Washington, DC: U.S. Government Printing Office.

shown over the last generation. This growth was driven by the two factors: changing employment mix and increasing need for household income.

When comparing participation rates internationally, the dominant variable is female participation. Table 1.4 illustrates that among advanced industrial economies the overall LFPRs are very similar for those with more or less the same female rates, but the rates tend to be much lower for these with significantly lower female rate (e.g., the LFPR of Italy). By inference, these results indicate a similarity among male participation rates.

At first view, Table 1.4 seems to indicate an unusual result. For one half of the countries the female participation rate is higher than the overall LFPR (to say nothing of the fact that the female participation rate for the United States is reported above its level in Table 1.2). But these oddities are easily explained. The overall data of Table 1.4 refer to all those over the minimum labor force potential age. The female data cuts off their potential at age 65, reinforcing an earlier point—the aging of the population depresses the labor force participation rate, as it is defined.

THE CHANGING WORKPLACE

The Changing Industrial Mix

The change in U.S. industrial production has gone in one direction for a century, away from goods to services. This movement shows no signs of slowing down. Before discussing this pattern and its causes in greater detail, it is fitting to examine the reasons why an extremely low percentage of workers are involved in the basic industry of agriculture. Farmers now make up less than 2% of the U.S. workforce and have been near that level for many years. The United States is not alone in having a small farm population; all advanced industrial economies share this pattern. In fact, if one were asked to

Table 1.4. Labor Force Participation Rates (LFPRs)—Overall and Female Rates among Selected Highly Developed Industrial Economies in 1994

Country	LFPR (%)	Female participation rate (%)
United States	66.6*	63.7
Australia	63.9	63.2
Canada	65.3	67.6
France	56.0	59.5
Germany	53.7	61.6
Italy	47.5	43.2
Japan	63.1	62.1
Netherlands	59.5	57.1
Sweden	63.9	74.4
United Kingdom	62.8	65.4

*All participation rates rounded to the nearest one-tenth.
SOURCE: U.S. Department of Commerce, Bureau of the Census, *Statistical Abstract of the United States* (1996), p. 84. Washington, DC: U.S. Government Printing Office.

determine whether a country was highly developed and were allowed to ask one indirect question before making that determination, one should ask what percentage of the country's workers are in agriculture. A country's stage of industrial development will be inversely related to the percentage of workers employed in farming.

Why is this so? The answer lies in significant advances in agricultural technology and even more in the substitutability of machines for human labor in agriculture. With development and industrial opportunities, every potential rise in farm wages leads to the use of machinery in place of labor, because, in agriculture, machinery and labor are easily substitutable.

The trend from goods to services seems to be accelerating, as seen in Table 1.5. Furthermore, the data understate the movement away from production to services. Within the goods-producing industries themselves, there are undoubtedly a growing number of workers who are in services—in market research, office work, technical writing, and so on.

We can dramatize the movement away from production by taking a close look at the basic goods-producing industry—manufacturing. In 1965, there were 18 million workers engaged in manufacturing. In 1996, this number remained the same. In 1965, this number represented 29.7% of nonfarm workers. In 1996, it represented only 15.3% of the labor force, or a decline of almost one half of its share of total employment.

Are we headed toward an economy in which no one makes anything? Will manufacturing consist of the 2% of the labor force as does agriculture? Probably not. But the same factors that reduced agricultural employment are at work lowering the number of workers making commodities—advanced technology. As a country increases its use of technology, its labor force moves from farming to making goods to professional and managerial services, for which there are fewer technological advances that permit the substitution of machines for these services.

Government work is an interesting service industry. It is a popular belief that the large number of workers in government services merely reflects a growing bureaucracy. Such is not the case. The term *bureaucracy* generally refers to a superfluous workforce of

Table 1.5. Percentage of Total Employment by Industry Group, 1950–1996

Year	Goods producing*	Service producing**
1950	40.9	59.1
1960	37.7	62.3
1970	33.2	66.8
1980	28.4	71.6
1990	25.1	74.9
1996	20.3	79.7

*Includes mining, construction, and manufacturing. **Includes transportation and public utilities, wholesale and retail trade, finance, insurance, real estate, and government. Source: U.S. Department of Labor, Bureau of Labor Statistics, *Employment and Earnings* (January 1997), p. 44. Washington, DC: U.S. Government Printing Office.

federal workers in redundant agencies. But the data on government employment do not substantiate this belief. In 1960, government workers accounted for just under 25% of all service workers, with federal workers at about 7% of the total, state workers under 5%, and local workers above 13%. In 1996, the overall percentage of all government workers was a little over 20% of the service industry, down somewhat from 1960. The federal, state, and local government workforces broke out at 2.9%, 4.8%, and 12.5%, respectively. Thus, the only significant relative loss of positions was among federal workers. Presently, over 60% of all government workers are employed at the local level.

The Changing Occupational Mix

As one would expect, just as employment has moved from production to services, the occupational pattern of the American labor force has shifted from jobs involved in making goods to those providing services. At the outset, we should note the differences between a *service industry* and a *service occupation*, as officially classified. The industrial classification of services is much broader; a hospital is listed as a service industry, a nurse is listed as a professional, and an orderly is classified as having a service occupation.

Table 1.6 presents the details of the altered patterns of the occupational mix by broad category over a 13-year period, 1983–1996. The trends that had been in place for decades prior to that period have not slowed down. The table shows a continued

Table 1.6. Percentage of Employment by Occupation, 1983–1996

	1983	1996
Total employed (millions)	100.8	126.7
Percent	100	100
Managerial and professions specialty	23.4	28.8
Executive, administrative, managerial	10.7	14.0
Professional specialty	12.7	14.8
Technical, sales, and administrative support	31.0	29.8
Technicians and related support	3.0	3.1
Sales occupation	11.7	12.2
Administration support, including clerical	16.3	14.5
Service occupations	13.7	13.6
Private household	0.9	0.6
Protective service	1.7	1.7
Other services*	11.1	11.3
Precision production, craft, and repairs	12.2	10.7
Operation, fabricators, and laborers	16.0	14.4
Machine operators, assemblers, and inspectors	7.7	6.2
Transportation and material moving occupation	4.2	4.2
Handlers, equipment cleaners, etc.	4.1	4.0
Farming, forestry and fishing	2.8	2.8

*Among other services the largest are food preparation and service, health aides, and building janitors and cleaners.
SOURCE: U.S. Department of Commerce, Bureau of the Census (1996), *Statistical Abstract of the United States*, pp. 405–407. Washington, DC: U.S. Government Printing Office; U.S. Department of Labor, Bureau of Labor Statistics (January 1997), *Employment and Earnings*, January, p. 170. Washington, DC: U.S. Government Printing Office.

movement toward managerial and professional fields away from lower-skilled production occupations.

An important feature of the labor market can be deduced from the occupational mix presented in Table 1.6. The decline in unionism is a current issue inherent within the context of the occupational patterns of the labor force.

The Decline in Unionism

Union membership grew from a low of about 7% of the labor force during the early 1930s to 25% in 1955. Growth was stimulated by prolabor legislation, specifically by the National Labor Relations Act (Wagner Act) passed in 1935, during the first administration of Franklin Roosevelt. No longer did union membership indicate boldness; in fact, in some settings that had closed shops (union membership required at hiring), nonmembership almost indicated irrational worker behavior.

From this high of 25%, the United States union membership gradually declined over the next 25 years to 20% in 1980. This slow attrition in union membership can be attributed to the changing occupational distribution of the labor force. Managers and professionals were (and are) not prime candidates for unionization. Workers who are— production workers in a large-scale manufacturing setting, for example—are a declining segment of the workforce. From 1980 to 1990 union membership in the United States fell to about 13% of the workforce before it stabilized. The gradual change in the occupational mix is not the single causal factor for this sharp decline from an already low level.

What was behind this recent membership decline was not new antiunion legislation, but the stricter application of old laws and court decisions under the promanagement administrations of the 1980s. For example, a 1938 Supreme Count decision allowed firms to replace striking workers with permanent replacements, not just strikebreakers. This replacement worker option was not practiced until the 1980s. Now, striking workers have an added worry to their loss of pay—loss of job.

Summary

Important features of labor force demographics include the relative stability of the overall participation rate for the workers over 40 years of age and the large growth in female participation in the work force (especially the unemployment rate among married women with children during times of greater prosperity).

An important feature of labor force demographics is the recent stability of the overall LFPR after a steady rise during the previous 40 years. At present, this rate is among the highest for advanced economies.

As for the strong growth in female participation, certainly changing industrial-occupational patterns and improved education opportunities for women entering the workforce have been important. But so too is the growing need for higher household income; witness the fact that the current participation rate for women with dependent children is higher than the overall rate for men in many age categories.

Important features of the changing nature of work are the shift from a goods-producing to a service-producing economy and the consequent occupational shift toward employment in managerial/professional and technical fields. As our economy continued on its inexorable path toward further development, it was inevitable that the production pattern would move more toward the servicing-producing and away from the goods-producing industries. (This movement reflects the path of developing countries, in general.) In fact, government data probably understate the change in as much as many workers in goods-producing industries are not production workers.

In keeping with these developments, the occupational mix has also changed, with a relative rise in employment of those in professional and managerial occupations.

The movement away from production work partially explains the decline of union membership in the United States. But this weakness in labor organization has also been caused by a recent promanagement climate that led to the application of long-dormant legal powers to weaken the union movement.

WORK DISABILITY

The epidemiology of work disability represents an area characterized by problems of definition, measurement, conceptualization, and methodology. Despite these problems, the data that do exist indicate that work disability in general is a prevalent problem (Feuerstein, 1991). The number of noninstitutionalized people in the United States with a work disability is estimated to be 16.9 million, which represents 10.1% of the working age population (16 to 64 years old). Work disability increases in frequency with age. For 16–24 years, 4.2% are work disabled; for 25–34 years, the proportion rises to 6.4%; for 35–44 years, 9.4%; from 45–54 years, 13.3%; and for 55–64 years, 22.9% are work disabled (LaPlante, 1995).

According to another data source, the National Health Interview Survey (1990–1992), the chronic health condition most frequently reported to cause work limitation is heart disease, 2.1 million conditions, followed by orthopedic impairment of the back or neck, 2.0 million; intervertebral disk disorders, 1.5 million; osteoarthritis and allied disorders, 1.3 million; and orthopedic impairment of the lower extremities at 861,000 (LaPlante, 1996).

Work-Related Disorders

Work-related disorders are typically conditions of multiple etiology in which work is a significant contributory factor in some or all cases. They may occur in a wide variety of working populations (Pheasant, 1991). The World Health Organization expert committee described "work- related" diseases as multifactorial, with the work environment and the performance of work contributing significantly, but as two of a number of factors to the causation of disease and disorders:

> They may be partially caused by adverse working conditions; they may be aggravated, accelerated or exacerbated by workplace exposures; and they may impair working capacity. It is important to remember that personal characteristics, other environmental and socio-cultural factors usually play a role as risk factors for these diseases. (WHO, 1985)

These factors have not been studied simultaneously with equal rigor in any scientific investigations. The identification of risk factors and causality remains a complex task.

Nevertheless, annual reports on occupational injuries and illnesses published by the

U.S. Department of Labor's Bureau of Labor Statistics present revealing information on the prevalence of work-related disorders associated with various occupational categories. The categories with the highest incidence and severity rates become the target and priority for intervention efforts aimed at identifying and eliminating risk factors that cause injury and illness.

Occupational Injuries and Illnesses

Occupational injuries and illnesses contribute to work disability. Over the past 20 years, the number of reported occupational injuries and illnesses has generally decreased, but the impact of these injuries and illnesses has greatly increased. In 1972, 10.9 cases of occupational injury or illness were recorded for every 100 full-time workers. By 1994, that incidence rate had dropped to 8.4 cases per 100 workers. In 1972, occupational injuries and illnesses caused 47.9 lost work days per 100 workers, whereas by 1991, the rate had increased to 86.5 lost workdays per 100 workers. Figure 1.1 graphically depicts these trends.

According to a 1995 survey by the Bureau of Labor Statistics, the incidence rates for injuries and illnesses (per 100 full-time workers) has declined in private industry over the past several years. Figure 1.2 shows the rates by industry division from 1992 thru 1995. Among goods-producing industries, manufacturing had the highest incidence rate in 1995 (11.6 cases per 100 full-time workers), followed by construction (10.6 cases per 100 full-time workers). Within the service-producing sector, the highest incidence rate in 1995 was reported for transportation and public utilities (9.1 cases per 100 full-time workers),

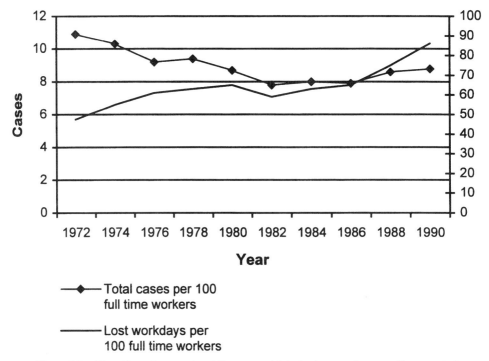

Figure 1.1. The effect of occupational illnesses and injuries increased over an 8-year period.

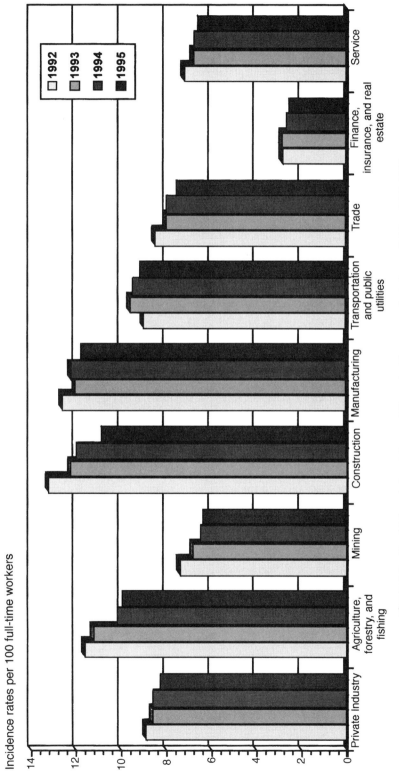

Figure 1.2. Nonfatal workplace injury and illness incidence rates by industry division, 1992–1995.

followed by retail and wholesale trade (7.5 cases per 100 workers). These records reflect not only the year's injury and illness experience, but also each employer's understanding of which cases were work-related under current record keeping guidelines set by the U.S. Department of Labor. The number of injuries and illnesses reported in any given year also can be influenced by changes in the level of economic activity, working conditions and work practices, worker experience and training, and the number of hours worked.

Injuries

In considering recent statistics, of the 6.6 million nonfatal injuries and illnesses that occurred in 1995, nearly 6.1 million were injuries that resulted in either lost work time, medical treatment other than first aid, loss of consciousness, restriction of work or motion, or transfer to another job. Injury rates generally were higher for midsize employers (50 to 249 workers) than for smaller or larger employers.

Illnesses

There were approximately 495,000 newly reported cases of occupational illnesses in private industry in 1995. Manufacturing accounted for slightly more than three fifths of these cases. Sixty-two percent (308,000) of the workplace illnesses were disorders associated with repeated trauma, such as carpal tunnel syndrome. This is slightly down from the 332,000 repeated trauma cases reported in 1994 (see Figure 1.3).

Lost-Work Time Injuries and Illnesses

Work-related disorders, such as carpal tunnel syndrome, hernias, amputations, fractures and sprains and strains, commonly keep workers off the job for several weeks. Table 1.7 provides a breakdown of the number of work-related cases and days away from work for each of these disorders from a 1995 survey by the United States Department of Labor's Bureau of Labor Statistics. The number of days away from work to recover from a particular type of injury largely reflects differences in the severity of injuries, individual recuperation times, and availability of light or restricted work activities.

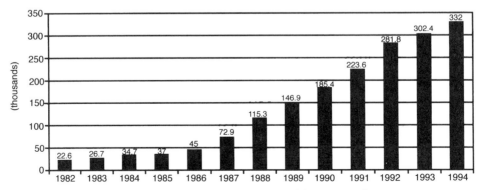

Figure 1.3. Repeated trauma cases reported by private industry.

Table 1.7. Selected Injuries or Illnesses:
Number of Work-Related Cases and Days Away from Work, 1995

Disabling condition	Total cases**	Percentage of total cases involving				Median days away from work*
		Under 3 days	3–10 days	11–20 days	21 days or more	
Total	2,040,929**	30†	34	11	24	5
Carpal tunnel syndrome	31,457	7	18	14	6	30
Hernia	30,482	5	16	25	54	22
Amputation	11,308	10	22	18	50	21
Fracture	124,601	14	25	14	46	18
Sprain, strain	876,792	27	38	12	23	5
Cut, laceration	153,193	43	35	10	13	3
Chemical burn	13,861	52	34	7	7	2

*Median workdays lost is the point at which half the injuries and illnesses involved more lost workdays and half involved fewer days. **The total number of cases involving days away from work includes data for disabling conditions in addition to the seven conditions shown separately. †Because of rounding percentages may not add to 100.
SOURCE: U.S. Department of Labor, Bureau of Labor Statistics (March 1998). *Occupational Injuries and Illnesses: Counts, Rates, and Characteristics, 1995.* Bulletin no. 2483. Washington, DC: U.S. Government Printing Office.

Gender and Occupation Relationships

Gender

Data on the four most disabling conditions shown in Table 1.7 can be further analyzed with respect to gender and occupation relationships. Men were more likely than women to experience three of the four types of severe injuries, but women suffering from carpal tunnel syndrome outnumbered men. Table 1.8 indicates that women workers make up the majority (seven tenths) of the lost-work-time cases involving carpal tunnel syndrome, compared with less than one tenth of the case totals for hernias and amputations and one fourth of all fractures. Surprisingly, the majority of women sustained carpal tunnel syndrome from operating machinery, performing assembly line tasks, and working in retail stores, as opposed to the most often thought of office environment. Nationally, women were about one third of the 2 million with injuries and illnesses in 1995 that caused days away from work.

Occupation

Workers' risks of sustaining injuries in occupations involving clerical and sales duties, operating or repairing machinery, making fabric products on assembly lines, moving material by hand or truck, cleaning and maintaining buildings, and staffing construction sites appear particularly high (see Table 1.9). Assemblers' share of total lost work time and illnesses (2.7%), for example, was twice their share of total private wage and salary employment (1.3%). Their share of carpal tunnel syndrome cases, however, was 8%.

A closer look at the survey data reveals differences in the manner in which workers sustain severe injuries (see Table 1.9). Virtually all cases of carpal tunnel syndrome resulted from stress or strain on a workers' wrists because of the respective nature of the tasks they perform. By contrast, about three fifths of work-related amputations are the

Table 1.8. Profiles for Four Types of Injuries Resulting in Lengthy Absences from Work, by Occupations Most Often Affected and Ways in Which Injury Occurred, 1995*

CARPAL TUNNEL SYNDROME		AMPUTATION	
Number of cases	31,457	Number of cases	11,308
Percent	100	Percent	100
Sex of injured	100	Sex of injured	100
Female	71	Female	9
Male	28	Male	90
Occupation	100	Occupation	100
Clerical and other administrative support	22	Machine operator	30
Data-entry keyer	4	Sawing machine	3
Secretary	3	Punching and stamping press	2
General office clerk	2	Precision production and craft	27
Machine operator	21	Carpenter	3
Sewing machine operator	4	Industrial machinery repairer	3
All other occupations	57	Butcher and meatcutter	2
Assembler	8	All other occupations	43
Laborer, exc. Construction	3	Laborer, exc. Construction	6
Cashier	2	Assembler	4
Sales supervisor	2	Truckdriver	3
Event or exposure	100	Construction laborer	8
Repetitive motion, all types	99	Event or exposure	100
Placing, grasping, exc. tool	26	Caught in, compressed by equipment,	
Typing or keyentry	22	machinery, or object(s)	61
Use of tool(s)	14	Struck by object(s)	19
All other events, exposures	1	Struck against object(s)	13
		All other events, exposures	8

HERNIA		FRACTURE	
Number of cases	30,482	Number of cases	124,601
Percent	100	Percent	100
Sex of injured	100	Sex of injured	100
Female	7	Female	25
Male	93	Male	74
Occupation	100	Occupation	100
Operator, fabricator, and laborer	45	Handler, helper, and laborer	16
Truckdriver	8	Laborer, exc. construction	6
Laborer, exc. construction	6	Construction laborer	4
Assembler	3	Transportation, material handling	12
Welder and cutter	3	Truckdriver	9
Precision procution, craft	27	Construction trade	10
Carpenter	3	Carpenter	3
Butcher and meatcutter	2	Machine operator	10
All other occupations	29	All other occupations	51
Cook	3	Janitor and cleaner	2
Janitor and cleaner	3	Assembler	2
Event or exposure	100	Miscellaneous food preparer	2
Overexertion, all types	86	Event or exposure	100
Lifting	60	Fall, all types	43
Pulling or pushing	13	Fall from ladder	5
Holding, carrying, turning	7	Struck against object(s)	27
All other events, exposures	14	Caught in, compressed by equipment,	
Bodily reaction (e.g., slip)		machinery, or object(s)	13
	5	All other events, exposures	17

*Each profile is a percent distribution of cases involving days away from work. The four disabling conditions are part of the BLS nature-of-injury-and-illness classification structure, issured in 1992. Because of rounding and omitted subcategories, percentages may not add to 100.
SOURCE: U.S. Department of Labor, Bureau of Labor Statistics (March 1998). *Occupational Injuries and Illnesses: Counts, Rates, and Characteristics, 1995*. Bulletin no. 2483. Washington, DC: U.S. Government Printing Office.

**Table 1.9. The Manner in Which Workers Sustained Injuries and Illnesses,
Resulting in Days Away from Work, 1992–1995**

Event or exposure*	Percentage of distribution (1995 cases)	Cases per 10,000 workers			
		1992	1993	1994	1995
Total	100**	305	286	277	250
Bodily reaction and exertion	43	135	128	121	109
Overexertion	27	86	81	76	69
Bodily reaction, e.g., slip, twist	10	34	32	30	26
Repetitive motion	4	12	12	12	10
Contact with objects and equipment	28	83	78	75	69
Struck by object(s)	13	39	37	36	33
Struck against object(s)	7	22	21	20	18
Caught in or compressed by equipment or object(s)	5	13	12	12	12
Fall	17	49	47	49	42
Fall on same level	11	31	31	33	28
Fall to lower level	5	15	14	14	13
Exposure to harmful substances(s) or environment(s)	5	15	14	14	13
Transportation incident	4	9	9	10	9
Highway accident	2	5	5	6	6
Assault and violent act	1	4	3	3	4
Assault by person(s)	1	3	3	3	3

*Total and broad event or exposure categories may include data for classifictions in addition to those shown separately.
**Because of rounding and because of classification not shown, percentages may not add to 100.
SOURCE: U.S. Department of Labor, Bureau of Labor Statistics (March, 1998). *Occupational Injuries and Illnesses: Counts, Rates, and Characteristics, 1995.* Bulletin no. 2483. Washington, DC: U.S. Goverment Printing Office.

result of a workers' fingers being caught in or compressed by machinery or an object such as a wire reel or printing press. Seven-eighths of all hernias were the result of an overexertion, primarily while lifting heavy objects.

CONCLUSION

The profile of a changing workforce and the overview of work-related disorders presented in this chapter require further analysis of associations between all the variables mentioned. Researchers are presently studying these perceived linkages in an effort to identify associated risk factors and ultimately prevent injuries and illnesses from occurring.

The occupational rehabilitation professional is better positioned to make informed decisions regarding the present nature and future of occupational rehabilitation by considering demographic changes in the workforce (e.g., an aging population and an increase in female participation) and occupational and employment trends (e.g., a shift from goods- to service-producing industries and a rise in the employment of a professional and managerial workforce) and the associations between these trends and work-related disorders.

REFERENCES

Economic Report of the Present (1996). *Annual report of the Council of Economic Advisors.* Washington, DC: U.S. Government Printing Office.

Feuerstein, M. (1991). A multidisciplinary approach to the prevention, evaluation, and rehabilitation of work disability. *Journal of Occupational Rehabilitation, 1*(1), 5-12.

LaPlante, M. (1995). *Chartbook on disability in the United States: An Info Use Report.* Washington, DC: National Institute on Disability and Rehabilitation Research.

LaPlante, M. (1996). *Data on disability from the National Health Interview Survey: 1990-1992. An Info Use Report.* Washington, DC: National Institute on Disability and Rehabilitation Research.

Pheasant, S. (1991). *Ergonomics, work and health.* Gaithersburg, MD: Aspen.

U.S. Department of Commerce, Bureau of the Census (1996). *Statistical Abstract of the United States.* Washington, DC: U.S. Government Printing Office.

U.S. Department of Labor, Bureau of Labor Statistics (1997). *Employment and earnings.* Washington, DC: U.S. Government Printing Office.

U.S. Department of Labor, Bureau of Labor Statistics (March, 1998). *Occupational injuries and illnesses: Counts, rates, and characteristics, 1995.* Bulletin No. 2483. Washington, DC: U.S. Government Printing Office.

World Health Organization. (1985). *Identification and control of work-related disorders* (Technical Report Services No. 714). Geneva: WHO.

2

Common Neuromusculoskeletal Disorders

Kurt T. Hegmann and J. Steven Moore

Neuromusculoskeletal disorders have high rates of prevalence and in composite are the most common reason to seek medical treatment. They are also commonly encountered in the occupational setting even without taking into account the potential contribution of workplace factors. Many of these problems appear clinically as acute disorders with a typically acute onset of symptoms. However, the pathophysiology of the disorders would indicate a chronic degenerative process. Thus, they appear best classified as diseases rather than injuries. Epidemiologic studies defining many of these disorders as occupational in etiology are weak or absent. Nevertheless, the inability to perform work often is a primary motivator for seeking medical care from occupational health professionals.

TRIGGER FINGER AND TRIGGER THUMB

The formal medical label for trigger finger or trigger thumb is stenosing tenosynovitis of the digits. Stenosing means that a structure is abnormally narrowed. Although tenosynovitis technically implies inflammation of a tendon sheath, the actual change is in thickness. Taken together, *stenosing tenosynovitis* means that part of the tendon sheath is narrowed secondary to thickening. Many tendon sheaths located throughout the body are susceptible to stenosing tenosynovitis. When stenosing tenosynovitis affects the flexor tendon sheath of one of the fingers, the condition is called *trigger finger*. When it affects the thumb, it is called *trigger thumb*.

Kurt T. Hegmann • Department of Preventive Medicine, Medical College of Wisconsin, Milwaukee, Wisconsin 53226.   **J. Steven Moore** • Department of Nuclear Engineering, School of Rural Public Health, Texas A&M University, College Station, Texas 77843-3133.

Sourcebook of Occupational Rehabilitation, edited by Phyllis M. King. Plenum Press, New York, 1998.

Anatomy and Function

The muscles that flex the fingers and one of the muscles that flexes the thumb are located on the flexor side of the forearm. The tendons that connect the ends of these muscles to the bones in the fingers are shaped like cords. For each finger, two flexor tendons run together along the palm side of the finger. The anatomy for the thumb is similar. A synovial sheath can be visualized as a tubular, balloon-like structure filled with a low-viscosity fluid (synovial fluid). The tendons (cords) are aligned with the balloon. As the cords are pressed into the balloon, the balloon wraps around the cords. As the cords move back and forth, the fluid inside the balloon reduces friction. In addition to the synovial sheath, there is a series of ligaments, called *pulleys*, that loop around the tendons and their synovial sheath. These pulleys hold the tendons close to the bones and joints. If you were on the tendon looking toward the pulley, you would see a tunnel. The underlying bone is the floor of the tunnel. The pulley makes up the walls and the roof of the tunnel. Stenosing tenosynovitis is a disorder that affects one of these tunnels. In particular, it affects the tunnel formed by the A1 pulley. The finger A1 pulleys are located approximately at the level of the distal crease in the palm.

Pathology

With trigger finger or trigger thumb, the A1 pulley appears thick and fibrous (Compere, 1933). As the pulley thickens, it reduces the cross-sectional area of the tunnel (stenosis). When the tunnel becomes too narrow, the tendons no longer move freely through the tunnel and may develop a nodular deformity (Compere, 1933; Zelle & Schnepp, 1936). Fibrocartilaginous metaplasia, a change characteristic of compression, has been observed (Sampson, Badalamente, Hurst, & Seidman, 1991). Because the flexor muscles are stronger than the extensor muscles, someone with trigger finger is usually able to flex the digit but has difficulty extending it. The result is snapping or locking (called *triggering*) that occurs when the flexed finger or thumb is straightened (Sperling, 1951).

Pathogenesis

Current theory suggests that the thickening of the A1 pulley is an adaptation to repeated or prolonged tension on the A1 pulley by the flexor tendons. According to biomechanical theory, this tension is primarily related to the degree of bending of the joint and the degree of tension (also called *loading*) in the tendon (e.g., loaded tendons turning corners) (Hume, Hutchinson, Jaeger, & Hunter, 1991). Maximum tensions in the A1 pulley appear to occur with extreme bending of the joint at the base of the finger (Hume et al., 1991). At this time, it is not known how high this pulley tension must be, how many times it must be experienced, or how long it must last before thickening of the A1 pulley begins.

Presentation, Symptoms, and Signs

For most people, trigger finger or trigger thumb develops gradually, but in some cases it may follow acute trauma (Compere, 1933; Sperling, 1951). Snapping, locking, or difficulty extending a flexed finger or thumb, often accompanied by discomfort or pain, are the most prominent symptoms (Compere, 1933). The snapping sensation may barely be perceptible without any actual triggering; or it may be painful, especially when a triggered digit is forcefully extended (Sperling, 1951). The triggering and pain are localized to an area in the palm where the digit joins the hand (Compere, 1933; Renard, Jacques, Chammas, Poirier, Bonifaci, Jaffiol, & Allieu, 1994; Sampson, Badalamente, Hurst, & Seidman, 1991; Sperling, 1956; Zelle & Schnepp, 1936). Some people report more difficulties in the morning compared with other times (Sperling, 1951). It may be possible for an examiner to feel a nodule on the tendon in the region of the A1 pulley as well as detect a clicking or snapping sensation with movement of the digit (Compere, 1933; Sperling, 1951).

DeQUERVAIN'S TENOSYNOVITIS

DeQuervain's tenosynovitis is a disorder that is very similar to trigger finger and trigger thumb. It is also a form of stenosing tenosynovitis, but it occurs along the thumb side of the wrist instead of the palm side of the finger or thumb.

Anatomy and Function

Most of the muscles that control the wrist and fingers anchor at the elbow or on the forearm bones. The tendons that connect these muscles to the bones out in the wrist and fingers are, like the finger flexor tendons, shaped like cords. As these tendons cross the wrist joint, they enter tunnels. On the extensor side of the wrist, the tendons crossing the wrist pass through six tunnels. These are called the six dorsal or extensor compartments. The first dorsal compartment is on the thumb side of the wrist. DeQuervain's tenosynovitis is stenosing tenosynovitis of the first dorsal compartment.

The tendon sheath for the first dorsal compartment is located at the end of the radius—the forearm bone on the thumb side. Two muscles that control the thumb, the abductor pollicis longus (APL) and extensor pollicis brevis (EPB), originate on the shaft of the radius in the forearm. The APL inserts on the backside of the first metacarpal bone (the bone that runs between the wrist and the thumb) just beyond the wrist. The EPB inserts on the backside of the proximal phalanx of the thumb (the first bone forming the shaft of the thumb) just beyond the MP joint (at the base of the thumb). These two muscles control the position and orientation of the thumb so the thumb can be used to grip, pinch, or press. These tendons normally glide freely through the tunnel of the first dorsal compartment.

Pathology

The primary change is a thickening of the roof of the tunnel (the extensor retinaculum) that results in narrowing of the tunnel (Conklin & White, 1960; Cotton, Morrison, & Bradford, 1938; Diack & Trommald, 1939; Eichoff, 1927; Finkelstein, 1930; Flörcken, 1912; Griffiths, 1952; Kelly & Jacobsen, 1964; Keppler, 1917; Lamphier, Crooker, & Crooker, 1965; Lipscomb, 1944; Michaelis, 1912; Muckart, 1964; Nussbaum, 1917; Patterson, 1936; Reschke, 1919–1920; Schneider, 1928; Stein, 1927; Younghusband & Black, 1963). Fibrocartilaginous metaplasia has also been observed (Troell, 1921; Wood, 1941). Functional impairment is believed to be caused by impaired gliding of the tendons within the tunnel (Cotton et al., 1938; Eichoff, 1927; Eschle, 1924; Finkelstein, 1930; Patterson, 1936; Reschke, 1919–1929; Wood, 1941).

Pathogenesis

Like trigger finger and trigger thumb, it is generally believed that the changes related to DeQuervain's tenosynovitis are a result of loaded tendons turning corners (Cotton et al., 1938; Eichoff, 1927; Griffiths, 1952; Moore, 1997; Wood, 1941). The APL and EPB tendons are loaded whenever the thumb is used. These tendons turn a corner when the wrist or the thumb is bent.

Presentation, Symptoms, and Signs

The onset of DeQuervain's tenosynovitis is usually gradual (Cotton et al., 1938; Diack & Trommald, 1939; Finkelstein, 1930; Lamphier et al., 1966; Muckart, 1964; Patterson, 1936; Schneider, 1928; Younghusband & Black, 1963). The most common symptom is pain localized on the thumb side of the wrist (Conklin & White, 1960; Cotton et al., 1938; Diack & Trommald, 1939; Finkelstein, 1930; Griffiths, 1952; Kelly & Jacobsen, 1964; Lamphier et al., 1965; Lipscomb, 1944; Muckart, 1964; Schneider, 1928; Stein, 1927; Troell, 1921; Younghusband & Black, 1963). The intensity of the pain varies, but it may be severe enough to keep a person awake at night (Cotton et al., 1938; Diack & Trommald, Finkelstein, 1930; Kelly & Jacobsen, 1964; Lamphier et al., 1965; Schneider, 1928; Stein, 1927; Troell, 1921). It also increases with pinching, grasping, sticking the thumb out to the side (the hitchhiking signal), and bending the wrist toward the little finger (Cotton et al., 1938; Diack & Trommald, 1939; Finkelstein, 1930; Griffiths, 1952; Kelly & Jacobsen, 1964; Muckart, 1964; Patterson, 1936; Schneider, 1928; Stein, 1927; Troell, 1921; Wood, 1941; Younghusband & Black, 1963). The pain may be severe enough to render the hand nonfunctional (Conklin & White, 1960; Cotton et al., 1938; Diack & Trommald, 1939; Finkelstein, 1930; Kelly & Jacobsen, 1964; Lamphier et al., 1965; Schneider, 1928; Troell, 1921; Younghusband & Black, 1963). There may be slight swelling at the thumb side of the wrist, and full but sometimes painful ranges of motion of the wrist and thumb (Cotton et al., 1938; Diack & Trommald, 1939; Finkelstein, 1930; Kelly & Jacobsen, 1964; Patterson, 1936; Schneider, 1928; Stein, 1927; Wood, 1941). Firm touching may result in tenderness at the thumb side of the wrist (Conklin & White, 1960; Cotton et al., 1938; Diack & Trommald, 1939; Finkelstein, 1930; Griffiths, 1952; Lamphier et al., 1965; Muckart, 1964; Patterson, 1936; Schneider, 1928; Stein, 1927; Wood, 1941; Younghusband & Black, 1963). There generally should be no sensation of creaking, called *crepitus*. Crepitus nearly always suggests a different disorder, called *peritendinitis*. Stretching or contraction of the APL or EPB muscles increases the pain (Cotton et al., 1938; Diack & Trommald, 1939; Finkelstein, 1930; Griffiths, 1952; Lamphier et al., 1965; Patterson, 1936; Schneider, 1928; Stein, 1927; Troell, 1921). A maneuver called *Finkelstein's test* is the most characteristic physical sign. This test is typically performed by having the patient flex the thumb and wrapping the other digits around the thumb; the health care provider then grasps the fist and deviates the wrist ulnarly (Finkelstein, 1930). Exquisite pain along the first dorsal compartment indicates a positive test.

PERITENDINITIS

The myotendinous junction is where a muscle joins its tendon. It is a specialized anatomical structure whose purpose is to transmit a muscle's tension to its tendon when it contracts. There is a myotendinous junction at the end of each muscle cell. The end of the muscle cell has numerous fingerlike projections that match up to similar projections from the tendon (Garrett & Tidball, 1988). This structure reduces stresses to the cell membrane of the muscle cells while maximizing the transmission of tension from the muscle to the tendon (Garrett & Tidball, 1988; Tidball & Daniel, 1986).

The myotendinous junction appears to be the structure involved in two types of conditions, muscle strains and peritendinitis. (Muscle strains will not be discussed here.) Peritendinitis is a condition that is widely recognized in other parts of the world but has not been discussed much in the United States since the 1940s. It appears that most cases of peritendinitis in the United States are mislabeled as "tendinitis" or "tenosynovitis."

More than half the cases of peritendinitis affect the same muscles involved in DeQuervain's tenosynovitis, the APL and EPB, but the location of the problem is more in the forearm (an inch or two toward the elbow) rather than at the wrist. Other commonly affected muscles are wrist extensors (also located on the back of the forearm).

Pathology

The problem is localized to the myotendinous junction. There is usually edema, hyperemia and inflammation (Howard, 1937, 1938; Rais, 1961; Thompson, Plewes, & Shaw, 1951). The surface of the muscle and tendon may be covered with a sticky substance called *fibrin* (Howard, 1937, 1938). The tendon and tendon sheath beyond the myotendinous junction appear normal (Howard, 1937, 1938; Rais, 1961; Thompson et al., 1951).

Pathogenesis

It is generally accepted that peritendinitis develops due to fatigue and exhaustion of selected muscle groups or direct trauma (Blood, 1942; Flowerdew & Bode, 1942; Howard, 1937, 1938; Rais, 1961; Thompson et al., 1951). Both factors lead to swelling, inflammation, and the deposition of fibrin around the myotendinous junction (Rais, 1961).

Presentation, Symptoms, and Signs

Pain, aching, soreness, and tenderness—sometimes severe—are the dominant symptoms (Flowerdew & Bode, 1942; Howard, 1937, 1938). These symptoms are localized to the mid-forearm, a few inches above the wrist (Blood, 1942; Flowerdew & Bode, 1942; Howard, 1937, 1938). Some patients may report crepitation in this area (Flowerdew & Bode, 1942; Howard, 1937, 1938; Thompson et al., 1951). Crepitation is a "creaking gate" noise or sensation associated with movement of the affected structures. The affected area may be swollen, red, warm, or tender to touch (Flowerdew & Bode, 1942; Garrett & Tidball, 1988; Howard, 1937, 1938; Thompson et al., 1951; Tidball & Daniel, 1986). It is usually painful to stretch or contract the affected muscle (Howard, 1937, 1938; Thompson et al., 1951).

LATERAL EPICONDYLITIS

The medical term for "tennis elbow" is *lateral epicondylitis.* The lateral epicondyle is the bony prominence located on the outer (lateral) side of the elbow when the arm is held along the side of the body and the palm facing forward. There is also a bony prominence on the inner (medial) side of the elbow called the medial epicondyle. When someone has pain localized to the medial epicondyle, the condition is called *medial epicondylitis* (also, "golfer's elbow"). Lateral epicondylitis is far more common than medial epicondylitis, and there is much less published information about medial epicondylitis; therefore, this section will focus on lateral epicondylitis.

Anatomy and Function

Two muscles primarily stabilize, extend, and deviate the wrist from side to side. The extensor carpi radialis longus (ECRL) originates just above the elbow and inserts on the backside of the base of the second metacarpal bone (just beyond the wrist). The extensor carpi radialis brevis (ECRB) originates primarily from the lateral epicondyle and inserts on the backside of the base of the third metacarpal bone (just beyond the wrist). Whenever the fingers are used to grasp or pinch something, there is simultaneous contraction of the wrist extensor muscles (cocontraction). This contraction stabilizes the wrist joint so that the wrist does not flex when the fingers forcefully grip or press on something.

Pathology

The pathology of lateral epicondylitis is not precisely known. The ECRB appears to be the most commonly involved structure. The tendon near the origin of the ECRB may appear normal from the outside but usually has some abnormal tissue on the underside (Goldie, 1964; Nirschl & Pettrone, 1979). A tear of the tendon is sometimes observed (Goldie, 1964; Nirschl & Pettrone, 1979). The nature of these changes as well as those observed under a microscope suggest that something rubs the underside of this tendon, frays some of the tendon's fibers, and the body tries to repair this damage (Chard, Cawston, Riley, Gresham, & Hazleman, 1994; Doran, Gresham, Rushton, & Watson, 1990; Goldberg, Abraham, & Siegel, 1988; Regan, Wold, Coonrad, & Morrey, 1992).

Pathogenesis

Why lateral epicondylitis develops is generally unknown. For cases that occur after blunt trauma to the elbow, it is believed that the trauma injured some of the fibers in the ECRB tendon. For nontraumatic cases, several researchers have postulated that microtears occur following repeated exertions (Dimberg, 1987; Kivi, 1982; Maffulli, Regine, Carrillo, Capasso, & Minella, 1990; Nirschl, 1974; Wadsworth, 1987). It has also been suggested that one of the forearm bones (the radial head) may rub the underside of the ECRB tendon (Moore, 1996). This action would most likely occur when the hand grasps an object, the elbow is extended, and the forearm rotates (pronates and supinates), as when using a screwdriver. Lateral epicondylitis does not appear to be a typical degenerative condition related to aging (Allander, 1947; Goldie, 1964), although some age-related influence may be present as the peak prevalences occur in the fourth and fifth decades of life.

Presentation, Symptoms, and Signs

Lateral epicondylitis usually presents as pain at the lateral side of the elbow (Coues, 1914; Dimberg, 1987; Goldberg et al,. 1988; Goldie, 1964; Hansson & Norwich, 1930; Kivi,

1982; Osgood, 1922; Wadsworth, 1987). The onset may be sudden or gradual (Coues, 1914; Dimberg, 1987; Goldie, 1964; Hansson & Norwich, 1930; Osgood, 1922; Wadsworth, 1987). The intensity of the pain varies (Coues, 1914; Goldie, 1964; Hansson & Norwich, 1930; Osgood, 1922). Relatively minor levels may be described as "discomfort," while more intense levels may be described as "sharp," "severe," or "lightning-like." The pain often limits activities of daily living (such as lifting a coffee cup or jar), leisure pursuits (gardening or sports), and work (both heavy and sedentary) (Coues, 1914; Duran et al., 1990; Goldie, 1964; Hansson & Norwich, 1930; Osgood, 1922; Wadsworth, 1987). There is usually tenderness localized at or near the lateral epicondyle (Coues, 1914; Duran et al., 1990; Goldie, 1964; Hansson & Norwich, 1930; Kivi, 1982; Osgood, 1922; Regan et al., 1992; Wadsworth, 1987). Gripping forcefully, pulling the wrist or long finger back against resistance (extension), having the elbow straight with the forearm turned inward and wrist bent forward, or resisting the rotation of the forearm inward and outward increases the pain (Coues, 1914; Duran et al., 1990; Goldie, 1964; Hansson & Norwich, 1930; Maffulli et al., 1990; Osgood, 1922; Wadsworth, 1987). Elbow extension or forearm pronation may be limited (Allander, 1947; Coues, 1914; Dimberg, 1987; Goldie, 1964; Hansson & Norwich, 1930; Maffulli et al., 1990; Moore, 1996; Osgood, 1922; Wadsworth, 1987). Grip strength and wrist extension strength may be reduced (Coues, 1914; Goldberg et al., 1988; Goldie, 1964; Kivi, 1982; Wadsworth, 1987).

CARPAL TUNNEL SYNDROME

Carpal tunnel syndrome is the most complex and controversial of the distal upper extremity disorders.

Anatomy and Function

The carpal tunnel is located on the palm side of the hand. The floor and walls are formed by the carpal bones; the roof is formed by a thick ligament, called the transverse carpal ligament. Normal contents of the carpal tunnel include two flexor tendons for each of the four fingers, one flexor tendon for the thumb, and the median nerve. As in other tunnels, these nine tendons within the carpal tunnel are covered by tendon sheaths.

Pathology

The tendon sheaths covering the nine tendons are often reported to be thickened (Cseuz, Thomas, Lambert, Love & Lipscomb, 1966; Lipscomb, 1959; Phalen, 1966; Phalen & Kendrick, 1957; Tanzer, 1957; Yamaguchi, Lipscomb, & Soule, 1965). The thickening appears to be related to swelling (edema) or scarring (fibrosis) within the tendon sheaths. Although these changes are often described as tenosynovitis, inflammation does not appear to be involved (Faithfull, Moir & Ireland, 1986; Fuchs, Nathan, & Myers, 1991; Neal, McManners, & Stirling, 1987; Schuind, Ventura, & Pasteels, 1990). The cause(s) of these changes are generally unknown and do not appear to differ whether the condition is believed to be work related or not.

The median nerve often looks normal, but individual nerve fibers inside the nerve may be affected. Most of the individual nerve fibers are covered by an insulation-like material called *myelin sheaths*. At the site of compression, this insulation appears pushed off the nerve fiber under the area of compression (Ochan & Marotte, 1973). Since this insulation is necessary for the fast conduction of nerve impulses, its loss contributes to slow (or delayed) nerve conduction, as measured during an electrodiagnostic test.

The symptoms of carpal tunnel syndrome are usually explained based on impaired circulation to the median nerve inside the carpal tunnel when intracarpal pressure is elevated (Cailliet, 1988; Dahlin & Rydevic, 1991; Dawson, Haillet, & Millender, 1990; Fullerton, 1963; Gilliatt & Wilson, 1953; Lundborg & Dahlin, 1989; Szabo & Gelberman, 1987; Thomas & Fullerton, 1963). When intracarpal pressure is elevated to a relatively high level for a sufficient period of time, circulation inside the nerve is stopped. Individual nerve fibers begin to spontaneously discharge and produce unusual sensations of numbness and tingling, called *paresthesias*. When intracarpal pressure is lowered, blood flow returns, spontaneous nerve discharges end, and the paresthesias end.

Pathogenesis

At this time, it is not possible to reliably state why carpal tunnel syndrome develops in a given person. There are several possible mechanisms that might be related to hand usage and numerous others that would include factors unrelated to hand usage (Moore, 1996). Some of the possible hand usage models include (1) thickening of the tendon sheaths inside the carpal tunnel, (2) hypertrophy (enlargement) of the tendons that pass through the carpal tunnel, (3) direct pressure on the median nerve by the flexor tendons when using the fingers with a flexed wrist, (4) retraction of some small hand muscles (lumbricals) into the carpal tunnel when forming a tight fist, (5) thickening of the transverse carpal ligament in response to tension from "loaded flexor tendons turning a corner" at the wrist (wrist flexion), (6) alterations within the nerve secondary to repeated or prolonged episodes of elevated intracarpal pressure, (7) traction or friction related to disproportionate movement of the tendons relative to the median nerve, and (8) bruising the median nerve within the carpal tunnel secondary to direct trauma or using the palm of the hand as a hammer. Which of these models is correct, if any, is currently unknown.

Presentation, Symptoms, and Signs

Excluding acute trauma, symptom onset is usually gradual and often related to unaccustomed activity (Bevin, 1986; Birkbeck & Beer, 1975; Brain, Wright, & Wilkinson, 1947; Cannon & Love, 1946; Crow, 1960; Eason, Belsole, & Greene, 1985; Gainer & Nogent, 1977; Garland, Bradshaw, & clark, 1957; Kendall, 1950, 1960; Nugent, 1980; Phalen, 1951, 1966, 1970, 1972; Phalan, Gardner, & La Londe, 1950; Rosenbaum & Ochoa, 1993; Tanzer, 1957; Upton & McComas, 1973; Vicale & Scarff, 1951; Yamaguchi et al., 1965). The dominant symptom is numbness or tingling, paresthesias (Bevin, 1986; Brain et al., 1947; Cannon & Love, 1946; Crow, 1960; Crymble, 1968; Dekel, Papaioannou, Rushworth, & Coates, 1980; Doyle & Carroll, 1968; Falck & Aarnio, 1983; Garland et al., 1957; Gelberman, Hergenroeder, Hargens, Lundborg, & Akeson, 1981; Goga, 1990; Hamlin & Lehman, 1967; Healthfield, 1957; Hybbinetee & Mannerfelt, 1975; Inglis, Straub, & Williams, 1972; Kaplan, Glickel, & Eaton, 1990; Katz, Larson, Sabra, Drarup, Stirrat, Sethi, Eaton, Fossel, & Liang, 1990; Kendall, 1950, 1960; Kremer, Gilliatt, Golding, & Wilson, 1953; Lipscomb, 1959; Love, 1955; Maslar, Hayesand, & Hyde, 1986; Nathan, Kenistion, Meyers, & Meadows, 1992; Newman, 1948; Nugent, 1980; Phalen, 1951, 1966, 1970, 1972;

Phalen et al., 1950; Phalen & Kendric, 1957; Rosenbaum & Ochoa, 1993; Shivde, Dreizin, & Fisher, 1981; Tanzer, 1957; Upton & McComas, 1973; Vainio, 1957; Vicale & Scarff, 1951; Yamaguchi et al., 1965). Pain or weakness is uncommon, although intense paresthesias may be reported as painful. Typically, the paresthesias affect the thumb, index, long, and part of the ring finger, but should spare the little finger (Doyle & Carroll, 1968; Falck & Aarnio, 1983; Hamlin & Lehman, 1967; Healthfield, 1957; Hybbinette & Mannerfelt, 1975; Katz & Stirrate, 1990; Kendall, 1950; Kremer et al., 1953; Lipscomb, 1959; Love, 1955; Nugent, 1980; Phalen, 1951, 1966, 1970, 1972; Phalen & Kendrick, 1957; Rosenbaum & Ochoa, 1993; Tanzer, 1957; Vainio, 1957; Vicale & Scarff, 1951). Symptoms may radiate into the forearm, elbow, arm, or shoulder (Crymble, 1968; Eason et al., 1985; Falck & Aarnio, 1983; Gainer & Nugent, 1977; Garland et al., 1957; Hamlin & Lehman, 1967; Healthfield, 1957; Kendall, 1960; Kremer et al., 1953; Lipscomb, 1959; Newman, 1948; Nugent, 1980; Phalen, 1966, 1970, 1972; Rosenbaum & Ochoa, 1993; Upton & McComas, 1973). Typically, the paresthesias occur at night or with static grasp and are usually relieved by changing position or shaking the affected hand(s) (Bevin, 1986; Doyle & Carroll, 1968; Falck & Aarnio, 1983; Goga, 1990; Hamlin & Lehman, 1967; Healthfield, 1957; Hybbinette & Mannerfelt, 1975; Kaplan et al., 1990; Kendall, 1960; Kremer et al., 1953; Lipscomb, 1959; Murray & Simpson, 1958; Newman, 1948; Nugent, 1980; Phalen, 1951, 1966, 1970, 1972; Phalen et al., 1950, 1951; Phalen & Kendrick, 1957; Rosenbaum & Ochoa, 1993; Vainio, 1957; Yamaguchi et al., 1965). Even though Phalen's test and Tinel's sign are commonly performed and reported, there are no physical findings considered reliable (Gelimers, 1979; Gellman, Gelberman, Tan, & Botte, 1986; Goodman & Gilliatt, 1961; Healthfield, 1957; Johnson, Wells, & Duran, 1962; Kaplan et al., 1990; Katz, Larson, Fossel, & Liang, 1991; Katz et al., 1990; Kendall, 1960; Lipscomb, 1959; Rosenbaum & Ochoa, 1993; Seror, 1987; Shivde et al., 1981; Stewart & Eisen, 1978; Tanzer, 1957; Thomas, Lambert, & Czeuz, 1967; Van Rossum, Kamphuisen, & Wintzen, 1980; Wand, 1990; Wertsch & Melvin, 1982; Yamaguchi et al., 1965). Phalen's test involves passive flexion of the wrists to 90° for 60 seconds. If the patient reports paresthesias in the median nerve distribution during this time interval, the test is considered positive. Tinel's sign involves tapping the skin overlying any peripheral nerve. For carpal tunnel syndrome, this tapping is done on the flexor side of the wrist and palm. Production of paresthesias in the distribution of the peripheral nerve is considered a positive test. Electrodiagnostic studies, often called *nerve conduction studies* or *EMGs*, are the best way to confirm the presence of carpal tunnel syndrome (American Academy of Electrodiagnostic Medicine et. al., 1993; Boniface, Morris, & Macleod, 1994; Buch-Jaeger & Foucher, 1994; Cioni, Passero, Paradiso, Giannini, Battistini, & Ruchworth, 1989; Dorwart, 1984; Falck & Aarnio, 1983; Goodman & Gilliatt, 1961; Goodwill, 1965; Johnson & Melvin, 1967; Johnson et al., 1982; Kimura, 1989; Nathan et al., 1992; Ross & Kimura, 1995; Seror, 1987; Stevens, 1987; Thomas et al., 1967; Van Rossum et al., 1980; Winn & Habes, 1990; Yamaguchi, Lipscomb, & Soule, 1965).

ULNAR NEUROPATHY AT THE ELBOW AND CUBITAL TUNNEL SYNDROME

Nontraumatic ulnar nerve neuropathies are substantially more common than radial nerve disorders, but less common than median nerve disorders (Mumenthaler, 1974). The two principal sites for ulnar neuropathies are at the elbow and at the wrist, although entrapment may occur at any point along the nerve.

Anatomy and Function

The ulnar nerve is located along the medial aspect of the elbow and crosses the elbow at the condylar groove prior to entering the cubital tunnel. The ulnar nerve generally supplies sensory function to the fifth digit, ulnar half of the fourth digit, and ulnar portion of the hand; exceptions are anatomical variants. The ulnar nerve is also the principal motor nerve for the hand, supplying the innervation for all but four muscles. The cubital tunnel, through which the ulnar nerve passes just distal to the elbow, is principally formed by the aponeurotic origins of the flexor carpi ulnaris. Unlike the carpal tunnel, the cubital tunnel does not have tendon and tendon sheaths occupying this space; the ulnar nerve is the only substantial occupant of this tunnel. Ulnar neuropathy at the elbow is likely to occur at either the retrocondylar groove or in the cubital tunnel.

Pathology

In contrast with carpal tunnel syndrome, there is a lack of significant research into the pathological bases for ulnar neuropathies at the elbow. Some researchers have reported finding evidence of fibers compressing the nerve proximal to the cubital tunnel, while others have reported finding compression distally (Inglis & Kinnett, 1978). Numerous case reports of neuropathy secondary to anatomic defects, including those resulting from trauma, ganglia, arthritides, and vascular anomalies, have been cited. The microscopic changes to the nerve fibers are believed to be the same as those for carpal tunnel syndrome (Ochoa & Marotte, 1973). One group of investigators reported an association with the anconeus epitrochlearis muscle or the cubital tunnel retinaculum, felt to be a remnant of the same muscle (O'Driscoll, Horii, Carmichael, & Morrey, 1991). The demyelination of the ulnar nerve is the change that is measurable by electrodiagnostic testing.

Symptoms are believed to develop in a manner similar to that of carpal tunnel syndrome. Impaired circulation is thought to result in paresthesias, while return of normal blood flow typically results in resolution of these symptoms.

Pathogenesis

Research into the development of ulnar neuropathies at the elbow is quite preliminary. Basic questions regarding occupational and nonoccupational risk factors have not been addressed. The previously outlined theoretical models for the development of carpal tunnel syndrome cannot be applied in nearly all instances because of the lack of tendons and tendon sheaths accompanying the nerve in the region of the elbow. Instead, the following theoretical models may be substituted: (1) recurrent subluxation (congenital or acquired) of the ulnar nerve out of the condylar groove upon elbow flexion (condylar groove ulnar neuropathy), (2) ulnar nerve compression or traction by flexing an elbow with a tight condylar groove (condylar groove ulnar neuropathy), (3) mechanical impingement of the edge of the flexor carpi ulnaris with simultaneous elbow flexion and exertion of force (cubital tunnel syndrome), (4) thickening of the flexor carpi ulnaris aponeurosis (cubital tunnel syndrome), and (5) external compression (ulnar nerve compression at both sites). As with carpal tunnel syndrome, the correct model(s) is (are) not known.

Presentation, Symptoms and Signs

Symptoms typically begin gradually with paresthesias in the distribution of the ulnar nerve. Occasionally, patients report awakening one specific morning with the symptoms and without resolution of the symptoms. Pain appears to be reported more frequently than it is in carpal tunnel syndrome, and radiation of pain from the elbow down to the wrist or fifth finger may occur. Nocturnal awakening occurs, but increased symptoms with static grasping are atypical. Physical examination findings (such as the elbow flexion test and Tinel's sign) are unreliable. The physical examination maneuver usually performed is the elbow flexion test (Buehler & Thayer, 1988). This test is performed by having the patient hyperflex the elbow while simultaneously extending the wrists to try to provoke the symptoms within 60 seconds. Weakness in the distribution of the ulnar nerve may occur, but it is typically a late finding (Vanderpool, Chalmers, Lamb, & Whiston, 1968).

Electrodiagnostic studies, particularly nerve conduction studies, are utilized to confirm the presence of an ulnar neuropathy at the elbow as well as to localize the area of delayed conduction to the condylar groove, cubital tunnel, or a much less common area.

ULNAR NEUROPATHY AT THE WRIST

Ulnar neuropathies at the wrist are less common than those of the elbow (Mumenthaler, 1974), and thus are far less common than carpal tunnel syndrome.

Anatomy and Function

The ulnar nerve is medial to and outside of the carpal tunnel. It is in close proximity to the ulnar artery, embedded in subcutaneous adipose tissue above the carpal tunnel and its flexor retinaculum. The ulnar nerve at the wrist is neither related to an anatomical tunnel nor is it accompanied by tendons and tendon sheaths as it crosses the wrist joint.

Pathogenesis

Many case reports on ulnar neuropathies at the wrist have focused on blunt trauma to the hypothenar eminence, sometimes repeated, as an etiology for this disorder. Other commonly found anatomical defects attributed to the development of these problems are ganglia, residua of trauma, and vascular anomalies. One of the pathophysiologic mechanisms is believed to involve a traumatic thrombosis of the ulnar nerve in this area, with resultant paresthesias, presumably on the basis of poor vascular supply to the nerve. The following theoretical models may be considered for nonacute traumatic ulnar neuropathy at the wrist: (1) repeated blunt trauma to the hypothenar area induces thrombosis or other vascular changes to impair blood flow to the ulnar nerve; and (2) repeated local mechanical compression deforms the nerve sheath.

Presentation, Symptoms, and Signs

Symptoms are usually the same as those for ulnar neuropathy at the elbow with the exceptions that pain in the area of the elbow is uncommon, and pain in the hypothenar eminence region may be present, particularly if there has been recurrent blunt trauma.

The physical examination is again generally unreliable, and electrodiagnostic studies are utilized to confirm the presence of an ulnar neuropathy at the wrist and to localize the precise area of delayed conduction (Urbaniak & Roth, 1982).

SHOULDER TENDINITIS

Rotator cuff tendinitis is perhaps the most vexing problem in neuromusculoskeletal medicine. Not only is it a progressive degenerative disorder, but it also tends to be recurrently symptomatic. From a clinical perspective, it is difficult to manage symptomatically. It is also difficult, if not impossible, to alter progression. It is the second most costly problem in workers' compensation systems, after low back pain.

Anatomy and Function

The rotator cuff complex of disorders is considered to include supraspinatus tendinitis, other rotator cuff tendinitides, subacromial bursitis, and the impingement syndrome. Some authors would include bicipital tendinitis of the long head of the biceps as part of this constellation of disorders. Despite these different names, these disorders are closely linked, and in some cases, probably synonymous.

There are four tendons and four respective muscles (supraspinatus, infraspinatus, teres minor, and subscapularis) that comprise the rotator cuff. They form an arc (cuff) of fibrous material (an aponeurosis) that connects and holds the arm to the torso and helps control rotation of the arm; thus, the composite anatomical structure is called the *rotator cuff*. From a medical standpoint, the supraspinatus is the key tendon, as nearly all pathological problems originate in this tendon (Codman, 1934; Cotton & Rideout, 1964; Keyes, 1935; Wilson & Duff, 1943). The subacromial bursa, normally a structure filled with a small amount of lubricating fluid, is located immediately above and adjacent to the supraspinatus tendon.

The supraspinatus tendon is prone to rupture from one to two centimeters from its insertion on the greater tuberosity of the humerus (Cotton & Rideout, 1964; Wilson & Duff, 1943). The reason for this propensity toward rupture is unclear, but it is believed to be related to vascular insufficiency (Lindblom, 1939; Rathbun & MacNab, 1970; Rothman & Parke, 1965). A competing theory suggests that the reason involves mechanical abrasion or impingement of the tissue between the bones of the shoulder joint (Neer, 1972, 1983).

Pathology

Numerous studies have consistently demonstrated that degeneration of the supraspinatus tendon and occurrence of supraspinatus tendon ruptures increase with age (Codman, 1938; Cotton & Rideout, 1964; Keyes, 1935; Wilson & Duff, 1943). Lifetime risk appears to be at least 30% (Cotton & Rideout, 1964), making this tendon rupture the most common, followed by the long head of the biceps, and rupture of the Achilles.

Gross anatomical changes observed in the rotator cuff include degeneration and fibrillation of the supraspinatus tendon (Codman, 1938; Cotton & Rideout, 1964; Keyes, 1935; Wilson & Duff, 1943). This change also appears to parallel abnormal morphology of the acromion process, which becomes progressively more abnormal as the degree of rotator cuff changes becomes more aberrant (Bigliani, Ticker, Flatow, Soslowsky, & Mow, 1991; Neer, 1972, 1983; Nicholson, Goodman, Flatow, & Bigliani, 1996). However, which condition leads to the other has not been established. Additional progressive changes that have been observed as part of this process are scarring (fibrosis) of the subacromial bursa, cellular degeneration, and deposits of calcium in the supraspinatus tendon (Rathbun & MacNab, 1970).

The microvascular anatomy of the supraspinatus has been found to be substantially deficient in adults; it decreases further with age in most studies performed (Lindblom, 1939; Rathbun & MacNab, 1970; Rothman & Parke, 1965), but not all (Moseley & Goldie, 1963) . The area of the tendon with the most deficient blood supply is located approximately two centimeters from the insertion on the humeral head, which coincides with the area prone to rupture. Thus, the disorder appears to be due, at least in part, to a deficient blood supply to the tendon. The bicipital tendon has also been found to have a deficient microvascular blood supply in its area of typical rupture (Rathbun & MacNab, 1970).

Pathogenesis

It is well known that any injured area with a poor blood supply does not heal well. Thus, it should not be surprising that a tendon without a sufficient blood supply is predisposed to progressive degeneration and rupture. This theory of rotator cuff tendinitis/rupture development could solely explain the disorder. However, another theory—the impingement theory (Neer, 1972, 1983)—is under consideration. This theory holds that there is a mechanical pinching of the tendon between the bones of the shoulder joint (head of the humerus and acromion process) (Neer, 1972, 1983). Impingement would require abduction or forward flexion of the shoulder to provoke the mechanical pinching of the supraspinatus tendon and the generation of the disorder. It is also possible that both theories are in part correct, and it is a combined effect that produces the pathological condition. This pinching might lead to disruption of the collagen fibers of the tendon, but healing is impaired by inadequate blood supply.

Presentation, Symptoms, and Signs

Rotator cuff tendinitis typically presents as a gradual onset of shoulder joint pain. The pain tends to be deep, boring, and aching. It generally does not cause neck symptoms or radiate beyond the upper arm. Paresthesias do not normally accompany the disorder. Sleep disturbance due to pain is common, and use of the arm above 90° of abduction or forward flexion is also painful, although not infrequently, pain also occurs with lesser degrees of abduction or forward flexion. Occasionally, a slight "catching" sensation is present, though true locking of the joint should be absent.

A complete tear of the supraspinatus tendon will generally occur in only one of three settings: (1) significant trauma, such as falling on the arm, particularly if the patient is over 40 years of age; (2) after a long history of rotator cuff tendinitis, whether symptomatic or not (necessitating older ages, particularly beyond 60 years, although occurring at younger ages); and (3) accompanying marked exertions, such as baseball pitchers (virtually excluding more typical occupational settings) (Codman, 1938; Neer, 1972).

If a complete rupture has occurred, it is usually accompanied by sudden muscular weakness and substantial pain. (The principle exception is gradual onset in the oldest age group.) Although supraspinatus tendinitis results in a slow improvement of symptoms with time, those with a ruptured tendon are particularly prone to a protracted course of recovery with poor improvement in symptoms and physical limitations.

Physical examination will often demonstrate a reduced range of motion limited by pain. Pain will occur with progressively greater abduction or forward flexion, although pain frequently occurs with internal and external rotation as well. Tenderness on palpation is unreliable. The most characteristic physical examination maneuver utilized is the supraspinatus test. This test involves resisted simultaneous forward flexion to 90° with abduction of 30°, complete internal rotation, and extended elbows; symptoms of shoulder joint pain equal to or possibly worse than that already experienced should be reproduced. The second physical examination procedure frequently used is the impingement sign. This test involves passive forward flexion of the arm while the spine of the scapula is fixed to prevent its movement. A positive test causes reproduction or magnification of pain. Neck motion is typically normal and pain free. Distal neurological functions, including muscle strength and deep tendon reflexes, should be normal.

In the case of a large, sudden rotator cuff tear, the patient may be completely unable to abduct the arm. With lesser tears, or those that occurred more gradually, symptoms may be less severe. The patient should be unable to perform the supraspinatus test or should demonstrate marked weakness.

REGIONAL LOW BACK PAIN

Regional low back pain, also referred to as a lumbar sprain, lumbar strain, lumbago, lumbosacral sprain/strain, pulled back muscle and low back pain, is the second most common reason to see a doctor after upper respiratory tract infections. More importantly, it is the most costly disorder for workers' compensation insurance. Despite the frequency and magnitude of the problem, much remains unknown, including the anatomic cause(s) of the disorder(s).

Anatomy and Function

The back performs several basic functions. First, it is a strong, weight-bearing structure (necessitating mineralization), which makes the carrying of heavy objects with the upper body as well as the attainment and maintenance of an upright posture possible. Second, it protects the spinal cord and spinal nerves. Third, the back also allows the attachment of other structures, such as the viscera.

The back is composed of a column of vertebral bodies. Each vertebra has three joints. The largest is the joint between the body of the vertebra and its adjacent neighbor, which is connected by a shock-absorbing, hockey-puck-shaped disc. The disc is filled with a gelatinous material (nucleus pulposus) and surrounded by a fibrous capsule, which contains the nucleus pulposus. The two other joints (facet joints, one on each side) are between the bony projections above and below each vertebra, are much smaller, and are located farther to the posterior. These facet joints are structurally more analogous to other joints in the body, such as those of the fingers.

Ligaments encapsulate the joints as well as connect the vertebral bodies at multiple points to provide additional stability.

The spinal cord and nerves are contained within the canal formed by the column of vertebral bodies. One nerve exits to each side at each vertebral level through a small canal called the foramen.

Multiple muscles constitute the back muscles. Some of these (erector spinae: spinalis, longissimus, and iliocostalis) are large and connect distant places in the back. However, most of the back muscles are quite small and connect at one or two vertebral levels (semispinalis, multifidus, rotatores brevis/longus, intertransversarius, interspinalis). Although most of these muscles are quite small, they also are quite powerful, allowing them to counteract the leverage created by the manual lifting of an object on the other side of the vertebral body.

Pathology

As aging occurs, there is a progressive rise in the appearance of pathological changes in the back, including decreased water content in the intervertebral discs, decreased resilience of the intervertebral discs, decreased intervertebral distance (narrowing), increased osteophytes (bony projections from the edges of the vertebral bodies), and bulging or ruptures of the intervertebral discs (Andersson, 1979; Bergquist-Ullman & Larson, 1977; Lawrence, 1969). There also is a concomitant rise in the numbers of individuals complaining of back pain as aging occurs, although it may decline somewhat in the elderly (Deyo & Tsui-Wu, 1987; Lawrence, 1969). Although there is basic agreement regarding the progression of changes that occur in the back with aging, there is not agreement on the source(s) of most low-back-pain problems. Some work has implicated disk degeneration as the primary problem (Caplan, Lester, & Connelly, 1966; Hult, 1954; Lawrence, 1969; Torgerson & Dotter, 1976), while others have not confirmed this hypothesis (Horal, 1969; Magora & Schwantz, 1976; Splitoff, 1953).

Pathogenesis

Because there is no consensus regarding the cause(s) of most cases of regional low back pain, there is not a shortage of hypotheses, which include the following: (1) disrupted myotendinous junction(s) of back muscles, (2) facet joint pain, (3) intervertebral disc degeneration, (4) ligamentous disruptions/tears, (5) abnormal posture, and (6) poor alignment or instability. (It may be instructive to observe that most cases of regional low back pain tend to have maximal pain and tenderness in the paraspinal areas of L4–S1, also the areas with most disk herniations.)

Presentation, Symptoms, and Signs

Most episodes of low back pain begin with an aching pain in the lower back area, either in the midline or slightly to one side or the other. A majority are attributed to overexertion, such as a heavy lift, or forceful push/pull. Symptoms are sometimes immediate, but other times occur gradually and progressively after such exertions. Some cases occur without an obvious attributable cause. Symptoms tend not to radiate, or if they do, generally do not radiate below the buttocks. Distal paresthesias do not occur. Maintenance of one posture, whether sitting, standing, or lying down, all tend to be markedly detrimental to the pain; many people experience the greatest pain arising the morning after the inciting event. There is no characteristic examination finding. Patients generally have tenderness in the paralumbar muscles, complain of pain with range of motion, and may demonstrate an antalgic gait. However, they should have normal muscle strength, deep tendon reflexes, and a straight-leg-raising test (Liang & Katz, 1991).

LUMBAR RADICULOPATHY

Anatomy and Function

Lumbar radiculopathy occurs when there is a significant pinching, tension, or irritation of a spinal nerve as it exits the spinal canal through its foramen. It is usually due to a lateral herniation of an intervertebral disc. The most common disc to herniate is L_5–S_1 with L_4–L_5 the next most common. The other discs are much less likely to herniate. Occasionally, lumbar radiculopathy may occur due to a large bulging disc (a disc that protrudes like a balloon but has not actually ruptured), although most bulging discs are thought to be asymptomatic. Another recognized cause of lumbar radiculopathy is excessive osteophytes that narrow the intervertebral canal.

Pathogenesis

The changes felt to be responsible for the development of the radiculopathy are the decreased resilience of the intervertebral disc combined with gradual tears in the ligamentous structure that contains the nucleus pulposus. These changes allow the herniation of the disc contents out of the disc on physical exertion, or in some cases, after no apparent exertion (Andersson, 1979; Bergquist-Ullman & Larson, 1977; Lawrence, 1969). The effect of aging appears more clear for disc degeneration, having a relatively clear linear relationship (Lawrence, 1969; Powell, Wilson, Szypryt, Symonds, & Worthington, 1986).

Presentation, Symptoms, and Signs

In contrast with regional low back pain, lumbar radiculopathy tends to present with a more severe pain and distal symptoms. The problem also may begin with a history of overexertion, although not infrequently, it will occur without such a history. The pain will typically radiate down the leg on the affected side beyond the knee. Paresthesias may occur, although pain is usually the predominant symptom. This characteristic presentation of pain is labeled *sciatica* because the sciatic nerve carries these sensations from the spine distally. Many patients experience excessive symptoms after sitting for any length of time, although some unfortunately experience symptom exacerbation on lying down.

The characteristic physical examination maneuver to elicit a finding of sciatica is the straight-leg-raising test. This maneuver is performed with the patient recumbent on the back. The lower extremity is raised with the knee extended. A positive test should elicit a reproduction of the symptoms of sciatica, typically in the position of 15°–40° of hip flexion. Other physical examination findings are more variable. Muscle weakness in a radicular pattern, reduction in sensation in a dermatomal pattern, and asymmetric deep tendon reflexes occur unreliably; when present, however, they are quite helpful in defining the affected nerve root. The Waddel's signs (Waddel, McCullock, Kummel, Venner, 1980) are sometimes used to evaluate for nonorganic back pain, such as a conscious or subconscious overreaction to innocuous stimuli (such as gentle pelvic rotation, or superficial palpation). The Waddel's signs were designed for evaluation of chronic low-back-pain patients; they have not yet been evaluated in a large study for acute low back pain although they have been evaluated in a modest-sized study (Gaines & Hegmann, in press).

Occasionally, a patient will develop lumbar stenosis. This is a condition, whether congenital or acquired, in which the spinal cord is compressed by a narrowed spinal canal. Such patients will typically present with pain that is more widespread, involving both lower extremities. They additionally will tend to complain of pain in the legs, including cramping of the calf muscles with walking. Such cramping is relieved with rest. Sometimes a stooped posture may be attained in an attempt to reduce symptoms as walking distance is increased.

CERVICAL RADICULOPATHY

The anatomy, pathology, and pathophysiology of cervical radiculopathy are generally thought to be analogous to those of lumbar radiculopathy. The anatomy is only modestly different: The cervical vertebral bodies are smaller in size than those of the lumbar region. This difference is not surprising because the only structure they support is the head. Research specifically related to cervical radiculopathy is, however, much more limited than that for lumbar radiculopathy. Very few epidemiologic studies have been performed. Aside from the traumatic setting, it is unclear if these are occupational disorders.

Presentation, Symptoms, and Signs

Cervical radiculopathy tends to be more difficult to diagnose than lumbar radiculopathy. It too tends to present with a more severe pain pattern than regional pain and typically causes distal upper extremity symptoms. A history of overexertion is usually not present. Neck pain is more unusual than typical. Generally, the patient has pain in the extremity in the distribution of the affected nerve root. Paresthesias are often present in the same distribution. Attainment of a comfortable position is often difficult for these patients, as it is for those with sciatica.

There is no characteristic physical examination finding for this disorder, which further complicates the difficulty in making a clinical diagnosis. The Sperling's test is usually attempted to reproduce the symptoms. This test involves flexion of the neck and simultaneous axial rotation of approximately 45°. (The patient is asked to touch the chin laterally to the midclavicle.) This maneuver theoretically results in narrowing of the foramen on the affected side and should result in reproduction or exacerbation of the symptoms. Other physical examination findings, including decrements in sensation in a dermatomal distribution, radicular muscle weakness, and asymmetric deep tendon reflexes, are more variable. Again, when present, however, these positive physical examination findings are highly helpful in defining the level impinged.

REFERENCES

Allander, E. (1947). Prevalence, incidence and remission rates of some common rheumatic diseases or syndromes. *Scandinavian Journal of Rheumatism, 3,* 94–97.

American Academy of Electrodiagnostic Medicine, American Academy of Neurology, and American Academy of Physical Medicine and Rehabilitation. (1993). Practice parameter for electrodiagnostic studies in carpal tunnel syndrome: Summary statement. *Muscle & Nerve, 16,* 1390-1391.

Andersson, G. B. J. (1981). Epidemiologic aspects of low-back pain in industry. *Spine, 6,* 53-59.

Bergquist-Ullman, M., & Larson, U. (1977). Acute low back pain in industry. *Acta Orthopaedica Scandinavica, 170*(Suppl.), 1-117.

Bevin, A. G. (1986). The carpal tunnel syndrome. *Seminars in Occupational Medicine, 1,* 131-139.

Bigliani, L. U., Ticker, J. B., Flatow, E. L., Soslowsky, L. J., & Mow, V. C. (1991). Die beziehung von akromial-architektur zu erkrannkungen der rotatorenmanschette. *Orthopade, 20,* 302-309.

Birkbeck, M. Q., & Beer, T. C. (1975). Occupation in relation to the carpal tunnel syndrome. *Rheumatology and Rehabilitation, 14,* 218-221.

Bjelle, A., Hagberg, M., & Michaelsson, G. (1979). Clinical and ergonomic factors in prolonged shoulder pain among industrial workers. *Scandinavian Journal of Work and Environmental Health, 5,* 205-210.

Blood, W. (1942). Tenosynovitis in industrial workers. *British Medical Journal, 2,* 468.

Boniface, S. J., Morris, I., & Macleod, A. (1994). How does neurophysiologic assessment influence the management and outcome of patients with carpal tunnel syndrome? *British Journal of Rheumatology, 33,* 1169-1170.

Brain, W. R., Wright, A. D., & Wilkinson, M. (1947). Spontaneous compression of both median nerves in the carpal tunnel. *Lancet, 1,* 277-282 .

Buch-Jaeger, N., & Foucher, G. (1994). Correlation of clinical signs with nerve conduction tests in the diagnosis of carpal tunnel syndrome. *Journal of Hand Surgery, 19B,* 720-724.

Buehler, M. J., & Thayer, D. T. (1988). The elbow flexion test: A clinical test for the cubital tunnel syndrome. *Clinical Orthopaedics and Related Research, 233,* 213-216.

Cailliet, R. (1988). *Soft tissue pain and disability.* Philadelphia, PA: F. A. Davis Company.

Cannon, B. W., & Love, J. G. (1946). Tardy median palsy; median neuritis; median thenar atrophy amenable to surgery. *Surgery, 20,* 210-216.

Caplan, P. S., Lester, L. M. J., Connelly, T. P. (1966). Degenerative joint disease of the lumbar spine in coal miners: A clinical and X-ray study. *Arthritis and Rheumatism, 9,* 693-702.

Chard, M. D., Cawston, T. E., Riley, G. P., Gresham, G. A., & Hazleman B. L. (1994). Rotator cuff degeneration and lateral epicondylitis: A comparative histological study. *Annals of the Rheumatic Diseases, 53,* 30-34.

Cioni, R., Passero, S., Paradiso, C., Giannini, F., Battistini, N., & Rushworth, G. (1989). Diagnostic specificity of sensory and motor nerve conduction variables in early detection of carpal tunnel syndrome. *Journal of Neurology, 236,* 208-213.

Codman, E. A. (1938). Rupture of the supraspinatus. *American Journal of Surgery, 42,* 603-626.

Compere, E. L. (1933). Bilateral snapping thumbs. *American Journal of Surgery, 97,* 773-777.

Conklin, J. E., & White, W. L. (1960). Stenosing tenosynovitis and its possible relation to the carpal tunnel syndrome. *Surgical Clinics of North America, 40,* 531-540.

Cotton, F. J., Morrison, G. M., & Bradford, C. H. (1938). DeQuervain's disease, radial styloid tendovaginitis. *New England Journal of Medicine, 219,* 120-123.

Cotton, R. E., & Rideout, D. F. (1964). Tears of the humeral rotator cuff. *Journal of Bone and Joint Surgery, 46B,* 314-328.

Coues, W. P. (1914). Epicondylitis (franke) or tennis elbow. *Boston Medicine Surgery Journal, 170,* 461-465.

Crow, R. S. (1960). Treatment of the carpal-tunnel syndrome. *British Medical Journal, 1,* 1611-1615.

Crymble B. (1968). Brachial neuralgia and the carpal tunnel syndrome. *British Medical Journal, 3*(616), 470-471.

Cseuz, K. A., Thomas, J. E., Lambert, E. H., Love, J. G., & Lipscomb, P. R. (1966). Long-term results of operation for carpal tunnel syndrome. *Mayo Clinical Proceedings, 41,* 232-241.

Dahlin, L. B., & Rydevic, B. (1991). Pathophysiology of nerve compression. In R. H. Gelberman (Ed.), *Operative nerve repair and reconstruction.* (pp. 847-866). Philadelphia, PA: J. B. Lippincott.

Dawson, D. M., Haillet, M., & Millender, L. H. (1990). Pathophysiology of nerve entrapment. In D. M. Dawson, M. Haillet, & L. H. Millender (Eds.), *Entrapment neuropathies,* (2nd eds., pp. 5-23). Boston: Little, Brown.

Dekel, S., Papaioannou, T., Rushworth, G., & Coates, R. (1980). Idiopathic carpal tunnel syndrome caused by carpal stenosis. *British Medical Journal, 1,* 1297-1299.

Deyo, R. A., & Tsui-Wu, Y.-J. (1987). Functional disability due to back pain. *Arthritis Rheumatism, 30,* 1247-1253.

Diack, A. W., & Trommald, J. P. (1939). DeQuervain's disease: A frequently missed diagnosis. *Western Journal of Surgery, 47,* 629-633.

Dimberg, L. (1987). The prevalence and causation of tennis elbow (lateral humeral epicondylitis) in a population of workers in an engineering industry. *Ergonomics, 30,* 573-580.

Gaines, W., & Hegmann, K. (in press). *Spine.*

Doran, A., Gresham, G. A., Rushton, N., & Watson, C. (1990). Tennis elbow. A clinicopathologic study of 22 cases followed for 2 years. *Acta Orthopaedica Scandinavica, 61,* 535-538.

Dorwart, B. B. (1984). Carpal tunnel syndrome: A review. *Seminars in Arthritis and Rheumatism, 14,* 134-140.

Doyle, J. R., & Carroll, R. E. (1968). The carpal tunnel syndrome. *California Medicine, 108,* 263-267.

Eason, S. Y., Belsole, R. J., & Greene, T. L. (1985). Carpal tunnel release: Analysis of suboptimal results. *Journal of Hand Surgery, 10B,* 365-369.

Eichoff, E. (1927). Zur Pathogenese der Tendovaginitis stenosans. *Bruns' Beiträge fur Klinischen Chirurgie, 139,* 746.

Eschle, A. (1924). Beitrag zur Kenntnis der stenosierenden fibrösen Tendovaginitis am Processus styloideus radii. *Schweizerische Medizinische Wochenschrift, 5,* 1006.

Faithfull, D. K., Moir, D. H., & Ireland, J. (1986). The micropathology of the typical carpal tunnel syndrome. *Journal of Hand Surgery, 11B,* 131-132.

Falck, B., & Aarnio, P. (1983). Left-sided carpal tunnel syndrome in butchers. *Scandinavian Journal of Work and Environmental Health, 9,* 291-197.

Feindel, W., & Stratford, V. (1957). Role of the cubital tunnel in tardy ulnar palsy. *Canadian Journal of Surgery, 1,* 287-300.

Feindel, W., & Stratford, V. (1958). Cubital tunnel compression in tardy ulnar palsy. *Canadian Medical Association Journal, 78,* 351-353.

Finkelstein, H. (1930). Stenosing tendovaginitis at the radial styloid process. *Journal of Bone and Joint Surgery, 12,* 509-540.

Flowerdew, R. E., & Bode, O. B. (1942). Tenosynovitis in untrained farm workers. *British Medical Journal, 2,* 367.

Flörcken, H. (1912). Zur Frage der stenosierenden Tendovaginitis am Processus styloideus radii (deQuervain). *München Medizinische Wochenschrift, 59,* 1378.

Fuchs, P. C., Nathan, P. A., & Myers, L. D. (1991). Synovial histology in carpal tunnel syndrome. *Journal of Hand Surgery, 16A,* 753-758.

Fullerton, P. M. (1963). The effect of ischaemia on nerve conduction in the carpal tunnel syndrome. *Journal of Neurosurgical Psychiatry, 26,* 385-397.

Gainer, J. V., & Nugent, G. R. (1977). Carpal tunnel syndrome: Report of 430 operations. *Southern Medical Journal, 70,* 325-328.

Garland, H., Bradshaw, J. P. P., & Clark, J. M. P. (1957). Compression of median nerve in carpal tunnel and its relation to acroparasthesiae. *British Medical Journal, 1,* 730-734.

Garrett, W., & Tidball, J. (1988). Myotendinous junction: Structure, function, and failure. In S. L.-Y. Woo & J. A. Buckwalter (Eds.), *Injury and repair of musculoskeletal soft tissues* (pp. 171-207). Park Ridge, IL: AAOS.

Gay, J. R., & Love, J. G. (1947). Diagnosis and treatment of the ulnar nerve. *Journal of Bone and Joint Surgery, 29,* 1087-1097.

Gelberman, R. H., Hergenroeder, P. T., Hargens, A. R., Lundborg, G .N., & Akeson, W. H. (1981). The carpal tunnel syndrome: A study of carpal tunnel pressures. *Journal of Bone and Joint Surgery, 63A,* 380-383.

Gellman, H., Gelberman, R. H., Tan, A. E., & Botte, M. J. (1986). Carpal tunnel syndrome: An evaluation of the provocative diagnostic tests. *Journal of Bone and Joint Surgery, 68A,* 735-737.

Gelmers, H. J. (1979). The significance of Tinel's sign in the diagnosis of carpal tunnel syndrome. *Acta Neurochirurgica, 49,* 255-258.

Gilliatt, R. W., & Wilson, T. G. (1953). A pneumatic-tourniquet test in the carpal tunnel syndrome. *Lancet, II,* 595-597.

Goga, I. E. (1990). Carpal tunnel syndrome in black South Africans. *Journal of Hand Surgery, 15B,* 96-99.

Goldberg, E. J., Abraham, E., & Siegel, I. (1988). The surgical treatment of chronic lateral humeral epicondylitis by common extensor release. *Clinical Orthopaedics and Related Research, 233,* 208-212.

Goldie, I. (1964). Epicondylitis lateralis humeris: A pathogenetical study. *Acta Chirurgica Scandinavica, 339*(Suppl.), 1-119.

Goodman, H. V., & Gilliatt, R. W. (1961). The effect of treatment on median nerve conduction in patients with the carpal tunnel syndrome. *Annals of Physical Medicine, 6,* 137-155.

Goodwill, C. J. (1965). The carpal tunnel syndrome: Long-term follow-up showing relation of latency measurements to response to treatment. *Archives of Physical Medicine, 8,* 12-21.

Griffiths, D. L. (1952). Tenosynovitis and tendovaginitis. *British Medical Journal, 1,* 645-647.

Hamlin, E., & Lehman, R. A. (1967). Carpal-tunnel syndrome. *New England Journal of Medicine, 276,* 849-852.

Hansson, K. G., & Norwich, I. D. (1930). Epicondylitis humeri. *Journal of the American Medical Association, 94,* 1557-1561.

Heathfield, K. W. G. (1957). Acroparæsthesiæ and the carpal-tunnel syndrome. *Lancet, 2,* 663–666.

Herberts, P., & Kadefors, R. (1976). A study of painful shoulders in welders, *Acta Orthopaedica Scandinavica, 47,* 381–387.

Herberts, P., Kadefors, R., Andersson, G., & Petersen, I. (1981). Shoulder pain in industry: An epidemiological study on welders. *Acta Orthopaedica Scandinavica, 52,* 299–306.

Herberts, P., Kadefors, R., Hogfors, C., & Sigholm, G. (1984). Shoulder pain and heavy manual labor. *Clinical Orthopaedics and Related Research, 191,* 166–178.

Ho, K. C., & Marmor, L. (1971). Entrapment of the ulnar nerve at the elbow. *American Journal of Surgery, 121,* 355–356.

Horal, J. (1969). The clinical appearance of low back disorders in the city of Gothenburg, Sweden. *Acta Orthopaedica Scandinavica, 118*(Suppl.), 9–109.

Howard, N. J. (1937). Peritendinitis crepitans: A muscle-effort syndrome. *Journal of Bone and Joint Surgery, 19,* 447–459.

Howard, N. J. (1938). A new concept of tenosynovitis and the pathology of physiologic effort. *American Journal of Surgery, 42,* 723–730.

Howard, N. J. (1941). Pathological changes induced in tendons through trauma and their accompanying clinical phenomena. *American Journal of Surgery, 51,* 689–706.

Huber, W. (1933). Histologische Befunde bei der Tendovaginitis stenosans. *Virchows Archiv für Pathologische Anatomie und Physiologie, 291,* 745–756.

Hult, L. (1954). Cervical, dorsal and lumbar spine syndrome. *Acta Orthopaedica Scandinavica, 17*(Suppl.), 1–102.

Hume, E. L., Hutchinson, D. T., Jaeger, S. A., & Hunter, J. M. (1991). Biomechanics of pulley reconstruction. *Journal of Hand Surgery, 16A,* 722–730.

Hybbinette, C. H., & Mannerfelt, L. (1975). The carpal tunnel syndrome. *Acta Orthopaedica Scandinavica, 46,* 610–620.

Inglis, A. E., Straub, L. R., & Williams, C. S. (1972). Median nerve neuropathy at the wrist. *Clinical Orthopaedics and Related Research, 83,* 48–54.

Johnson, E. W., & Melvin, J. L. (1967). Sensory conduction studies of median and ulnar nerves. *Archives of Physical Medicine and Rehabilitation, 48,* 25–30.

Johnson, E. W., Wells, R. M., & Duran, R. J. (1962). Diagnosis of carpal tunnel syndrome. *Archives of Physical Medicine and Rehabilitation, 8,* 414–419.

Kaplan, S. J., Glickel, S. Z., & Eaton, R. G. (1990). Predictive factors in the non-surgical treatment of carpal tunnel syndrome. *Journal of Hand Surgery, 15B,* 106–108.

Katz, J. N., Larson, M. G., Fossel, A. H., & Liang, M. H. (1991). Validation of a surveillance case definition of carpal tunnel syndrome. *American Journal of Public Health, 81,* 189–193.

Katz, J. N., Larson., M. G., Sabra, A., Krarup, C., Stirrat, C. R., Sethi, R., Eaton, H. M., Fossel, A. H., & Liang, M. A. (1990). The carpal tunnel syndrome: Diagnostic utility of the history and physical examination findings. *Annals of Internal Medicine, 112,* 321–327.

Katz, J. N., & Stirrat, C. R. (1990). A self-administered hand diagram for the diagnosis of carpal tunnel syndrome. *Journal of Hand Surgery, 15A,* 360–363.

Kelly, A. P., & Jacobsen, H. S. (1964, August). Hand disability due to tenosynovitis. *Industrial Medicine and Surgery,* 570–574.

Kendall, D. (1950). Non-penetrating injuries of the median nerve at the wrist. *Brain, 73,* 84–94.

Kendall, D. (1960). Aetiology, diagnosis and treatment of paraesthesiae in the hands. *British Medical Journal, 2,* 1633–1640.

Keppler, W. (1917). Zur Klinik der stenosierenden Tendovaginitis am Processus styliodeus radii. *Medizinische Klinik, 13,* 1014.

Keyes, E. L. (1935). Anatomical observations on senile changes in the shoulder. *Journal of Bone and Joint Surgery, 17,* 953–960.

Kimura, J. (1989). *Electrodiagnosis in diseases of nerve and muscle: Principles and practice.* Philadelphia, PA: F. A. Davis.

Kivi, P. (1982). The etiology and conservative treatment of humeral epicondylitis. *Scandinavian Journal of Rehabilitation Medicine, 15,* 37–41.

Kremer, M., Gilliatt, R. W., Golding, J. S. R., & Wilson, T. G. (1953). Acroparæsthesiæ in the carpal-tunnel syndrome. *Lancet, 2,* 590–595.

Lamphier, T. A., Crooker, C., & Crooker, J. L. (1965). DeQuervain's disease. *Industrial Medicine and Surgery,* 847–856.

Lawrence, J. S. (1969). Disc degeneration: Its frequency and relationship to symptoms. *Annals of Rheumatic Diseases, 28,* 121–137.

Liang, M. H., Katz J. N. (1991). Clinical evaluation of patients with a suspected spine problem. In J. W. Frymoyer (Ed.), *The adult spine: Principles and practice* (pp. 223–239). New York: Raven Press.

Lindblom, K. (1939). On pathogenesis of rupture of the tendon aponeurosis of the shoulder joint. *Acta Radiologica, 20*, 563–577.

Lindblom, K., & Ivar, P. (1939). Ruptures of the tendon aponeurosis of the shoulder joint—the so-called supraspinatus rupture. *Acta Chirurgica Scandinavica, 82*, 133–142.

Lipscomb, P. R. (1944). Chronic nonspecific tenosynovitis and peritendinitis. *Surgical Clinics of North America, 24*, 780–797.

Lipscomb, P. R. (1959). Tenosynovitis of the hand and wrist: Carpal tunnel syndrome, DeQuervain's disease, trigger digit. *Clinical Orthopedics, 13*, 164–180.

Love, J. G. (1955). Median neuritis or carpal tunnel syndrome: Diagnosis and treatment. *North Carolina Medical Journal, 16*, 463–469.

Lundborg, G., & Dahlin, L. B. (1989). Pathophysiology of nerve compression. In R. M. Szabo (Ed.), *Nerve compression syndromes–Diagnosis and treatment* (pp. 15–39). Thorofare NJ: Slack.

Macnab, I. (1973). Rotator cuff tendinitis. *Annals of the Royal College of Surgeons of England, 53*, 271–287.

Macnicol, M. F. (1979). The results of operation for ulnar neuritis. *Journal of Bone and Joint Surgery, 61B*, 159–164.

Maffulli, N., Regine, R., Carrillo, F., Capasso, G., & Minella, S. (1990). Tennis elbow: An ultrasonographic study in tennis players. *British Journal of Sports Medicine, 24*, 151–155.

Magora, A., & Schwantz, A. (1976). Relation between low back pain syndrome and X-ray findings: 1. Degenerative osteoarthritis. *Scandinavian Journal of Rehabilitation Medicine, 8*, 115–125.

Masear, V. R., Hayesand, J. M., & Hyde, A. G. (1986). An industrial cause of carpal tunnel syndrome. *Journal of Hand Surgery, 11A*, 222–227.

Michaelis, P. (1912). Stenosierende Tendovaginitis im Bereiche des Processus styloideus radii. *Zeitschrift für Orthopadie Chirurgie, 30*, 192.

Moore, J. S. (1996). Proposed pathogenetic models for specific distal upper extremity disorders. *Proceedings of the International Conference on Occupational Disorders of the Upper Extremities*, Ann Arbor, MI.

Moore, J. S. (1997). DeQuervain's tenosynovitis. *Journal of Occupational and Environmental Medicine, 39* (10), 999–1002.

Moseley, H. F., & Goldie, I. (1963). The arterial pattern of the rotator cuff of the shoulder. *Journal of Bone and Joint Surgery, 45B*, 780–789.

Muckart, R. D. (1964). Stenosing tendovaginitis of abductor pollicis longus and extensor pollicis brevis at the radial styloid (DeQuervain's disease). *Clinical Orthopedics, 33*, 201–208.

Mumenthaler, M. (1974). Charakteristische krankheitsbilder nicht unmittelbar traumatischer peripherer nervenschaden, *Nervenarzt, 45*, 61–66.

Murray, I. C. P., & Simpson, J. A. (1958). Acroparæsthesia in myxoedema. *Lancet, 1*, 1360–1363.

Nathan, P. A., Keniston, R. C. Meyers, L. D., & Meadows, K. D. (1992). Longitudinal study of median nerve sensory conduction in industry: Relationship to age, gender, hand dominance, occupational hand use, and clinical diagnosis. *Journal of Hand Surgery, 17A*, 850–857.

Neal, N. C., McManners, J., & Stirling, G. A. (1987). Pathology of the flexor tendon sheath in the spontaneous carpal tunnel syndrome. *Journal of Hand Surgery, 12B*, 229–232.

Neer, C. S. (1972). Anterior acromioplasty for the chronic impingement syndrome in the shoulder. *Journal of Bone and Joint Surgery, 54A*, 41–50.

Neer, C. S. (1983). Impingement lesions. *Clinical Orthopaedics and Related Research, 173*, 70–387.

Newman, P. H. (1948). Median nerve compression in the carpal tunnel. *Postgraduate Medical Journal*, 264–269.

Nicholson, G. P., Goodman, D. A., Flatow, E. L., & Bigliani, L. U. (1996). The acromion: Morphologic condition and age-related changes. A study of 420 scapulas. *Journal of Shoulder and Elbow Surgery, 5*, 1–11.

Nirschl, R. P. (1974). The etiology and treatment of tennis elbow. *Journal of Sports Medicine, 2*, 308–323.

Nirschl, R. P., & Pettrone, F. A. (1979). Tennis elbow: The surgical treatment of lateral epicondylitis. *Journal of Bone and Joint Surgery, 61A*, 832–839.

Nixon, J. E., & DiStefano, V. (1975). Ruptures of the rotator cuff. *Orthopedic Clinics of North America, 6*, 423–447.

Nugent, G. R. (1980). Identifying carpal tunnel syndrome. *Hospital Medicine, 1*, 48–49.

Nussbaum, A. (1917). Beitrag zur Tendovaginitis stenosans fibrosa des Daumens (deQuervain). *Bruns' Breiträge fur Klinischen Chirurgie, 104*, 140.

Ochoa, J., & Marotte, L. (1973). The nature of the nerve lesion caused by chronic entrapment in the guinea pig. *Journal of Neurological Science, 19*, 491–495.

O'Driscoll, S. W., Horii E., Carmichael, S. W., & Morrey, B. F. (1991). The cubital tunnel and ulnar neuropathy. *Journal of Bone and Joint Surgery—British Volume, 73*, 613-617.

Osgood, R. B. (1922). Radiohumeral bursitis, epicondylitis, epicondylalgia (tennis elbow). *Archives of Surgery, 4*, 420-433.

Patterson, D. C. (1936). DeQuervain's disease: Stenosing tendovaginitis at the radial styloid. *New England Journal of Medicine, 214*, 101-102.

Phalen, G. S. (1951). Spontaneous compression of the median nerve at the wrist. *Journal of the American Medical Association, 145*, 1128-1132.

Phalen, G. S. (1966). The carpal-tunnel syndrome. *Journal of Bone and Joint Surgery, 48A*, 211-228.

Phalen, G. S. (1970). Reflections on 21 years experience with carpal-tunnel syndrome. *Journal of the American Medical Association, 212*, 1365-1367.

Phalen, G. S. (1972). The carpal tunnel syndrome. *Clinical Orthopedics, 83*, 29-40.

Phalen, G. S., & Kendrick, J. I. (1957). Compression neuropathy of the median nerve in the carpal tunnel. *Journal of the American Medical Association, 164*, 524-530.

Phalen, G. S., Gardner, W. J., & La Londe, A. A. (1950). Neuropathy of the median nerve due to compression beneath the transverse carpal ligament. *Journal of Bone and Joint Surgery, 32A*,109-112.

Powell, M. C., Wilson, M., Szypryt, P., Symonds, E. M., & Worthington, B. S. (1986). Prevalence of lumbar disc degeneration observed by magnetic resonance in symptomless women, *Lancet, 2*, 1366-1367.

Rais, O. (1961). Heparin treatment of peritenomyosis (peritendinitis) crepitans acuta. *Acta Chirurgica Scandinavica, 268*(Suppl.), 1-88.

Rathbun, J. B., & MacNab, I. (1970). The microvascular pattern of the rotator cuff. *Journal of Bone and Joint Surgery, 52B*, 540-553.

Regan, W., Wold, L. E., Coonrad, R., & Morrey, B. F. (1992). Microscopic histopathology of chronic refractory lateral epicondylitis. *American Journal of Sports Medicine, 20*, 746-749.

Renard, E., Jacques, D., Chammas, M., Poirier, J. L., Bonifaci, C., Jaffiol, C., & Allieu, Y. (1994). Increased prevalence of soft tissue hand lesions in type 1 and type 2 diabetes mellitus: Various entities and associated significance. *Diabetes and Metabolism, 20*, 513-521.

Reschke, K. (1919-1920). Zur stenosierenden Tendovaginitis (deQuervain). *Archiv für Klinische Chirurgie, 113*, 464.

Rosenbaum, R. B., & Ochoa, J. L. (1993). *Carpal tunnel syndrome and other disorders of the median nerve.* Boston: Butterworth-Heinemann.

Ross, M. A., & Kimura, J. (1995). AAEM Case Report 2: The carpal tunnel syndrome. *Muscle & Nerve, 18*, 567-573.

Rothman, R. H., & Parke, W. W. (1965). The vascular anatomy of the rotator cuff. *Clinical Orthopaedics, 41*, 176-186.

Sampson, S. P., Badalamente, M. A., Hurst, L. C., & Seidman, J. (1991). Pathobiology of the human A1 pulley in trigger finger. *Journal of Hand Surgery, 16A*, 714-721.

Schneider, C. C. (1928). Stenosing fibrous tendovaginitis over radial styloid (deQuervain). *Surgery Gynecology and Obstetrics, 64*, 846-850.

Schuind, F., Ventura, M., & Pasteels, J. L. (1990). Idiopathic carpal tunnel syndrome: A histologic study of flexor tendon synovium. *Journal of Hand Surgery, 15A*, 497-503.

Seror, P. (1987). Tinel's sign in the diagnosis of carpal tunnel syndrome. *Journal of Hand Surgery, 12B*, 364-365.

Shivde, A. J., Dreizin, I., Fisher, M. A. (1981). The carpal tunnel syndrome: A clinical-electrodiagnostic analysis. *Electromyography Clinical Neurophysiology, 21*, 143-153.

Sperling, W. P. (1951). Snapping finger: Roengten treatment and experimental production. *Acta Radiologica, 37*, 74-80.

Splitoff, C. A. (1953). Lumbosacral junction: Roentgenographic comparison of patients with and without backache. *Journal of the American Medical Association, 152*, 1610-1613.

Stein, H. C. (1927). Stenosing tendovaginitis. *American Journal of Surgery, 3*, 77-78.

Stevens, J. C. (1987). AAEE Minimonograph26: Electrodiagnosis of carpal tunnel syndrome. *Muscle & Nerve, 10*, 99-113.

Stewart, J. D., & Eisen, A. (1968). Tinel's sign and the carpal tunnel syndrome. *British Medical Journal, 2*, 1125-1126.

Szabo, R. M., & Gelberman, R. H. (1987). The pathophysiology of nerve entrapment syndromes. *Journal of Hand Surgery, 12A*, 880-884.

Tanzer, R. C. (1957). The carpal tunnel syndrome: A clinical and anatomical study. *Journal of Bone and Joint Surgery, 41A*, 626-634.

Thomas, J. A., & Fullerton, P. M. (1963). Nerve fibre size in the carpal tunnel syndrome. *Journal of Neurology, Neurosurgery and Psychiatry, 26,* 520-527.

Thomas, J. A., Lambert, E. H., & Czeuz, K. A. (1967). Electrodiagnostic aspects of carpal tunnel syndrome. *Archives of Neurology, 16,* 635-641.

Thompson, A. R., Plewes, L. W., & Shaw, E. G. (1951). Peritendinitis crepitans and simple tenosynovitis: A clinical study of 544 cases in industry. *British Journal of Industrial Medicine, 8,* 150-160.

Tidball, J. G., & Daniel, L. (1986). Myotendinous junctions of tonic muscle cells: Structure and loading. *Cell and Tissue Research, 245,* 315-322.

Troell, A. (1921). On tendovaginitis and tendinitis stenosans. *Acta Chirurgica Scandinavica, 54,* 7-16.

Upton, A. R. M., & McComas, A. J. (1973). The double crush in nerve-entrapment syndrome. *Lancet, 2,* 359-362.

Urbaniak, J. R., & Roth, J. H. (1982). Office diagnosis and treatment of hand pain. *Orthopedic Clinics of North America, 13,* 477-495.

Vainio, K. (1957). Carpal canal syndrome caused by tenosynovitis. *Acta Rheumatologica Scandinavica, 4,* 22-27.

Van Rossum, J., Kamphuisen, H. A. C., & Wintzen, A. R. (1980). Management in the carpal tunnel syndrome. *Clinical Neurology and Neurosurgery, 82*(3), 169-176.

Vanderpool, D. W., Chalmers, J., Lamb, D. W., & Whiston D. B. (1968). Peripheral compression lesions of the ulnar nerve. *Journal of Bone and Joint Surgery, 50B,* 792-803.

Vicale, C. T., & Scarff, J. E. (1951). Median neuritis owing to the compression in the carpal tunnel in the absence of osseous disease at the wrist. *Transactions of the American Neurological Association,* 187-191.

Waddell, G., McCullouch, J. A., Kummel, E., Venner, R. M. (1980). Nonorganic physical signs in low-back pain. *Spine, 5,* (2), 117-125.

Wadsworth, T. G. (1987). Tennis elbow: Conservative, surgical, and manipulative treatment. *British Medical Journal, 294,* 621-624.

Wand, J. S. (1990). Carpal tunnel syndrome in pregnancy and lactation. *Journal of Hand Surgery, 15B,* 93-95.

Welti, E. (1896). Ein Fall con sogen. Chronischer Tendovaginitis. *Cor-Bl f schweiz Aertze, 26,* 300.

Wertsch, J. J., & Melvin, J. (1982). Median nerve anatomy and entrapment syndromes. *Archives of Physical Medicine Rehabilitation, 63,* 623-627.

Wilson, C. L., & Duff, G. L. (1943). Pathologic study of degeneration and rupture of the supraspinatus tendon. *Archives of Surgery, 47,* 121-135.

Winn, F. J., & Habes, D. J. (1990). Carpal tunnel area as a risk factor for carpal tunnel syndrome. *Muscle & Nerve, 13,* 254-258.

Wood, C. F. (1941). Stenosing tendovaginitis at the radial styloid process. *Southern Surgeon, 10,* 105-110.

Yamaguchi, Y. M., Lipscomb, P. R., & Soule, E. H. (1965, January). Carpal tunnel syndrome. *Minnesota Medicine,* 22-33.

Younghusband, O. Z., & Black, J. D. (1963). DeQuervain's disease: Stenosing tenovaginitis at the radial styloid process. *Canadian Medical Association Journal, 89,* 508-512.

Zelle, O. L., & Schnepp, K. H. (1936). Snapping thumb: Tendovaginitis stenosans. *American Journal of Surgery,* 321-322.

3

Regulatory Agencies and Legislation

Thomas M. Domer

Whether in an individual capacity or as part of a rehabilitation team, on a daily basis occupational rehabilitation professionals are faced with decisions on employee hiring, placement and retention, employee safety and injury avoidance, and for more severely disabled individuals, vocational rehabilitation and benefits entitlement. This chapter addresses five specific areas of regulation and legislation:

- The Americans with Disabilities Act (ADA)
- The Occupational Safety and Health Administration (OSHA)
- The Rehabilitation Act of 1973 (as amended)
- Social Security Disability
- Workers' Compensation

This chapter also provides advice on litigation and serving as an expert witness. Rehabilitation professionals must know the following, for example:

- Whether a physically impaired person is a "qualified individual with a disability" and, further, the "essential functions" of that individual's job to help determine whether or to what extent an employee's request for accommodation must be followed.
- Whether OSHA regulations dictate rules for use of office and factory equipment (such as vibrating tools for individuals complaining of cumulative trauma injuries)
- What benefits are available to work-injured employees, and the circumstances under which the employer has an obligation to rehire
- What vocational opportunities exist when an employee cannot return to former employment under the vocational rehabilitation laws
- Under what circumstances rehabilitation professionals testify or provide advice as experts in court and administrative proceedings

Thomas M. Domer • Shneidman, Myers, 700 West Michigan Avenue, Milwaukee, Wisconsin 53201-0442.

Sourcebook of Occupational Rehabilitation, edited by Phyllis M. King. Plenum Press, New York, 1998.

THE AMERICANS WITH DISABILITIES ACT (ADA)

Over 40 million Americans have difficulty performing one or more basic physical activities. These activities include seeing, hearing, speaking, walking, using stairs, lifting or carrying, getting in and out of bed, and getting around outside or inside. Currently, people with disabilities represent the largest minority in the United States. However, they are largely a hidden minority. People with disabilities often are afraid and reluctant to participate in society. The ADA was designed in part to address these fears.

Purpose

The ADA is a federal antidiscrimination law intended to eliminate employment discrimination and remove architectural and communication barriers for disabled Americans. The ADA contains five titles, each with a specific purpose. *Title I* provides that no employer may discriminate against a qualified individual with a disability in the terms and conditions of employment. *Title II* protects qualified individuals with disabilities from discrimination on the basis of disability in governmental services, programs, and activities and applies to all activities of public entities, including their employment practices. *Title III* pertains to the provision of public transportation by a private entity. (Title II deals with the provisions of public transportation by a public entity.) Title III also prohibits discrimination against individuals with disabilities in all places that serve the public. *Title IV* covers telecommunications and mandates that communication services be made available to all people, specifically requiring that companies offering telephone services to the public provide phone relay systems to individuals who use telecommunications devices for the deaf or other similar devices. *Title V* addresses miscellaneous provisions.

Coverage

Table 3.1 describes who is covered by the ADA. The employment provisions of the ADA (Title I) pertain to employers with 15 or more employees. The ADA does not pre-empt state antidiscrimination laws. Where conflict exists, the applicable law is that which provides the greatest protection to the individual employee. Where conflict exists between ADA and state provisions, the ADA will generally prevail although employees may proceed in both forums.

Interviews, Hiring, and Medical Exams

Under ADA pre-employment inquiry is a delicate subject. Recently revised guidelines promulgated by the Equal Employment Opportunities Commission (EEOC) do allow questions about accommodations in three specific situations during the initial interview stage:

1. The employer reasonably believes the applicant will need reasonable accommodation because of an obvious impairment. For example, an applicant with obvious blindness is asked by the employer if reasonable accommodations will be necessary to perform a job involving computer work. The applicant replies, "No." The employer may press no further on the topic of accommodation although the

applicant may be asked to describe or even demonstrate how essential functions will be performed, even if other applicants are not asked to do so.

2. The employer believes that the applicant will need reasonable accommodations because of a hidden disability that the applicant has voluntarily disclosed to the employer. For example, an applicant volunteers that she has diabetes. The employer may ask if reasonable accommodations are needed. The applicant suggests the need for periodic breaks to take medications. The employer may seek further clarification regarding how frequent the breaks will be necessary and for how long.

3. The applicant has voluntarily disclosed to the employer that he or she needs a reasonable accommodation to perform the job. For example, the applicant discloses that he will need customized software to increase the size of text. The employer may seek clarification regarding the specific product needed, compatibility with existing hardware, and the like. The employer may not ask questions regarding the applicant's underlying impairment.

The revised guidelines resulted from legitimate employer complaints about the unrealistic interviewing processes that resulted from the more restrictive original guide-

Table 3.1. Americans with Disabilities Act: Who Is Covered?

Title	Private sector	Public sector	Exemptions
Title I: Employment	Employers with 15 or more employees Employment agencies Labor organizations Joint labor-management committees	Congress (House, Senate, and their instrumentalities)	Employers with fewer than 15 employees United States government and wholly owned government corporations Native American tribes Private membership clubs
Title II: Public services; public transportation by public entities	N/A	State and local government (no minimum number of employees) Departments, agencies, special purpose districts of state or local government (no minimum number of employees) AMTRAK	Public schools (buses) U.S. government
Title III: Public accommodations	Place of public accommodations Private businesses providing public transportation	N/A	Private clubs Religious organizations Lodgings with 5 or fewer rooms Air transportation
Title IV: Telecommunications (telephone and television)	Common carriers providing interstate or intrastate communications by wire or radio	Federally funded or produced television public service announcements	N/A

lines. Except for these limited circumstances; however, all disability-related inquiries—including questions directed to the applicant (or others) about health status, health history, workers' compensation histories, or medical examination—must be deferred until a conditional offer of employment has been made.

Under ADA, all health-related inquiries, including medical examinations, are unlawful prior to an offer of employment. Exceptions exist for drug testing and fitness for duty examinations. Pre-employment medical examinations are allowed provided that (a) they occur only following a conditional offer of employment; (b) they are required of all employees entering into the same job classification; and (c) the results are kept confidential and used only in accordance with ADA regulations.

Medical examinations for current employees, however, are severely restricted and must be job-related and consistent with business necessity.

Filing Requirements and Enforcement

ADA Title I is enforced by the EEOC, which must investigate claims filed within 300 days of the alleged discriminatory act (i.e., termination, refusal to hire, denial of benefits, etc.). If the EEOC finds probable cause that discrimination occurred, it may prosecute. Alternatively, the EEOC may issue the employee a "right to sue" letter that allows the employee to retain a private attorney and proceed in federal court. The employee is then entitled to a jury trial and the possibility of corrective action and compensatory and punitive damages if the employer is found guilty. Monetary caps on damages exist and vary from $50,000 to $300,000, depending on the size of the offending company. However, the EEOC is currently understaffed, and it may take as long as a year before complaints are resolved. Because of this situation, it behooves individuals who wish to file Title I complaints to consider additionally available avenues of redress (i.e., state equal rights acts, workers' compensation, or state Family and Medical Leave Act provisions). Table 3.2 provides specific information related to implementation of the ADA.

Definition of Disability

Remedies under the employment discrimination provisions of the ADA are reserved for "qualified individuals with a disability." To have an ADA-based disability, a person must have a *physical or mental impairment that substantially limits the performance of one or more major life activities*. Temporary or chronic conditions or those with little long-term impact are not disabilities under ADA. However, individuals are also disabled if they have a history of or are regarded as having a substantially limiting impairment.

The definition of the term *qualified individual with a disability* reflects the principle of equal opportunity to work and the broad remedial purposes of the ADA. It focuses on what an individual with a disability can do, rather than on what she or he cannot do. Reflecting the act's focus on individual rather than group characteristics, the definition requires an individualized assessment of a person's abilities. Moreover, the definition looks at whether an individual with a disability is qualified for the specific position at issue, not at whether he or she is qualified for work in general.

The determination of whether an individual with a disability is qualified should be made in two steps. The first step is to determine if the individual has the education, training, skills, experience, and other job-related credentials for the position. The second step is to determine whether the individual can perform the essential functions of the

Table 3.2. Americans with Disabilities Act: Implementation

Title	Responsible agency	Effective date	Regulations
Title I: Employment	Equal Employment Opportunity Commission (EEOC)	July 26, 1992: employers with 25 or more employees and other covered entities July 26, 1994: employers with 15 or more employees	29 C.F.R. Part 1630, 56 Fed. Reg. 36,725 (July 26, 1991)
Title II: Public services	Department of Justice (DOJ)	January 26, 1992	28 C.F.R. Part 36, 56 Fed. Reg. 35,694 (July 26, 1991)
public transportation by public entities	Department of Transportation (DOT)	New vehicles: August 26, 1990 Rail systems: July 26, 1993 (extensions up to 20 or 30 years) Paratransit: January 26, 1992	49 C.F.R. Part 37, 55 Fed. Reg. 40,762 (Oct. 4, 1990) 49 C.F. Parts 27, 37 and 38, 56 Fed. Reg. 45,584 (Sept. 6, 1991)
Title III: Public transportation by private entities	Department of Transportation (DOT)	Existing vehicles: January 26, 1992 New vehicles; August 26, 1990 Rail, over-the-road buses: July 26, 1996 (large providers) July 26, 1997 (small providers)	49 C.F.R. Parts 27, 37 and 38, 56 Fed. Reg. 45,584 (Sept. 6, 1991)
public accommodations	Department of Justice (DOJ)	January 26, 1992 (new construction) January 26, 1993	28 C.F.R. Part 36, 56 Fed. Reg. 35,544 (July 26, 1991)
Title IV: Telecommunications (telephone and television)	Federal Communications Commission (FCC)	July 26, 1993	49 C.F.R. Parts 0 and 64, 56 Fed. Reg. 36,729 (Aug. 1, 1991)

position held or desired with or without accommodation. The second step's purpose is to ensure that individuals with disabilities who can perform essential job functions are not denied employment opportunities simply because they are not able to perform the position's marginal or peripheral functions.

The determination of whether a person is a qualified individual with a disability requires an individualized case-by-case assessment of the specific abilities of the person, the specific requirements of the position, and the manner in which the person may be able to meet those requirements. The issue is whether a particular individual with a disability is qualified for a particular position, not whether the individual or group of individuals with a particular disability is qualified for a class of positions.

Essential Functions of the Job

The employer must determine whether the individual can perform the essential functions of the position held or desired. The EEOC has a three-factor analyses for determining essential functions. Not all functions that employees actually perform in their particular jobs constitute essential functions. A job duty rises to the level of being essential when loss of that function fundamentally alters the position. The EEOC regulations identify three types of job functions that may be considered essential for purposes of the ADA.

1. The reason that the position exists is to perform the particular function.
2. There are a limited number of employees available among whom the performance of the job function can be distributed.
3. The function is highly specialized so that the incumbent in the position is hired for his or her expertise or ability to perform the particular function.
   a. Where a position exists to perform a particular function, that function is clearly essential. For example, a security guard who checks identification cards requires the ability to read as an essential function. The only reason the position exists is to have the identification cards checked.
   b. The second factor pertains to the number of other employees available to perform the job function. This is an important factor when the total number of employees is low and each employee may be called upon to perform a number of different functions. In such a situation, an employee's ability to perform each function becomes critical, and the options available to the employer are limited.
   c. The third factor is the degree of expertise or skill required to perform the job function. In a certain highly skilled position or profession, an employee may be hired for his or her expertise or ability to perform a specific job function in that situation. The ADA regulations provide that specialized task is an essential function.

Under ADA Title I, the individual must meet the definition of "qualified individual with the disability." The *qualified* employee is one who can perform the essential functions of the job. The employee must meet all the qualification standards (education, experience, specific vocational preparation) that are job-related and consistent with business necessity. *Essential functions* are fundamental duties of the position and include such considerations as time involvement, impact, and relationship to the job's purpose.

Employer's Duty to Accommodate

The duty to make a reasonable accommodation to a qualified individual with a disability lies at the heart of the ADA. An employer in appropriate circumstances may need to take affirmative steps to accommodation a person with a disability in order to provide equal opportunity in all aspects of the employment relationship.

Exactly what constitutes reasonable accommodation is not explicitly defined in the statute. EEOC regulations suggest that accommodation consists of any change in the work environment that enables an individual with a disability to enjoy equal employment opportunity. The regulations specify a three-part definition of the term *reasonable accommodation* as meaning any modification or adjustment to (a) the job application process, (b) the work environment, and (c) the enjoyment of equal benefits and privileges of employment.

The most common types of accommodations an employer may be required to provide include the following: job restructuring; part-time or modified work schedules;

reassignment to vacant positions; acquisition or modification of equipment or devices; adjustment or modification of examinations, training, or policies; providing qualified readers or interpreters as aides to disabled workers and altering the existing facility. Court decisions have indicated that an employer is not required to achieve *identical conditions* for disabled and nondisabled employees to fulfill reasonable accommodation obligations (*Vande Zande v. Wisconsin Department of Administration*, 1995).

Definition of Undue Hardship

The definition of the term qualified individual with a disability expressly requires consideration of whether the individual can perform essential functions when reasonably accommodated. The ADA requires employers to provide reasonable accommodation to the known physical or mental limitations of otherwise qualified individuals with disabilities unless doing so would result in undue hardship. This reasonable accommodation requirement is critical to achieve the goals of the ADA.

Other Forms of Accommodation

In general, a reasonable accommodation is any change in the work environment or in the way processes are customarily done that enables an individual with a disability to enjoy equal employment opportunities. Some of the most common accommodations an employer may be required to provide include job restructuring, part-time or modified work schedules, and modifications of equipment or devices. Most importantly, the assessment of whether an individual with a disability is qualified should be based on the capabilities of that individual at the time of the employment decision. Speculation that the individual may become incapacitated in the future is inappropriate.

Direct Threat to Health or Safety of the Individual or Others

An employer's qualification standards may include a requirement that an individual not pose a direct threat to the health or safety of other individuals in the workplace. The employer may take steps to protect the rights of employees and other individuals in the workplace; these steps may include not hiring a job applicant, assigning an employee to a particular job, or terminating an existing employee. Before an employer may take any of these steps, that employer must determine that the individual with the disability would pose significant harm to his or her own health or safety or that of others, and also determine that this harm could not be eliminated through reasonable accommodation.

Public Accommodation and Facilities Operated by Private Entities (Title III)

Most of the focus of employment discrimination is in the provisions of Title I of the ADA. However, because Title III of the ADA prohibits discrimination in public accommodations and facilities operated by private entities, it is also of concern to employers. Unlike Title I, which focuses on employees, Title III focuses on customers, clients, and visitors. New construction and alteration of virtually all privately owned nonresidential facilities must meet the requirements of Title III and the ADA Accessibility Guidelines for Buildings and Facilities. Although the employment discrimination provisions of Title I do not apply to employers with less than 15 employees, there is no such limitation to Title III's coverage. In addition, Title III prohibits discrimination on the basis of disability by public accommodations, which encompasses virtually all private businesses that serve the public. Providing public accommodations requires making reasonable modifications in policies, practices, and procedures where necessary to insure that individuals with disabilities are provided integrated and equal access to activities, goods, and services. Such modifications may include the provision of auxiliary communication aids and services, the immediate removal of architectural barriers in existing facilities, and the removal of transportation barriers in shuttle services for clients or customers.

Role of Occupational Rehabilitation Professional

The skills and expertise of the occupational rehabilitation professional are especially helpful in enforcing the ADA. He or she may be called on to perform the following:

1. Determine essential functions of a job and consult in the hiring process.
   The DA provides fertile ground for the employment, expertise, and professional talents of the rehabilitation specialist. Analyzing written job descriptions and observing workers can help occupational rehabilitation professionals determine the essential functions of a job—as distinguished from the marginal or peripheral functions.
2. Provide accommodation alternatives, ergonomics, and workplace modification.
   Equally as significant is the input of rehabilitation professionals in suggesting accommodation alternatives. Providing input on how jobs can be restructured—through part-time or modified schedules or, more specifically, through the modification of equipment and devices—is a significant opportunity for the rehabilitation professional. Ergonomic design and workplace modifications also provide specific opportunities.
   Often overlooked because of the focus on Title I are opportunities to provide suggestions regarding public accommodations and facilities—in areas as diverse as customer service and architectural design.
3. Provide expert testimony regarding undue hardship, reasonableness of accommodation, and job dangers.

THE OCCUPATIONAL SAFETY AND HEALTH ADMINISTRATION (OSHA)

The Occupational Safety and Health Act became law December 29, 1970. Its goal is "to assure as far as possible every working man and woman in the nation safe and healthful working conditions and to preserve our human resources" (preamble).

All businesses are covered under the Occupational Safety and Health Administration (OSHA) with no exclusion from coverage because of the number of workers on the payroll. The scope of coverage includes federal and state employees in every sector of employment in America. Only self-employed individuals and family farms are not covered.

Under the act it is the employer's duty to furnish employment free from "recognized hazards" that cause or are likely to cause death or serious harm to workers. Each employer must comply with the OSHA standards promulgated by the secretary of labor.

Employees' duties are simply to comply with the safety and health standard rules, regulations, and orders that apply to the employee under the act.

Administration of the Act

The secretary of labor publishes standards in the *Federal Register* that have the effect of law. These rules apply to such areas as requirements for record keeping, posting of notices, citations for violations, and information employers and employees of their rights under the act. The act also provides rules covering requirements for recording and reporting of occupationally caused deaths, accidents, and illnesses; notice of hearings; internal administrative procedures; and any interpretation of the provisions that require the publication of rules.

Many states administer their own plans, assuming responsibility for enforcement of standards. The secretary of labor monitors the operations of each state under an approved plan.

The research function of OSHA is performed under the National Institute for Occupational Safety and Health (NIOSH). NIOSH is directed to do research, experiments, and demonstrations; publish a list of toxic material; and establish criteria for the development of occupational safety and health standards. NIOSH is authorized to require that workplaces be monitored for occupational exposures, measuring toxic substances, and requiring the physical examinations of workers for the effects of those exposures.

Adoption of Standards

An occupational safety and health standard is a uniform set of required conditions or practices, methods, and operations or processes established in order to provide safe and healthful employment in the workplace. OSHA is authorized to set these standards on an interim, permanent, or emergency basis. Standards governing the exposure of workers to toxic materials or harmful physical agents must adequately assure that workers regularly exposed to such hazards will not suffer material impairment of health or the ability to function.

Inspection

OSHA inspectors are given the right of entry into all workplaces under the act, although directed to inspect "at reasonable time, during regular work hours, within reasonable limits and within a reasonable manner." The act directs that a representative of the employer and a union representative be given an opportunity to accompany the inspector on rounds of the workplace to aid the inspection. A special inspection may occur in response to an employee's request if there is imminent danger of a violation of a standard that could cause serious physical harm. Either before or during a regular inspection, employees or their representatives can notify OSHA in writing of any alleged violation of the act.

Citations for Violation

If the inspector believes that an employer has violated a standard rule, the inspector will issue a written citation setting a reasonable time for correcting the violation. Several kinds of violations of the act carry civil and criminal penalties, including standards violations willful or repeated violations, and failure to correct a cited violation.

Record Keeping and Reporting

Before the act became effective, no centralized and systematic method existed for monitoring occupational safety and health problems. Statistics on job injuries and illnesses were collected by some states and private organizations. Hence, projections of national figures were not reliable. With OSHA standards came the first basis for consistent nationwide procedures, a vital requirement for gauging and solving problems.

The act requires employers maintain records of occupational injuries and illnesses as they occur. The purpose of keeping records is to permit the Bureau of Labor Statistic to survey and compile material to help define high-hazard industries and to inform employees of the status of their employers' records.

An occupational injury is any injury such as a cut, fracture, sprain, or amputation that results from a work-related accident or from a single incident involving exposure in the work environment. An occupational illness is any abnormal condition or disorder, other than one resulting from an occupational injury caused by exposure to environmental factors, associated with employment. Included are acute and chronic illnesses that may be caused by inhalation, absorption, ingestion, or direct contact with toxic substances or harmful agents. All occupational illnesses must be recorded regardless of severity. All occupational injuries must be recorded if they result in death, one or more lost work days, restriction of work or motion, loss of consciousness, transfer to another job, or medical treatment other than first aid.

Record-Keeping Forms

Forms must be maintained and available for inspection by representatives of OSHA, including OSHA 200, a log and summary of occupational injuries and illnesses, and OSHA 101, a supplementary record of injuries that contains more detail about each injury or illness. This latter form must be completed within six working days from the time the employer learns of the work-related injury or illness (a substitute for OSHA 101, such as an insurance or workers' compensation form, may be used if it contains all required information).

Posting Requirements

A copy of the information on injuries, including total number of injuries, must be posted at each establishment, whenever notices to employees are customarily posted. Employers are responsible for keeping employees informed about OSHA and the various safety and health matters with which they are involved. Additional postings must include information on job safety and health protection, advising employees of their rights and responsibilities.

Employee Protection and Nondiscrimination

The act forbids any employer from discharging or otherwise discriminating against any employee who has filed a complaint, requested a special inspection, testified at a hearing on standard adoption, or at any other enforcement hearing. The protection extends to requesting an occupational history, accompanying an inspector on a walk-around inspection, or any other rights under the act.

Worker Rights Under the OSHA Act

Among important employee rights are the following:

- The right to request information from employers on safety and health hazards in their work areas
- The right to ask for an inspection of the workplace by NIOSH or OSHA to see if safety or health hazards exist
- The right to remain anonymous in this request
- The right to protection from being fired or punished in any way for exercising these rights under the act
- The right to have an employee representative accompany inspectors on plant safety and health inspections
- The right to know the results of an inspection report
- The right to appeal certain OSHA findings or orders
- The right to become part of certain legal proceedings in which an employer appeals OSHA findings or orders
- The right to obtain a copy of OSHA standards and other rules, regulations, and requirements
- The right to a safe and healthful workplace

State Jurisdiction and State Plans

OSHA is not solely a federal occupational safety and health program. OSHA also sets forth the conditions whereby states may administer and enforce their own programs and receive federal matching grants. Many states have administrative codes that "mirror" federal OSHA provisions.

The Role of the Occupational Rehabilitation Professional

Rehabilitation professionals assist in the establishment and running of safety committees, reading and interpreting NIOSH research and OSHA standards and implementing those standards in the workplace. Occupational nurses and ergonomic specialists assist in record keeping and accident reporting and insure that OSHA standards are met.

THE REHABILITATION ACT OF 1973 (AS AMENDED)

Many of the concepts contained in the Americans with Disabilities Act (ADA) have as their origin the Rehabilitation Act of 1973 and the case law that construed the various provisions of that act. Basic grounding in the Rehabilitation Act is helpful in understanding how the more expansive ADA is interpreted and enforced.

Although significant, the 1973 Rehabilitation Act is a law limited in scope. By its terms, the statute prohibits discrimination only by federal agencies, entities that have contracts with the federal government, and recipients of federal financial assistance. Three major classes of recipients of federal funds are (a) public school systems, (b) colleges and other institutions of higher learning, and (c) health, welfare, and social service providers. Until the ADA, no federal law prohibited discrimination by employers in the private sector, places of public accommodation, or state and local government agencies that do not receive federal aid.

Enforcement

The Department of Justice is in charge of coordinating each agency's enforcement of Section 504. For federally assisted programs, regulations provide for grievance procedures and administrative complaints, but the agency procedures require complaints file within 180 days of the date of the discriminatory act. Remedies, which include the termination of federal funding to the grant recipient, are subject to judicial review. Under Section 504, private employees have a right of action against employers receiving federal funding. These employees need not exhaust administrative remedies prior to bringing a court suit.

Rehabilitation Act General Provisions

The act covers private and public employment. In 1992, the Rehabilitation Act was amended so that its terms would conform to those set forth in the ADA. The Rehabilitation Act amendment substituted the term *disability* for *handicap* in the statute.

Section 501 of the act applies to all federal departments and agencies and is aimed at preventing agencies of the federal government from discriminating against applicants and employees with disabilities. The language of Section 501 requires federal agencies to take affirmative action to hire and retain employees with disabilities. Section 501 is enforced initially through the Equal Employment Opportunities Commission (EEOC) administrative process, but claimants also can initiate action.

Section 503 governs federal contractors, while Section 504 applies to programs conducted by private entities receiving federal financial assistance and to programs conducted by executive agencies.

Section 503(a) specifically provides that parties contracting with the federal government must implement affirmative action programs to accommodate individuals with disabilities under the following conditions: Any contract in excess of $10,000 entered into by an federal department or agency purchasing personal property and nonpersonal services for the United States must contain a provision requiring that the party contracting with the United States take *affirmative action* to employ and advance in employment qualified individuals with disabilities. The Department of Labor is responsible for administering Section 503. The act provides an administrative remedy through the Department of Labor's Office of Federal Contract Compliance Program (OFCCP).

Section 504 prohibits discrimination under any program or activity that receives federal financial assistance and prohibits discrimination against individuals with disabilities employed by executive agencies. Section 504 requires reasonable accommodation, but no affirmative action.

Relationship Between the Rehabilitation Act and the ADA

Section 501 of the ADA specifically provides that the ADA and the Rehabilitation Act are to be considered in tandem. The ADA prevents the provisions of the Rehabilitation Act. Similarly, following the passage of the ADA, Congress amended Section 504 to provide that the standards used to determine violations of employment discrimination shall be the standards applied under the ADA.

1992 Amendments—Vocational Rehabilitation Services

Declaration of Policies

Congress found that work is a valued activity to individuals and society, and that as a group individuals with disabilities experience staggering levels of unemployment and poverty. Discrimination and lack of accessible and available transportation, fear of loss of health coverage, and a lack of education and training are reasons that a significant number of individuals with disabilities do not secure work at levels commensurate with their abilities and capabilities.

State Plans

Each state submits to the commissioner of the Rehabilitation Services Administration a plan for vocational rehabilitation and assigns a state agency to administer or supervise the plan.

Individualized Written Rehabilitation Program (IWRP)

The 1992 amendments to the Rehabilitation Act presume that an individual can benefit in terms of an employment outcome from vocational rehabilitation services unless the designated agency can demonstrate by clear and convincing evidence that such an individual is incapable of benefitting from such services. Each IWRP should be designed to achieve an employment objective consistent with the individual's unique strengths, resources, priorities, concerns, abilities, and capabilities and include a statement of the long-term rehabilitation goals and of the intermediate rehabilitation objectives. The IWRP must include a statement of the specific vocational rehabilitation services to be provided, projected dates for the initiation and duration of each service, specific rehabilitation technology services to be provided to assist in the implementation of the goal, and the specific one-the-job and related personal assistance services to be provided.

Scope of Vocational Rehabilitation Services

The Rehabilitation Act of 1973 provides for training and community rehabilitation programs (Section 301). The act authorizes grants and contracts to insure that skilled personnel are available to provide rehabilitation services to individuals with disabilities through vocational, medical, social, and psychological rehabilitation programs and through supported employment programs, independent living services programs, and client assistant programs. The grants and contracts exist to provide training and information to individuals with disabilities and to their parents, families, guardians, advocates, and authorized representatives. The law authorizes grants for special projects and demonstrations that hold the promise of expanding or otherwise improving rehabilitation services to individuals with disabilities. The general grant and contract requirements are contained in Section 306.

Rights and Advocacy

The original law and amendments establishes within the federal government an Interagency Committee on Handicapped Employees to provide a focus for federal employment of individuals with disabilities and other employment opportunities, and to review in cooperation with the Equal Employment Opportunities Commission the adequacy of hiring, placement, and advancement practices with respect to individuals with disabilities by each department and agency of the government. This committee also insures that the special needs of such individuals are being met. The law also provides for the establishment of community service employment pilot programs for individuals with handicaps and for the coordination of these projects with industry. The act further provides for supported employment services, business opportunities, and independent living services and centers for individuals with severe disabilities.

Opportunities for Occupational Rehabilitation Professionals under the Rehabilitation Act of 1973 (with 1992 Amendments)

Vocational rehabilitation professionals have many opportunities under this act. Grant writing, project coordination, and community rehabilitation program coordination are only a few. The vocational retraining provisions of the act and specifically of the IWRP call for skilled vocational rehabilitation counselors whose training in occupational rehabilitation is particularly useful in this process.

SOCIAL SECURITY DISABILITY

The Social Security Act established a social insurance program designed to provide guaranteed income to individuals with disabilities when they are found to be generally incapable of gainful employment. Its purpose is to provide a basic level of financial support for people who cannot support themselves because of disability. Social Security retirement benefits date back to 1935 and the New Deal. In adding disability as a basis for benefits administered by the Social Security Administration in the mid-1950's, Congress recognized society's obligation to provide assistance to people whose disabilities prevent them from achieving economic self-sufficiency.

Social Security Administration Programs

The Social Security Act (SSA) provides for several disability benefit programs administered by the SSA, including the Social Security Disability Insurance (SSDI) and Supplemental Security Income (SSI) programs. The SSDI program provides benefits to disabled workers, dependents, and widows/widowers if the worker is insured under the provisions of the program. The SSI program provides benefits to disabled individuals whose incomes and assets fall below a specified level (Social Security Act, 1954). Although the eligibility criteria under the two programs are different (SSDI is insurance based and SSI is based on need), their determinations of disability are virtually identical.

Eligibility Determination

To receive SSA disability benefits, an individual must prove that she or he is disabled under the SSDI or the SSI program. According to the Social Security Disability Act, the essential requirement for both programs is that the claimant be unable to engage in

> any substantial gainful activity by reason of any medically determinable physical or mental impairment which can be expected to result in death or which has lasted or can be expected to last for a continuous period of not less than 12 months (sec 42 USC §423(d)(1)(a); 20 CFR §404,1505).

Under the statute, a person is entitled to disability benefits if the impairment is of such severity that he or she is not only unable to do his or her previous work but cannot, considering age, education, and work experience, engage in any other kind of substantial, gainful work that exists in the national economy. Work that exists in the national economy means jobs within the individual's limitations must exist in significant numbers either in the region where the individual lives or in several regions of the country. Isolated jobs that exist only in limited numbers and at relatively few locations outside the region where the claimant lives are not considered as work that exists in the national economy.

Social Security and Work Efforts

The Social Security Act itself, however, recognized that an individual may be unable to engage in substantial gainful activity and yet still be able to work. Although the SSA program is designed to provide a guaranteed income to individuals who are found to meet SSA disability eligibility criteria, Congress has recognized the importance of encouraging individuals with disabilities to work whenever possible. Accordingly, the Social Security Act contains numerous work incentive programs. For example, the SSA has a trial work period that allows beneficiaries to work for nine months while their benefit entitlement and payment levels remain unchanged. Similarly, the SSA has an extended period of eligibility that provides individuals who return to work with benefits in any month in which earnings fall below a statutory level. Thus, even the SSA does not view a person who meets the definition of disabled as someone who is totally unable to work.

SSA Definition of Disability Process

A sequential evaluation process is used to determine if an individual meets the SSA definition of disabled. This five step process requires the SSA to ask the following questions:

1. Is the claimant currently engaging in substantial gainful activity? If the answer is yes, the claim is denied; if the answer is no, the claim continues to the next step.
2. Does the claimant have a severe impairment? If the answer is no, the claim is denied; if the claimant has an impairment that significantly limits his or her ability to work—that is it is "severe," the claim continues to Step 3.
3. Does the claimant have an impairment that is equivalent to any impairment the SSA has listed as so severe that is automatically precludes substantial gainful activity? If the claimant has an impairment that is medically the equivalent of a listed impairment, the claimant is presumed disabled by the SSA, and benefits are

granted. (Some examples of impairment are asthma, ischemic heart disease, and affective disorders.) If the claimant does not have a listed impairment, the claim proceeds to Step 4.

4. Does the impairment prevent the claimant from performing his or her "past relevant work"? If the claimant can perform this past relevant work, the claim is denied. If the claimant cannot perform such work, the claim continues to Step 5.

5. Does the impairment prevent the claimant from performing any other type of work? If the SSA determines that the claimant is able to perform other work that exists in the national economy, the claim is denied. If the SSA determines that the claimant is unable to perform any work considering age, education, and past work experience, benefits are granted. A grid that considers past work, age, and education is used in this process to help determinations of disability (see Figure 3.1). For example, a 59-year-old worker (advanced age) with a sedentary lifting limitation, an unskilled job background, and no post–high school education would be considered disabled under this grid. However, if that same individual were 45 years old or had light duty restrictions, the grid presumption would be against disability, and SSA benefits would be denied unless another combination of factors were shown.

SSA Interplay with ADA

The SSA acknowledges the differences between its standards and those of other statutory schemes. In that regard, SSA regulations note that a decision by any other entity about whether the individual is disabled is based on the other entity's rules and may not be the same as the SSA's determination based on Social Security law. For example, a determination of permanent and total disability under workers' compensation based on a state statute would not compel the SSA to reach a similar determination.

The SSA determination of disability is inherently different from the ADA definition of qualified individual with a disability. First, while the ADA always requires an individualized inquiry into the ability of a person to meet the requirements of a particular position, the SSA permits general presumptions about an individual's ability to work. In that regard, the SSA considers some conditions to be presumptively disabling. If a claimant has an impairment that is medically the equivalent of a listed impairment, for example, then the SSA presumes that the disorder is so severe as to prevent the claimant from doing any substantial, gainful activity—without considering his or her age, education, or past work experience. Thus, an individual can have a disability under the SSA definition and yet still be able to work.

Second, in determining whether a person meets the SSA definition of disability, the SSA looks at the customary requirements of jobs as usually performed in the national economy without focusing on the essential functions of a particular position. All tasks required to perform the job are considered with no distinction made between fundamental and peripheral or marginal functions. Thus, a person who is able to perform the essential but not the marginal functions of a particular position may be found to be unable to work and eligible for disability benefits. Accordingly, the SSA's determination that a person is unable to engage in any substantial, gainful activity in the national economy does not mean that there is no job the person can perform. The person may still be able to perform the essential functions of a particular position.

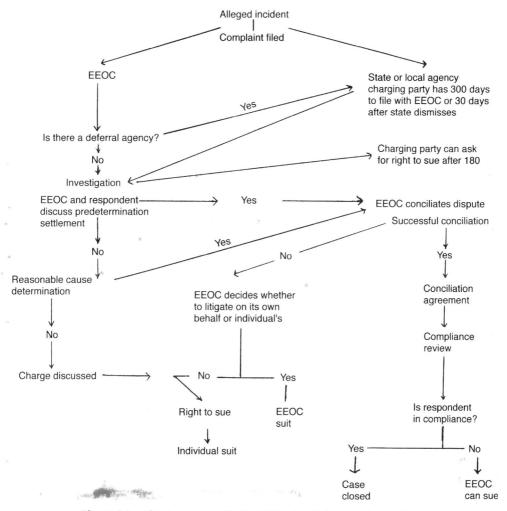

Figure 3-1.   The Americans with Disabilities Act: Enforcement procedures.

Third, unlike the ADA definition, the SSA definition does not consider whether the individual can work with a reasonable accommodation. The EEOC Enforcement Guidance on Disability Representations (2-12-97) addressing the effect of the ADA or SSA's disability determination process states the following:

> The fact that an individual may be able to return to a past relevant job, provided that the employer makes accommodations, is not relevant to the issue to be resolved. Hypothetical inquiries about whether an employer would or could make accommodation that would allow return to a prior job would not be appropriate. (p. 5)

Thus, the SSA may find that a person is unable to do any of the work that exists in the national economy even though he or she can work with a reasonable accommodation. In those instances, the individual is categorized as a person with a disability under the SSA and a qualified individual with a disability under the ADA. Accordingly, a person claiming to be disabled or found to be disabled under the SSA programs still may be entitled to protection under the ADA.

Procedures

Because occupational rehabilitation professionals are used as resources by persons with disabilities who may qualify for SSDI, a brief overview of the procedures is appropriate. An application form for total disability can be obtained at any Social Security office. The form should be submitted as soon as it appears likely that the claimant cannot perform any substantial, gainful work for at least a year. If the disability claim is approved, monthly checks will generally start on the sixth full month of disability. If the sixth month has already passed, the first check will include back payments. Benefits are retroactive for up to a year from the date of application. Thus, a disabled individual should not wait longer than a year before processing an application for benefits.

If the initial determination is unfavorable, the claimant should always appeal the decision by a simple letter to the claimant's local Social Security office. The next step is a "reconsideration determination." If that decision is unfavorable, the claimant should always appeal. Thereafter, the claimant will be given a hearing before an administrative law judge. At the hearing level, the claimant should always be represented by counsel. An attorney or representative can charge up to 25% of the past-due benefits as a fee. If that hearing provides live testimony before an administrative law judge, it may involve the participation of a vocational expert to provide assistance to the judge in making vocational determinations. Denials of claims after a hearing may be appealed to the Appeals Council (again within 60 days) and, further, to a federal district court.

Benefits

Recipients of SSA benefits receive monthly checks, as do dependents under 18 years of age. Monthly benefit amounts depend on the SSA's calculation of average earnings during the claimant's work history. Recipients are also entitled to Medicare benefits (Type A, hospitalization; Type B, physician's care).

SSDI payments and workers' compensation disability payments can be collected at the same time, subject to certain reductions in total benefits, depending on the amount of past earnings.

Role of the Occupational Rehabilitation Professional in the SSA Process

Initially, occupational rehabilitation professionals can be used by claimants and claimants' attorneys as experts to help determine eligibility. Although an administrative law judge will likely make eligibility findings according to the five-step process, if the matter proceeds to a hearing, the claimant's vocational expert can assist the claimant and the claimant's representative with proof that the claimant can perform neither past relevant work nor any other work available in the national economy. Additionally, the vocational expert may assist the claimant or his or her representative in suggesting ways to meet the criteria of the "grid," consisting of past relevant work, education, age, and training.

An additional role for the occupational rehabilitation professional is as a designated vocational expert in SSA hearings. Vocational experts are hired by the SSA (usually for several successive hearings in "whole-day blocks") to provide vocational testimony at hearings. The role of a vocational expert at an SSA hearing is to review the medical file of the claimant, the claimant's vocational history, age, education, and experience and assist the administrative law judge if the judge presents hypothetical examples to the expert as a way of determining the claimant's eligibility for SSA benefits. The vocational expert must be familiar with SSA rulings and vocational guidelines if she or he were to serve as an expert in this capacity. Familiarity with the *Dictionary of Occupational Titles* and labor market statistics in the local and national labor markets is also required. For example, the judge may hypothetically ask the vocational expert, "Assuming a sedentary lifting limitation, a high school education, an age of 55, and a past relevant work history of unskilled jobs, does work exist in the national economy (and in what numbers) for the claimant?" The qualified vocational expert should have a ready response.

WORKERS' COMPENSATION

Coverage and Statutory Framework

Workers' compensation is a no-fault insurance system that pays benefits to employees for accidental injuries or diseases related to the employee's work. Workers' compensation provides financial benefits to employees injured on the job, including payment of medical bills related to the injuries, benefits to the dependents of employees who die from work-related injuries or diseases. Beginning with Wisconsin in 1911, all states have adopted workers' compensation laws. The workers' compensation remedy is exclusively for work-related injuries. Under worker's compensation employees cannot sue their employers. At the same time, an employee's negligence will not preclude recovery based on a statutory schedule of benefits.

Disability in Workers' Compensation

The workers' compensation definitions of "disability" reflect the purposes of workers' compensation laws. They provide a system for securing a prompt and fair settlement of employees' claims against employers for occupational injury and illness. Procedurally, an administrative hearing takes the place of a court case. Claims are routinely handled in a speedier manner than through the clogged state court system.

The laws require employers to compensate employees who are injured in the course of employment for the resulting loss of earning capacity and medical care expenses. Thus, workers' compensation provides benefits to individuals whose earning capacity has been reduced because of a work-related injury. Because of the emphasis on lost earning capacity, the workers' compensation definitions of disability (as contrasted with the ADA) generally focus on what a person can no longer do rather than on what he or she is still capable of doing with or without reasonable accommodation.

Eligibility

To receive workers' compensation benefits, an employee generally must prove that he or she has a compensable disability as defined by the applicable workers' compensation statute. The term *disability* in this context most commonly means the loss of reduction of earning power that results from a work-related injury. The injury can stem from a traumatic event (most commonly a workplace accident) or a prolonged exposure to work that results in an occupational disease. Mental injuries are also routinely compensated—whether they stem from the mental effects of a traumatic injury (post-traumatic stress disorder) or are nontraumatically induced as a result of extraordinary stress. Considerations of employee or employer fault are irrelevant (although such a finding can increase or decrease benefits). Some statutes do not define disability in terms of lost earning capacity. Instead, under these statutes an injured worker has a disability if his or her physical efficiency has been substantially reduced (compensation is determined according to a "schedule of benefits," with the loss or injury of each body part correlated with a number of weeks of disability).

Although workers' compensation laws vary from state to state, the typical statute ordinarily provides the following four classifications of disability, determined by duration (permanent or temporary) and severity or extent (partial or total):

- Temporary partial disability
- Temporary total disability
- Permanent partial disability
- Permanent total disability

Generally, a disability is partial rather than total when the claimant is still capable of gainful employment, even though the disability may prevent a return to his or her former employment. Conversely, a worker generally is considered totally disabled when the injury is found to render the worker temporarily or permanently unable to do any kind of work for which there is a reasonably stable labor market.

Compensation Payment

Temporary total disability is routinely paid over a "healing period" during which the applicant is convalescing, still healing, and unable to work. Benefits are paid as a percentage of gross pay (normally two thirds) subject to a weekly cap (see Figure 3.2—the Wisconsin "model"). Once an individual reaches a healing plateau, a physician generally assesses a percentage of permanent partial disability. These permanent partial disability benefits are paid at a reduced rate for a prescribed number of weeks according to a schedule of benefits. An individual can be permanently and totally disabled if he or she cannot do any work for which there is a reasonably stable employment market. This scenario will provide lifetime benefits for the disabled employee and at some point will usually require the testimony or opinion of a vocational rehabilitation expert.

Choice of Physician

In most states, an employee can choose any physician, chiropractor, psychologist, podiatrist, or dentist for treatment. The insurance carrier will be liable for the medical expenses incurred from the work-related injury. An employee's choice of physician is sometimes limited, however, unless a prior agreement with the employer had been reached. Insurance carriers and employers have a right to call for medical examinations at reasonable intervals.

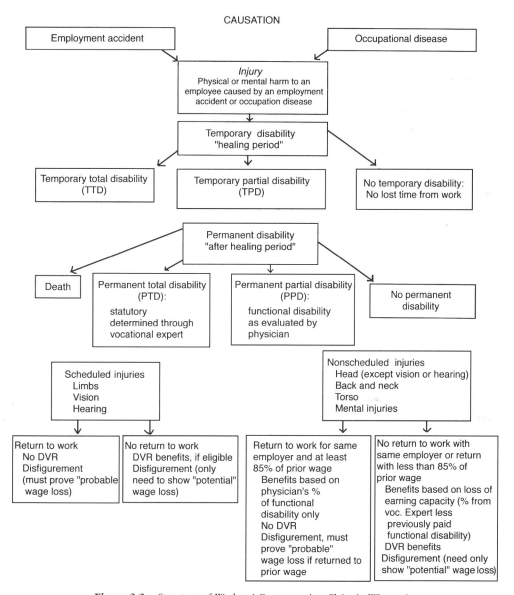

Figure 3-2. Structure of Workers' Compensation Claim in Wisconsin.

Payment of Medical Bills

In most states, payments of workers' compensation to medical providers exceed 50% of the total workers' compensation dollars. If the medical expenses incurred are related to the work injury, the insurance carrier is liable for all medical expenses. Many states have initiated a process by which an insurance carrier can challenge the reasonableness or necessity of the medical services. This process is separate and distinct from the applicant's indemnity claim for disability benefits.

Return-to-Work Issues in Vocational Rehabilitation

Significance of Physician's Assessment of Permanent Limitations

The treating physician's assignment of permanent limitations triggers the employer's responsibility to return the work-injured employee to work if a job exists. Unlike the ADA, however, most workers' compensation statutes do not require any reasonable accommodation. If a job does not exist within the permanent limitations of the employee as assigned by the employee's treating physician, the employer has no obligation under workers' compensation to modify a position to accommodate the employee.

Unlike the ADA definition of qualified individual with a disability, the workers' compensation definitions of disability do not distinguish between marginal or essential functions and do not consider whether an individual can work with reasonable accommodation. In many workers' compensation cases, a person has a total disability when he or she is unable to do certain tasks, even if those tasks are marginal functions or if he or she could perform them with reasonable accommodation. Thus, a person may be totally disabled for workers' compensation purposes and yet still be able to perform the essential functions of the job with or without reasonable accommodation.

Disability under ADA versus Workers' Compensation

A person can receive workers' compensation benefits for a temporary total disability from which he or she is expected to recover if during the time of incapacitation he or she is unable to perform the duties in the occupation in which he or she was employed at the time of injury. The person is found to have a temporary total disability even if the duties he or she cannot perform are marginal functions, or he or she could perform those duties with reasonable accommodation. Further, some statutes permit a finding of total disability when a person can work, but the work that he or she can do is of such limited availability that a reasonably stable and continuous market for such labor does not exist.

A determination under a workers' compensation statute that a person cannot do any kind of work for which a reasonably stable employment market exists and therefore is totally disabled does not necessarily mean that there is no job that the person can perform. Accordingly, an individual receiving workers' compensation benefits still may be entitled to protection under the ADA.

Return to Work Decisions

If the employer decides to re-employ the work-injured employee, even with permanent restrictions, the most significant workers' compensation benefits are foreclosed. Loss of earning capacity benefits, which are the most significant benefits in workers' compensation, are also precluded if the employer rehires the employee at the same or similar wage rate.

Refusal to Rehire Issue and Employer Penalties

In many states, if the employer refuses to rehire a work-injured employee because of the work injury, the employer is liable to pay a penalty of up to one year's wages. Reinstatement, however, is not contemplated in a workers' compensation recovery. An employee must look to the state's fair employment laws for an order to reinstate if the employer has discriminated on the basis of a handicap.

State Division of Vocational Rehabilitation Requirements

Under the Rehabilitation Act of 1973, 29 USC 701 to 7976, as amended through the 1992 amendments, state designated agencies operate a comprehensive coordinated program of vocational rehabilitation for individuals with disabilities, including those with work-related disabilities. Work-injured individuals who apply for rehabilitation benefits under state departments designated to provide vocational rehabilitation services are assessed by the state agency in the same way that any other person with a disability is.

Development of an Individualized Written Rehabilitation Program

If an initial interview and a preliminary and comprehensive assessment determine that a client is eligible for an individual written rehabilitation program (IWRP), one is drafted. For workers' compensation clients, the state agency must notify the time-of-injury employer to determine whether work is available for that employee. The IWRP can focus on job placement or academic retraining. If transferrable skills exist, a job search is required before the state agency will sponsor academic retraining tuition and book expenses.

Under workers' compensation, if a work-injured client who is sponsored by the state vocational rehabilitation agency is enrolled in school under an IWRP, the workers' compensation insurance carrier must pay maintenance benefits for the duration of his or her schooling at a temporary total disability benefit rate.

Significance of Testing, Transferrable Skills, and Job Search

The state agency must follow its own procedures in order to insure that the workers' compensation insurance company will be liable for maintenance benefits for the duration of academic training for the work-injured client. Most state agency procedure manuals require contact with the time-of-injury employer, the workers' compensation carrier, and other interested parties. If transferrable skills exist, most insurance carriers require that reasonable efforts at job placement be made before accepting liability for an academic retraining program.

Restoring Lost Earnings

The state vocational rehabilitation agency has as its primary purpose the restoration of earning capacity for work-injured employees. When this goal is not achievable, however, or only partially achievable, many work-injured employees are also eligible for a loss of earning capacity for specific kinds of injuries.

Loss of Earning Capacity

State workers' compensation laws differentiate between scheduled and unscheduled injuries. In some states, a differentiation is made between scheduled (limb injuries, sight and hearing loss) and unscheduled (torso, back, systemic problems) injuries. Because benefits for scheduled injuries are built in, no loss of earning capacity assessment is available. For unscheduled injuries, many states also allow a loss of earning capacity component.

The majority of states allow a loss of earning capacity evaluation in the event that the work-injured employee cannot return to his time-of-injury employer, whether the injury is to a "scheduled" or "unscheduled" part of the body.

Use of Vocational Experts and Criteria

A physician's assessment of a percentage of functional disability is only one component of a loss of earning capacity claim. A vocational expert is regularly employed to determine the loss of access to the labor market due to the claimant's work-injury limitations. In making that determination, vocational experts routinely rely on such factors as the following:

- Age
- Education
- Training
- Previous work experience
- Previous earnings
- Present occupation and earnings
- Likelihood of a future suitable occupational change
- Efforts to obtain suitable employment
- Willingness to make a reasonable change in a residence to secure suitable employment
- Success of and willingness to participate in reasonable physical and vocational rehabilitation programs
- Other pertinent evidence

For work-injured employees whose work injuries are so severe that a stable labor market does not exist, permanent and total disability is warranted. These employees can be characterized as permanently and totally disabled under an "odd lot" doctrine that suggests that the combination of vocational factors listed here so limits them that the quality, quantity, and stability of remaining jobs places them in an "odd lot" category. Hence, they should be paid permanent and total disability.

Lawyer Involvement

Attorneys are allowed contingent fees in workers' compensation matters (regularly 20% of benefits). These fees are paid from the proceeds recoverable by the applicant not in addition to them. Workers' compensation claims can be resolved by a stipulation wherein the insurance carrier agrees to pay a certain percentage of permanent disability and duration of disability, by a compromise that forecloses the applicant's claim, or by a limited compromise that forecloses some claims and leaves others open. States have varying statutes of limitation in workers' compensation claims, ranging from 2 to 12 years.

The Occupational Rehabilitation Professional's Role in the Workers' Compensation Process

The occupational rehabilitation professional can play many roles in the workers' compensation process in the interest of the applicant and that of the workers' compensation insurance carrier. Insurance carriers use job placement specialists and job modification experts to prevent work injuries *before* they occur. Occupational nurses and job safety and ergonomics experts can provide information to employers to assist in preventing injuries. After work injuries occur, insurance carriers continue to use rehabilitation nurses and job placement experts in an attempt to return work-injured employees to productive employment (with a secondary purpose of reducing their liability). Rehabilitation nurses can help treating physicians determine what limitations may be appropriate for a particular work setting, limiting the insurance company's liability for ongoing temporary disability. Additionally, as discussed earlier, many occupational rehabilitation professionals work for the Division of Vocational Rehabilitation, devising rehabilitation plans for work-injured employees who seek help through the designated state vocational agency.

Lastly, injured workers and insurance carriers employ rehabilitation professionals. Vocational counselors must be familiar with the local labor market, *Dictionary of Occupational Titles* criteria, and workers' compensation laws.

REFERENCES

Social Security Disability Act, 42 U.S.C. §413 (1954).
Vande Zande v. Wisconsin Department of Administration, 44 F. 3d, 538 (1995).

4

Health Care Reform

Linda Ogden Niemeyer

WHY THE NEED FOR REFORM

In the early 1990s, the workers' compensation reimbursement system began spiraling toward financial disaster. In 1985, medical costs per case averaged $3,673, and indemnity or nonmedical costs averaged $7,773. Five years later, these figures almost doubled to $6,611 and $12,833 respectively. There were more than eight consecutive years of unprofitability for workers' compensation insurers, during which costs exceeded premium income by as much as 23%. Medical cost inflation was blamed on a number of factors. First, most reimbursement had been on a fee-for-service basis. The more services that were rendered, the more procedures that were performed, the more fees that could be billed. This system created a disincentive for being a cost-effective health care provider. Second, the growth of medical technology led to more expensive diagnostic and surgical procedures. Once a new procedure was in use, it influenced accepted standards of care. Third, as reimbursement from Medicare and employee benefit plans became more limited due to stringent cost management, health care providers attempted cost shifting, charging workers' compensation insurers more to make up differences (Curtis, 1993). Finally, the definition of compensable injury was expanded to include claims related to difficult-to-treat cumulative trauma, other repetitive motion disorders, and psychological stress on the job (Dent, 1990).

In addition to the growing financial burden, there was the problem of poor rehabilitation outcomes. In at least 20–25% of cases, injured workers were unable to successfully return to work within projected time frames. For these individuals, functional improvement was slow, degree of disability seemed out of keeping with the original diagnoses, and many developed chronic pain syndrome. The problem was termed *delayed recovery* (Derebery & Tullis, 1983). Several studies found that cases characterized by delayed recovery incurred 80%–90% of the costs of workers' compensation (Arm-

Linda Ogden Niemeyer • Rehabilitation Technology Works, 2195 Club Center Drive, Suite G, San Bernardino, California 92408.

Sourcebook of Occupational Rehabilitation, edited by Phyllis M. King. Plenum Press, New York, 1998.

strong & Silverstein, 1987; Frymoyer, 1988; Louis, 1987; Philips, Grant, & Berkowitz, 1991; Pope, Andersson, Frymoyer, & Chaffin, 1991; Spengler, Bigos, Martin, Zeh, Fisher, & Nachemson, 1986). Psychologists and other health care professionals focused on the injured workers as the source of the problem and conducted studies to determine ways to identify and deal with "malingering," "symptom magnification," and "abnormal (or inappropriate) illness behavior." Others in the health care industry focused on the workers' compensation system and discovered a growing win–lose mentality; the competing and conflicting interests of health care providers, legal representatives, organized labor, legislators, claimants, employers, and compensation or insurance agencies were being served at the expense of the whole. Poor rehabilitation outcome was attributed to the cumulative result of conflicting messages and agendas from different sectors, which bogged down rehabilitation efforts, a phenomenon sometimes called *comalingering* (LeClair & Mitchell, 1992).

Escalating medical costs, fraud and abuse, and the complexities and inefficiencies associated with the administration of claims and benefits fueled the movement toward health care reform in workers' compensation. In an attempt to direct resources to cost-effective interventions and increase accountability for the quality and effectiveness of care, workers' compensation payers began following the precedent set by other health care delivery systems, namely making the transition from fee-for-service reimbursement to managed care (Cerne, 1994).

HISTORY AND DEFINITION OF MANAGED CARE

As early as the 1940s, Kaiser Steel established a precursor of the managed care approach, a health maintenance organization that served its own employees. However, the main impetus for managed care was a retrospective utilization review process set up in the mid-1960s to determine whether government funds under Medicare were being spent only on medically necessary services. The alarming growth in health care expenditure that resulted from the federal government's becoming a major financier of the health care needs of the elderly forced a greater emphasis on cost containment. Hospitals, extended care facilities, and other delivery systems participating in Medicare were required by the government to conduct retrospective utilization reviews. However, this type of review process had little impact on clinical practice or the cost of care (Giles, 1991; Tischler, 1990).

Amendments to the Social Security Act passed in 1972 established a nationwide network of voluntary, nonprofit professional standard review organizations (PSROs). PSROs were charged with the task of determining by means of retrospective review whether government funds were being spent only on medically necessary services rendered in appropriate settings in accordance with accepted standards of practice. Then in 1982, Congress enacted laws replacing PSROs with utilization and quality control peer review organizations (PROs). Peer review organizations were given stronger sanctioning authority; practitioners and providers who failed to meet professionally recognized standards of care could be fined or excluded from Medicare (Tischler, 1990).

These activities in the public sector firmly endorsed the concept of peer involvement in judgments regarding the appropriateness, necessity, and quality of care. Many private health insurance carriers followed suit, developing their own independent peer and utilization review systems and incorporating retrospective review into the claims processing. Health insurance carriers in the private sector, however, went one step farther. In the late 1970s, they began implementing *prior* review techniques, such as preadmission certification, case management, concurrent review, second surgical opinions, and discharge planning (Tischler, 1990).

The considerable growth and change that occurred in managed care over the next decade resulted in three major types of managed care insurance plans: managed indemnity programs, health maintenance organizations (HMOs), and preferred provider organizations (PPOs). In each approach, prior review techniques were included as part of the cost management package to reduce the unnecessary use of patient services and assess the appropriateness of care. Managed indemnity programs are traditional insurance plans in which an enrolled individual can seek care from any licensed provider and receive the same level of benefit. However, a major trend has been the use of preferred provider networks, a practice that has been adopted by HMOs and PPOs. An HMO is an integrated, comprehensive health care system composed of a limited number of doctors, hospitals, and other providers who give care to enrolled members. Premiums are based on a community rating process usually not tied to utilization. A staff model HMO employs its own physicians and acquires its own hospitals. In the individual practice association (IPA) model, an HMO contracts with physicians who have an existing private practice to provide care to its membership. Except for emergencies, individuals are covered for their care only if they use an HMO-affiliated provider, although open-ended HMOs offer limited reimbursement for services received from nonaffiliated providers (Managed Care Communications, 1992).

A PPO is a health care plan that contracts with a comprehensive network of health care providers who show cost-effective practice patterns. Enrollees receive HMO-level benefits when they use doctors and hospitals that are affiliated with the PPO. The benefit level drops when an individual chooses to receive care from outside licensed sources, so there is a financial incentive encouraging enrollees to use providers associated with the network. Point-of-service plans are a hybrid that combine characteristics of HMOs and PPOs and offer more freedom of choice. A network of contracted preferred providers is used, but enrollees have the option of selecting a primary care physician to act as a gatekeeper who controls referrals (Managed Care Communications, 1992).

In summary, managed care in the 1990s offers integrated financing and delivery systems for health care benefits, using preferred provider networks. There are selection standards for providers, contracted payer–provider relationships, an organized system for ongoing utilization review, and formal processes for monitoring provider cost-effectiveness. Major insurers such as Aetna and Cigna have established managed care preferred provider networks for workers' compensation policyholders in a growing number of states.

THE MANAGED CARE DILEMMA

The recent history of managed care has been fraught with ethical dilemmas. These dilemmas occur because managed care is a system of providing health care in an integrated manner while at the same time *controlling costs*. Costs are controlled by transferring health care decisions from the patient and health care provider to a gatekeeper, who is likely to be a primary care physician, adjuster, or case manager. Part of the gatekeeper's mission is to limit the type, length, and frequency of a medical evaluation or treatment to that which is deemed necessary and appropriate. The gatekeeper works within certain guidelines and cost-saving incentives handed down from administration. The ethical dilemma occurs when cost management begins to override the provision of quality care. There have been a growing number of cases of alleged abuses stemming from the way managed care organizations have influenced the practice of health care. These abuses include delaying or denying needed care, discharging patients from care prematurely, instituting "gag rules" that restrict providers from discussing certain policies or health care options, overruling clinical decision makers, and threatening to exclude providers who do not adhere to administration policies. As a result, there has been a regulatory backlash as federal and state lawmakers have introduced legislation to guard the public interest (Berg, 1997). For example, on the federal level, Representative Charles Norwood (R-GA) has introduced the Patient Access to Responsible Care Act (PARCA) to establish a regulatory framework and provide consumers with important protections (Pontzer, 1997).

As managed care insurers enter the workers' compensation arena, they bring with them many of the same managed cost policies and practices, for example, a focus on reducing expenditures through short-term cost containment and contracting with providers who offer the lowest fee-for-service. However, workers' compensation is a different ball game. While traditional managed care insurance covers only medical and rehabilitative care, workers' compensation additionally covers temporary disability payments while the individual is unable to work and vocational rehabilitation if the worker is unable to return to his or her usual and customary job. Insurers are learning that dollars saved initially lead to increased overall costs and that these policies therefore become self-defeating. This is the managed care dilemma for workers' compensation.

Here is a scenario that occurs when a workers' compensation delivery system is focused on short-term cost containment, particularly with soft-tissue injures, such as sprains, strains, or tendinitis. In this kind of delivery system, patients are sent to emergency care or industrial clinics where they are taken off work and receive rest and conservative medical treatment for up to several months. If the injured worker does not show sufficient improvement after that time, he or she may then be referred for therapy and/or specialized medical evaluation, which may lead to surgery. In addition, providers who offer the best discounts are selected. To the insurance adjuster, money is saved by putting off referral to specialized services until they are absolutely necessary and paying the lowest fees possible. Yet this approach to managing care not only needlessly prolongs a case, but it also decreases the likelihood of a successful return to work.

How does short-term cost containment contribute to the decreased likelihood of return to work? For one thing, the most effective providers are not necessarily those offering the lowest rates, and forced discounting may actually put the better providers out of business. This factor, plus delays in receiving specialized care, can lead to an inadequately diagnosed and undertreated injury that simply does not improve. But it is often the psychosocial issues that crop up during time off work that present the real barriers to successful job reentry. The longer the case goes on, the longer the worker will have been exposed to deconditioning, forced dependency, financial losses, marital problems, and other life stresses related to not working. Interpersonal problems on the job that were unsolved at the time of injury become more difficult to resolve. Psychopathologies like depression, anxiety, and alcoholism can either develop or be exacerbated. Marginal coping skills can be tested to the limit. An injury that does not get better, in addition to all of the above psychosocial stresses, can lead to an attitude change, including perceived loss of control over one's life, loss of self-esteem, and hostility. All these factors increase the length and complexity of rehabilitation and decrease the chance that intervention will be successful. Evidence suggests that when an injured employee is absent from work for six months or more, the likelihood of a successful return is 40% or less (Frymoyer, 1988).

Once an acute industrial injury progresses to a condition involving chronic pain and an ongoing disability of six months or longer, that is, a delayed recovery (Derebery & Tullis, 1983), the cost of workers' compensation increases dramatically. Delayed recovery is a case manager's nightmare; it is a consequence of short-sighted and disorganized managed care with little concern for follow-up. The total cost of workers' compensation can only be kept under control if the incidence of delayed recovery is low. Ironically, it is more cost effective in the long run to pay for appropriate services during the first 30 days of a claim in order to expedite an employee's return to work. The solution, therefore, to the managed care dilemma in workers' compensation is a paradigm shift to a coherent, comprehensive guiding philosophy that looks at the broader picture.

THE PARADIGM SHIFT FOR THE 1990s

The philosophical shift currently under way in workers' compensation managed care involves modification of three traditional payer assumptions (Foto & Niemeyer, 1993). The first assumption is that the costs of claims can be controlled by negotiating lower rates. Tom Chapman, former CEO of Kemper International Risk Management Services, has noted that the trend in the market is to look for good providers who demonstrate meaningful outcomes, not just providers who give meaningful discounts (Foto & Niemeyer, 1993; Framrose, 1995). The second assumption is that a clinical report based solely on measures of impairment is an accurate indicator of an employee's ability to return to work. In actuality, medical impairments generally have a low correlation with actual work capacity. Increasingly, the industry is asking for reporting based on improvement in work-related function rather than just reduction in impairment.

The third assumption is that limiting the dollars spent within the first 30 days will control overall case costs. In actuality, we have seen that this practice contributes to the incidence of delayed recovery. The more correct assumption supports an injured worker-centered approach with early case management and timely specialized care for injured workers whose cases appear to have some complicated aspects. In addition, case managers serve as worker advocates to provide support and minimize feelings of alienation.

A second aspect of the paradigm shift has to do with modifying the traditional adversarial "vendor–vendee" relationships between players in the workers' compensation system and creating partnerships or *partnering* (Framrose, 1995; Niemeyer & Foto, 1994; Simental, Niemeyer, & Foto, 1994). As discussed earlier in this chapter, poor rehabilitation outcomes among injured workers have arisen from the cumulative effects of conflicting messages and agendas from different sectors. This comalingering has contributed to the detriment of the disability compensation system (LeClair & Mitchell, 1992). Partnering involves sharing information and a coordinated effort that allows all players to win. In other words, the injured worker returns to his or her job, everybody gets paid, and costs are controlled. Within workers' compensation, partnering can lead to creative transdisciplinary teams committed to the process and working together for the common good. An example of this kind of partnering is a *disability prevention* program, implemented through cooperation of the employer, insurer, physicians, and rehabilitation providers. Disability prevention is defined as a proactive process of developing policies and procedures related to employee health and rehabilitation care (1) to identify health and safety practices or disability risks in order to minimize the future impact of injury in the workplace, and (2) to minimize the impact and cost of work injury and encourage return to work (Habeck, 1994; LeClair & Mitchell, 1993). In the partnering arrangement, players clarify their roles and agree on coordinated claim management, case management, and return-to-work strategies. Creative solutions that partnering makes possible include skilled early triage and integrated case management, global treatment planning, on-site therapy at the workplace, modified work programs, and procedures for tracking outcomes. The partnering philosophy is the key to effective disability prevention; in the long run, disability prevention is the key to controlling costs.

REIMBURSEMENT SYSTEMS IN MANAGED CARE

The polar extremes of reimbursement in a managed care environment are discounted fee-for-service and capitation (National Association of Occupational Health Professions, 1994). Though discounted fee-for-service may help to rein in rising costs, it provides few incentives for health care providers to produce desired outcomes at the least cost in the shortest possible time. Capitation, on the other hand, forces providers to continually improve efficiency and performance if they are to survive (Pollock, 1993). There are different types of capitation, though the basic premise is that a single rate is paid per patient or per subscriber. A capitation rate is calculated on the basis of loss experiences with a particular large population; this information is used to project future "reasonable and allowable" costs for that group (McDonald, 1994). Medicare, a major leader in the managed care movement, established a capitation system for rehabilitation and other specialty hospitals by means of the 1982 Tax Equity and Fiscal Responsibility Act (TEFRA). Under TEFRA, a provider is paid actual costs up to a maximum reimbursement limit per patient discharge; the limit is the same for all patients regardless of clinical differences (Harada, Kominski, & Sofaer, 1993). The reasonable cost limit per discharge under TEFRA is established separately for each participating facility based on the average cost per discharge during a base year, so that TEFRA limits vary widely among providers. With capitated physician reimbursement, for example, within a Medicare-reimbursed health maintenance organization (HMO), a physician is paid a set rate per month for all members covered under a plan, whether he or she sees them or not.

Despite its success in reducing overutilization, there have been problems with capitation in the larger managed care industry. For any individual provider, capitation works best when there is a large volume of business with a relatively low number of high-cost events and a case mix of patients that represent a close match to the insurer's reference population. If the volume of patients is small, and there is a disproportionate number of difficult cases or even a few very costly cases or "outliers," their care can quickly exhaust capitation earnings, and the provider stands to take a loss (McDonald, 1994). Providers have some options for handling the risk of capitation losses. For example, they can let the payer withhold a portion of the capitation rate, which goes into stop-loss insurance coverage purchased by the payer, or they can take the full capitation amount and buy their own coverage (Pallerito, 1994). Nevertheless, incentives to minimize capitation losses can create a serious selection bias because providers may avoid taking on individuals with higher-cost health care needs (Newhouse, 1994).

Straight capitation may not be feasible for workers' compensation because of these problems. First, establishing valid rates is more difficult due to the lack of good data and wide variations in claims. Capitated rates must take into consideration factors such as industry type, socioeconomic class mix, and geographic location (Cerne, 1994). Second, one of the best ways to reduce workers' compensation costs is to better manage the approximately 20% of "difficult cases" involving chronic pain and disability who incur 80% of the cost (Niemeyer & Foto, 1994; Philips, Grant, & Berkowitz, 1991). The ideal handling of such cases requires early involvement in interdisciplinary rehabilitation programs that include work-focused functional activity (Feuerstein, Menz, Zastowny, & Barron, 1994). Under capitation, providers who are willing to incur the expense of developing and maintaining such programs and, in addition, take on an overall lower volume of clients to care for a higher proportion of difficult cases would be severely penalized.

A case-rate prospective payment system provides a middle-ground alternative. Case-rate agreements define costs for specific claims up front. The process of negotiation between payer and provider can work rather simply. The carrier channels the case to a provider and a case rate is established after an initial evaluation. Interactive case management is initiated when unforeseen developments during the course of treatment mandate renegotiation of the case rate, for example, when the diagnosis changes, a medical or psychological complication arises, or new surgery is required (National Association of Occupational Health Professionals, 1994). With a prospective lump-sum payment, the provider shares risk because the actual cost of providing therapy could exceed the agreed-on reimbursement, but there is more flexibility in planning and carrying out a course of treatment. There is incentive to keep the length and complexity of any given program within bounds, but allowance is made for the greater cost of more severe or complicated cases by assigning these a higher case rate. Case rates allow smaller providers to subcontract for ancillary specialized services when such need is anticipated (e.g., psychological counseling or job modification consultation) to speed the progress of a patient toward return to work. Provider risk can be reduced through (1) a system of internal case management to expedite each client's progression through his or her program, (2) a stop-loss contractual agreement similar to those used to handle the risk of capitation losses (Pallerito, 1994), and (3) quality care that promotes patient satisfaction which will lead to the desired outcome (i.e., early return to work) of building payer loyalty.

Developing a workable prospective payment system based on case rates requires a mechanism for accurately classifying patients by projected cost of care. In the traditional managed care insurance industry, patients are grouped by category of diagnosis. For example, in Medicare's case-based prospective payment system for patients admitted to acute care hospitals, reimbursement is linked to diagnostic-related groups (DRGs). The question is whether classification by diagnostic factors alone will be adequate as the basis for setting case rates for workers' compensation. With medicare patients undergoing rehabilitation, for instance, diagnostic category alone accounts for only 7%–15% of the variance in length of stay (McDonald, 1994; Stineman, Escarce, Goin, Hamilton, Granger, & Williams, 1994).

Recent studies have set a precedent by which research by the provider can be applied in order to establish valid case rates. The advantage is that the provider has access to a broader spectrum of clinical information than is available from billing statements to the insurer. These studies were aimed at developing alternative schemes for more accurately grouping patients receiving Medicare by similar resource use. The goal in each project was to establish a means to adjust capitation rates so that they more closely reflected actual cost of care. Adjusting rates would protect against enrollment bias and reduce providers' financial risks in accepting patients with special health service needs.

Manton and colleagues (Manton, Newcomer, Vertrees, Lowrimore, & Harrington, 1994) statistically generated six discrete case-mix profiles that differed in terms of the cost of care for acute Medicare inpatients. Different provider sites could then be compared in terms of distribution of the six profiles. For example, the authors found that HMO enrollees were healthier and less frail than those remaining in the Medicare fee-for-service system. Two separate studies (Harada, Kominski, & Sofaer, 1993; Stineman, Escarce, Goin, Hamilton, Granger, & Williams, 1994) statistically partitioned medical rehabilitation patients receiving Medicare based on diagnostic, functional, and other clinical data to form subgroups with similar length of stay. Functional status at admission was found to be strongly associated with rehabilitation length of stay, so the subgroups were labeled *function-related groups* or *FRGs*. Classification based on age, diagnosis leading to disability, and functional status at admission explained from 20% to 30% of the variance in rehabilitation length of stay.

The case-rate reimbursement approach, also called *stratification* and *levels of care* (Salcido, 1995), is a viable option for workers' compensation providers practicing within the managed care framework. Considerable groundwork must be laid before it can be implemented successfully, however. This kind of reimbursement needs the partnering context. Developing an accurate classification system and valid case rates requires information sharing. Insurer, physician, employer, and provider must come to an agreement regarding such issues as the provider's authority to determine level of care required, what the desired outcome or endpoint of care is, how far the provider's responsibility for ensuring that outcome extends, and how much latitude the provider has in treatment planning. Within an adversarial climate, for example, insurance companies or physicians might override the provider's recommended case rate for an injured worker, claim that the provider has continued responsibility for providing treatment when an extraneous factor has prevented a return to work, or forbid use of psychological counseling.

FUTURE TRENDS

Managed care companies during the 1990s have been scrambling to develop workers' compensation products, and they will continue to do so. Two innovative programs emerged in mid-1994. PacifiCare Health Systems in California and Liberty Mutual Insurance Group in Boston formed a strategic alliance and developed a product, Compremier, that billed itself as the nation's first capitated workers' compensation HMO. Employers pay a fixed capitated fee per employee for medical services. The financial risk for getting the employee well and back to work within these payment parameters rests with Compremier and its contracting providers. Health Net in California, an HMO, developed an alternative solution to straight capitation with a worker's compensation managed care product called Comp•24. Health Net used data from the fee-for-service system to develop case rates based on "care paths" that represented the most cost-effective treatment for the top workers' compensation injuries in terms of dollar volume

(Cerne, 1994; National Association of Occupational Health Professions, 1994). The viability of these managed care options as compared with discounted fee-for-service is being tested in current markets.

Another upcoming trend is integrated coverage or "24-hour care." Under such a plan, one insurance policy provides managed care to a group of employees or a particular employer for their workers' compensation disability and regular health benefits (Framrose, 1995). Basically, there is a single source managing all aspects of care, regardless of the occupational or nonoccupational nature of a health problem. The industry has created several new partnerships to administrate this comprehensive product. For example, in 1994, Blue Cross of California bought UniCARE Insurance Company, a workers' compensation carrier and launched an integrated program called UniCARE Source One (Clifton, 1996). In 1995, Kaiser Permanente of California forged a strategic alliance with State Compensation Insurance Fund, a state-sponsored, nonprofit workers' compensation carrier, to provide unified coverage (Hall, 1995). These insurance behemoths are marketing to employers the concept of a single health plan that will cover workers around the clock.

There are some good reasons why attempts are being made to combine these two systems. First, it would streamline the paperwork involved in administering two separate health plans. Joint administration would unite cost containment strategies, and claim submission would be simplified. An employer would not have to require employees to go to one network for a health claim and another for workers' compensation. Second, it would reduce the errors and abuses that are the results of two separate bureaucracies processing medical bills. For example, if a provider is treating a patient for a work-related back injury as well as a non-work-related knee injury, they are billing one carrier for workers' compensation and another for the health claim. In the processing of these medical bills, information is not being shared by both payers. This opens the door for such fraudulent practices as "double dipping," whereby claims are submitted to both insurers for the same injury.

There are pitfalls, however, in merging what are essentially two cultures, and the mission could backfire. According to a study by the California Workers' Compensation Institute in San Francisco (Haggerty, 1994), low-intensity, long-duration treatments, which placed greater reliance on the natural healing process, were common in group medical practice. In contrast, medical care for work injuries involved an aggressive approach with greater frequency and intensity of treatment to speed recovery and return to work. The two systems must recognize these fundamental differences or revisit the workers' compensation dilemma of trading lower medical for higher disability costs. Furthermore, initial efforts to integrate benefits could become hung up in complex administrative requirements and financial arrangements until the two bureaucratic structures can be logically melded (Aron, 1996).

The most accelerated trend by far lies in the managing and processing of information (Framrose, 1995; Niemeyer & Foto, 1994). In all segments of the health care industry, on local and national levels, insurance companies are tracking courses of care and outcomes on computer databases drawn from billing documents. These documents yield many megabytes of data on clinical encounters, including every date of service, procedure code, charge, and diagnosis. One of the primary uses of this information is in the performance-based assessment of individual practitioners, known as provider or practice profiling. A provider's track record in terms of such dimensions as the quality of care, use of services, and cost is compared with community standards. Those providers who deviate in key ways from these standards may be excluded from managed care contracts. The practice of provider profiling is being contested, particularly when it is used to make decisions about hiring, firing, disciplining, and paying practitioners. Billing data alone may not be relevant or adequate in representing clinical performance. It may fail to disclose information that is linked to outcome—such as baseline functional status, co-existing illnesses, patient compliance, and desire for care—as well as important outcomes, such as quality of life (Kassirer, 1994).

Information drawn from insurance databases is also used to set guidelines for treatment or case management. Insurers are able to supply course-of-care and outcome data to staff people with medical expertise who then can assess what would be considered a good treatment plan for any given diagnosis. These treatment guidelines are then stored on-line for various diagnostic codes (Niemeyer & Foto, 1994). Case management software is also being developed. For instance, the *Medical Disability Advisor* (Reed, 1994) projects expected disability duration based on such factors as age, comorbidity, educational background, language barriers, and workplace issues to help set a target return-to-work date. The payer's goal is to evaluate the efficacy and cost-effectiveness of the health care they are paying for and eliminate unnecessary services. As in the case of provider profiling, there is concern that limitations in data derived from billing may inadequately portray an injured worker's clinical picture and course of treatment.

CHALLENGES TO HEALTH CARE PROVIDERS

We have seen that billing data collected by insurance companies are being used to project care needs and outcomes ranges and develop care paths for injured workers. Given both the growth and limitations of information technology in the insurance industry, it is apparent that the most critical challenge to providers is to embrace the new technology. The process of facilitating the quality and cost-effectiveness of care would be greatly enhanced by the kinds of information traditionally found in clinicians' charts but not in insurance records. Practitioners who have the talent to put the massive data that computers can capture into meaningful formats will gain a competitive advantage in the marketplace (Framrose, 1995). There are four aspects to accomplishing this mission (Niemeyer & Foto, 1995): (a) clinicians must determine what variables or data elements are important and relevant for their areas of practice; (b) they must adopt appropriate measures or indicators of key variables, such as functional and psychosocial status; (c) they must develop a system of coding the data for entry into the computer; and finally (d) practitioners have to implement a user-friendly and cost-efficient way to gather, enter, and process the data.

One notable example of such an effort is the UE NET (Upper Extremity Network) national database project developed through the collaboration of the American Society of Hand Therapists (ASHT), Rehabilitation Technology Works (RTW), and Greenleaf Medical Systems. Greenleaf Medical is a leading developer of medical software, and RTW is a free-standing therapist-owned outpatient rehabilitation provider in San Bernardino, California, which served as a primary clinical testing site. The Outcomes Reporting and Clinical Analysis (ORCA) software was developed to capture in a uniform manner the complex clinical data generated during treatment of hand and upper-extremity acute injuries and cumulative trauma disorders. Therapists input evaluation, daily treatment, and functional outcome data directly into specially programmed handheld computers (Apple Newtons) by "pen-tapping" on the screen. Additional data can be typed in using a plug-in keyboard. This information is then sent via infrared beam communication from the handheld devices to a clinic server, which is a desktop computer with the capability of generating reports and billing statements and also compiling data to be sent to the UE NET national database. An individual clinic can access its own data from the server by using a relational database application, such as Fox Pro or Microsoft Access.

It can be seen that partnering is an essential ingredient in these kinds of projects. Within each discipline, cooperation and sharing of information can lead to the kind of uniformity of process that lends itself to multicenter or even national data acquisition projects. Once transdisciplinary data-handling capabilities and partnerships are well established, the stage is set to develop a powerful, integrated model for managing care. The richer data pool would lend itself to more useful and valid ways of measuring outcomes, generating care paths and systems of classification, managing resources, and ensuring continuity of care. All players in the workers' compensation system, including injured workers, employers, providers, and insurers, can then receive the high-quality information they need to make the best decisions.

According to Tom Chapman, "Payers expect practitioners to be partners with them … to be accountable for what they're doing" (Framrose, 1995, p. 52). A second critical challenge revolves around this accountability issue. Providers must now demonstrate the quality of the product for which they expect the insurer to pay. There are a number of strategies that help ensure objective and demonstrable effectiveness and efficiency of care when built into a practice (Foto & Niemeyer, 1993). Outcomes orientation entails meeting the final goal—returning and successfully sustaining the injured worker at the job site. Ideally, the planning process for achieving the final goal begins during the acute postinjury phase. The plan should include a projection of the duration of treatment, number of visits, and complexity and intensity of care. Once the level of care is established, this information is communicated to the carrier and can be used to negotiate a case rate if desired. At the end of treatment, the actual outcome and care provided are documented and compared with the projections.

A protocol for internal case management is the second provider strategy. Internal case management parallels and supports the case management provided by the workers' compensation insurer. Its purpose is to provide ongoing monitoring of an injured worker in-house to ensure that he or she is receiving the most effective treatment and is progressing in a timely manner. The final strategy is a system for internal utilization management to analyze outcomes, determine patterns of deviation from projected levels of care, and recognize contributory factors, success rates, and cost–benefit ratios.

The marketplace for health care services is shifting. Being able to respond to these changes constitutes the third critical challenge. Providers need to be alert as to who the customer truly is; in other words, who brings in the business? Traditionally, the patient was the primary customer. For rehabilitation providers, the physician was also a customer. Then, with the growth of managed care, the insurance carriers moved into the driver's seat. More recently, employers are becoming self-insured and have a vested interest in injury prevention and in directing workers who do become injured to effective programs. Marketing to employers means developing products for disability prevention, including ergonomic assessment, fitness programs for workers, early intervention, on-site therapy, and modified work.

In conclusion, proactive and balanced health care reform that makes everybody a winner is within our grasp. The key ingredients are managing *care* not *costs*, embracing information technology, and forming partnerships.

REFERENCES

Armstrong, T. J., & Silverstein, B. A. (1987). Upper extremity pain in the workplace—role of usage in causality. In N. M. Hadler (Ed.), *Clinical concepts in regional musculoskeletal illness* (pp. 333-354). Orlando, FL: Grune & Stratton.

Aron, L. J. (1996). Testing 24-hour coverage. *Case Review*, *2*(3), 18.

Berg, J. (1977). Unbridled growth of managed care fuels cry for regulation. *OT Week*, *11*(14), 14-15.

Cerne, F. (1994). Lowering the boom on workers' compensation. *Hospitals & Health Networks*, *68*, 50.

Clifton, D. W., Jr. (1996). Where is managed care with workers' compensation? *Case Review*, *2*(3), 22.

Curtis, N. M. (1993). Managed care and workers' compensation. *Hand Clinics*, *9*(2), 373-377.

Dent, G. L. (1990). *Return to work-by design: Managing the human and financial costs of disability*. Stockton, CA: Martin-Dennison Press.

Derebery, V. J., & Tullis, W. H. (1983). Delayed recovery in the patient with a work compensable injury. *Journal of Occupational Medicine*, *25*, 829-835.

Feuerstein, M., Menz, L., Zastowny, T., & Barron, B. A. (1994). Chronic back pain and work disability: Vocational outcomes following multidisciplinary rehabilitation. *Journal of Occupational Rehabilitation*, *4*, 229.

Foto, M., & Niemeyer, L. O. (1993). Working partners. *Risk & Benefits Journal*, *3*(3), 24-25, 30-31.

Framrose, A. (1995). 24-hour managed care. A conversation with Tom Chapman. *Rehab Management*, *8*(2), 51-52, 54, 56-57, 131.

Frymoyer, J. W. (1988). Back pain and sciatica. *New England Journal of Medicine*, *318*, 291-300.

Giles, T. R. (1991). Managed mental health care and effective psychotherapy: A step in the right direction? *Journal of Behavior Therapy and Experimental Psychiatry*, *22*, 83-86.

Habeck, R. V. (1994). Examining the disability management model for rehabilitation service delivery. *Work Injury Management Digest*, *3*(10), 1-6.

Haggerty, A. G. (1994, August 22). Group medical: WC mix could backfire. *National Underwriter*, A2.

Hall, C. T. (1995, June 1). Kaiser returns to roots: Venture to offer unified coverage. *San Francisco Chronicle*, B3.

Harada, N. D., Kominski, G., & Sofaer, S. (1993). Development of a resource-based patient classification scheme for rehabilitation. *Injury*, *30*, 54-63.

Kassirer, J. P. (1994). The use and abuse of practice profiles. *The New England Journal of Medicine*, *330*(9), 364-365.

LeClair, S., & Mitchell, K. (1992). *Rehabilitation in industry: Staff mentoring and development program resource manual*. Worthington, OH: National Industrial Rehabilitation Corporation.

LeClair, S., & Mitchell, K. (1993). *Work disability: Corporate assessment, program development, cost reduction—a resource manual for employers*. Columbus, OH: National Rehabilitation Planners.

Louis, D. S. (1987). Cumulative trauma disorders. *Journal of Hand Surgery 12A*, 823-925.

Managed Care Communications. (1992). *The Employer's Guide to Managed Health Care*. Boston, MA: Author.

Manton, K. G., Newcomer, R., Vertrees, J. C., Lowrimore, G. R., & Harrington, C. A. (1994). Method for adjusting capitation payments to managed care plans using multivariate patterns of health and functioning: The experience of social/health maintenance organizations. *Medical Care*, *32*, 277-297.

McDonald, W. H. (1994). The big gamble capitation forces on you. *Medical Economics*, *71*, 47.

National Association of Occupational Health Professions. (1994, October 3). Case rates: Middle-ground approach. *Workers' Compensation Managed Care Bulletin*, 1 (newsletter).

Niemeyer, L. O., & Foto, M. (1994). Partnering in workers' compensation. *Rehab Management*, *7*(4), 138-139, 141.

Niemeyer, L. O., & Foto, M. (1995). Using outcomes data. *Rehab Management*, *8*(3), 105-106.

Newhouse, J. P. (1994). Patients at risk: Health reform and risk adjustment. *Health Affairs-Millwood*, *13*, 132.

Pallerito, K. (1994). Covering the risks of capitation. *Modern Healthcare*, *24*, 44.

Philips, H. C., Grant, L., & Berkowitz, J. (1991). The prevention of chronic pain and disability: A preliminary investigation. *Behaviour Research and Therapy*, *29*, 443.

Pollock, W. M. (1993). Succeeding under capitation. *Medical Group Management Journal*, *40*, 6.

Pontzer, K. (1997). Rep. Norwood's managed care act gets AOTA vote. *OT Week*, *11*(14), 16-17.

Pope, M. H., Andersson, G. B. J., Frymoyer, J. W., & Chaffin, D. B. (1991). *Occupational low back pain: Assessment, treatment, and prevention* (pp. 95–113). St. Louis, MO: C. V. Mosby.

Reed, P. (1994). *The medical disability advisor: Workplace guidelines for disability duration.* Denver, CO: Reed Group.

Salcido, R. (1995). Sorting & saving. *Rehab Management, 8*(2), 33–34, 36–37, 131.

Simental, L., Niemeyer, L. O., & Foto, M. (1994). The workers' comp team. *Rehab Management, 7*(6), 105–107.

Spengler, D. M., Bigos, S. J., Martin, N. A., Zeh, J., Fisher, L., & Nachemson, A. (1986). Back injuries in industry: A retrospective study: I. Overview and cost analysis. *Spine, 11*(3), 241–245.

Stineman, M. G., Escarce, J. J., Goin, J. E., Hamilton, B. B., Granger, C. V., & Williams, S. V. (1994). A case-mix classification system for medical rehabilitation. *Medical Care, 32,* 366.

Tischler, G. L. (1990). Utilization management and the quality of care. *Hospital Community Psychiatry, 41,* 1099–1102.

Whitehead, W. (1995, March 13). A more immediate solution: Managing costs of group health and work comp. *Business Insurance,* 12 (newsletter).

5

Functional Capacity Matching

Designing the Continuum of Care

Susan J. Isernhagen

Occupational health professionals serve industry and workers in a unique manner. They have the ability to design a continuum of care from *prehire to retire* (see Figure 5.1). Their educational backgrounds and functional points of view can be developed into competency-based products to be utilized for, in, and with business and industry.

Two specific skills form the foundation of the continuum of services. The first skill is the ability to functionally analyze the capacity of the human worker. The second is the ability to evaluate the functional demands of a job. With these two unique skills, occupational health professionals can serve employees and employers by continuously matching the worker with the work.

Commonly utilized strategies are forms of this matching. Ergonomics is designing work to fit the worker (Rodgers, 1988). Prework screening utilized in hiring practices emphasizes choosing the worker to fit the work (Himmelstein, 1988). These strategies emphasize opposite points of intervention. The occupational health professional blends the two: the need of the worker to be able to do safe, productive work, and the need of the employer to have productive, fit workers.

Occupational health professionals recognize that neither work nor workers are static entities. Work continually changes through quality improvements, production requirements, and product designs (Pope, Andersson, & Chaffin, 1991). Workers constantly change through conditioning, deconditioning, aging, illness, or injury (Nygard, Suurnakki, & Ilmarinen, 1988). Therefore, the work of the occupational health professional in matching work with the worker is ongoing. The employer who seeks a "one time solution" to productivity and safety will find that today's solution will not fit tomorrow's needs. Workers who feel capable of doing their jobs may find that in the course of a decade many of their capacities have changed, and they are either more or less able to meet changing job demands.

Susan J. Isernhagen • Isernhagen & Associates, 1015 E. Superior Street, Duluth, Minnesota 55802.

Sourcebook of Occupational Rehabilitation, edited by Phyllis M. King. Plenum Press, New York, 1998.

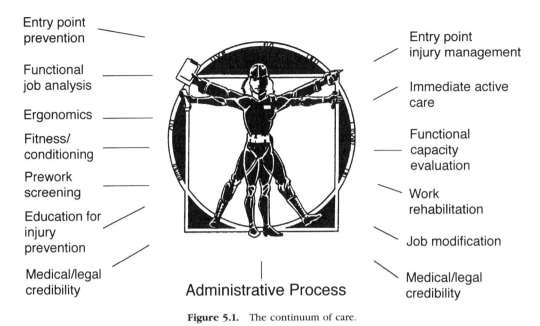

Entry point
prevention

Functional
job analysis

Ergonomics

Fitness/
conditioning

Prework
screening

Education for
injury
prevention

Medical/legal
credibility

Entry point
injury management

Immediate active
care

Functional
capacity
evaluation

Work
rehabilitation

Job modification

Medical/legal
credibility

Administrative Process

Figure 5.1. The continuum of care.

Designing a continuum of care using occupational health professionals requires constant matching of a worker's functional abilities with ongoing analysis of the requirements of the job. When either the requirements of the job grow to be too great, or the ability of the worker to handle the job begins to slip, remedial action can be instituted. Conditioning, educating, and modifying work for the worker can result in higher capability levels (Darphin, Smith, & Green, 1992). Ergonomics technique training and quality improvement reduce work's physical stressors. And both actions can improve productivity. The model set forth in this chapter brings together the concept of ongoing functional capacity matching.

STRUCTURING THE AGREEMENT FOR DESIGNING THE CONTINUUM

The occupational health professional creates an agreement with the employer to provide all or certain components of the Work INjury MAnagement and Prevention (WINMAP) continuum (see Figure 5.2). WINMAP has components that can be utilized individually, but when utilized together provide an integrated continuum of care. However, there must be an understanding of the purpose, outcomes, and methods of the system in order to determine utilization of components or implementation of the entire system (Clifton, 1992; Isernhagen, 1992a).

Individuals involved in initial planning may include the following:

- Management
- Worker and/or union representatives
- Safety directors
- Human resources coordinators
- Hiring directors

An interactive innovative corporation dedicated to optimize industrial productivity and safety through matching the demands of work and the capacities of workers.

Isernhagen Ltd. was founded by work function specialists who believe that work injury management and prevention is an interactive continuum of programs.

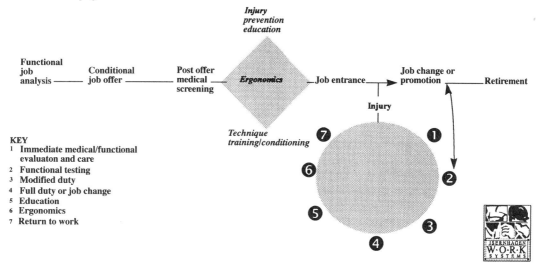

Figure 5.2. The WINMAP concept.

- Disability managers
- Ergonomists or engineers
- Financial officers
- Occupational health consultants
- Occupational medicine physicians
- Occupational health nurses

The team works together to discuss all concepts. The continuum of care includes prevention and injury management components. The employer pays the prevention portion in almost all cases. These are the proactive steps that the employer takes to maximize productivity and minimize the cost of work injury, illness, or disability. For effectiveness, implementation of the system requires interaction with workers and their "buy in" of the process (Baum, 1995). The planning and understanding of the components and concepts by all parties is critical.

The first step is to educate all team members. The employer will educate the consultant about current practices, problems, and opportunities. The consultant will educate the employer and other team members on components of the continuum.

The education leads to the second step—the opportunity to choose appropriate WINMAP components. The full WINMAP system is often preferred because it provides methods to not only solve current problems, but also to form building blocks for future issue resolution.

A written proposal will delineate the components that will be implemented and the methods by which they will be implemented. It will be designed to meet the needs identified during the evaluation process. The occupational health consultant should present the written WINMAP plan to the employer (the payer). The employer should sign a letter of agreement authorizing the implementation of the plan. The plan should include measurable goals, time lines, and costs.

Ongoing Consultation

The occupational health professional acts as a manager of the implementation plan. In implementation, however, the process is dynamic and all parties communicate to problem solve, troubleshoot, and improve the process. The work changes as worksite adaptations are made and workers change. These changes require a constant matching of workers and work through meetings, consultations, further evaluations, and quality outcome measurement.

THE TWO CORNERSTONES OF THE CONTINUUM OF CARE

Functional Job Analysis

The role of the functional job analysis (FJA) in the continuum of care is to provide a quantitative and qualitative description of the demands of work (see Figure 5.3). It is more comprehensive than merely recording times, distances, repetitions, and angles. It includes the analyses of work methods, techniques of task performance, body positioning, and identification of stressors in the workplace that may interfere with productivity or safety (Anderson, 1995; Benz, 1995; Bullock, 1990; Hart, Matheson, & Isernhagen, 1993b; Isernhagen, 1992b; Pheasant, 1991; Rodgers, 1988).

The two primary components are work and worksite variables. Work requirements may include the following:

- Force
- Repetition

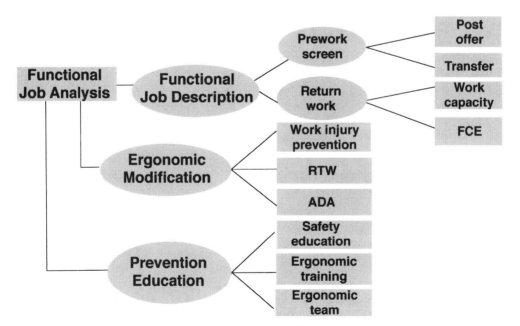

Figure 5.3. Functional job analysis: Three core outcomes.

- Angle of body parts
- Hold time versus rest time (static positioning)
- Impact and vibration
- Cold, heat, humidity
- Variation of work (shifts and time between breaks)

In addition to the work factors, the worksite is analyzed for the following components:

- Sitting and standing postures and supports (chair, cushioning)
- Tools
- Product and product materials
- Integration with a team
- Sensory components (light, noise, temperature)

These two aspects, the stressors of the work and the aspects of the workplace, form the framework within which the human performs productive activity.

Outcomes of functional job analysis depend on the factors evaluated. If recommendations are implemented, outcome measurement can be instituted to compare preintervention statistics with postintervention data (e.g., injury rate, productivity, job satisfaction). The following list delineates many of the most common categories of recommendations.

- Ergonomic adaptations
- Redesign or design of worksites
- Tool evaluation and recommendations
- Improved work patterns
- Rest and/or stretch breaks
- Education for injury prevention/body mechanics
- Technique training
- Job rotation

One outcome of the FJA is the functional job description (FJD). The FJD is a written baseline for compliance with the Americans with Disabilities Act (ADA) because it delineates and validates the essential functions of the job (see Figure 5.4). It is written after the job analysis and validated by employees and employer.

The ADA does not require that employers have written functional job descriptions. Yet, if ADA violations are suspected, a validated functional job description can become part of the defense for the employee. Inaccurate, incomplete or nonvalidated job descriptions can become tools of the plaintiff (usually an employee) (EEOC, 1992b).

An employer who desires accuracy in placement, ergonomics, or return-to-work issues will insist on accurate, up-to-date, and valid job descriptions as the foundation of all other aspects of WINMAP.

Functional Capacity Evaluation

For functional evaluation experts, such as physical and occupational therapists, and functional performance practitioners, the ability to evaluate quantitative and qualitative aspects of human performance becomes critical. Guidelines for professionals emphasize objectivity, accuracy, and purpose (Hart, Matheson, & Isernhagen, 1993).

```
┌─────────────────────────────────────────┐
│                                           │
│        Functional Job Description         │
│                                           │
│     1.  Job objective                     │
│     2.  Essential functions               │
│     3.  Worksite measurements             │
│     4.  Equipment/product utilized        │
│     5.  Critical physical demands         │
│                                           │
│                 Process                   │
│     1.  Quantitative evaluation           │
│     2.  Qualitative evaluation            │
│     3.  Worker input                      │
│     4.  Validation                        │
│                                           │
└─────────────────────────────────────────┘
```

Figure 5.4. The functional job description.

The Department of Labor in the *Dictionary of Occupational Titles* (*DOT*) delineated the physical parameters that are most often utilized in work. Most practitioners, through their own use of the *DOT*, have utilized and adapted this list. (Figure 5.5 presents an example that has expanded some components.)

The evaluator recognizes the need to expand the physical performance analysis to better describe aspects of work tasks. For example, "lift" is listed as one of the physical aspects. Yet, there are three distinctly different lifts. It is clear to the educated practitioner that a lift from the floor has different biomechanical stresses and neuromuscular performance aspects from a lift that is performed from waist height to overhead. The lift at waist level is most effective and strongest because the weight is at the body's center of gravity, and upper and lower extremities are not disadvantaged by vertical excursion. Also, the muscle groups used are different in the three lifts. The metabolic demands are different. Stresses on joints are different. Ergonomic body mechanics differ. Capacities and endurance are different.

Therefore, in this one simple listing—lifts—there are numerous complex lifting patterns. The practitioner who does not utilize expertise in evaluating the lift components just explained will miss options in identifying how a worker does his or her work. For example, a weakness in the quadriceps or dysfunction in the knee will disadvantage the worker in the performance a floor lift, but will not disadvantage her or him in performing an overhead lift. Conversely, rotator cuff tendinitis will affect overhead lifting more than lifting from lower levels.

The kinesiophysical approach to functional evaluation utilizes the professional competencies that bring functional evaluation to its highest level. Knowledge of anatomy, pathology, physiology, and kinesiology come together to evaluate healthy workers in a preplacement situation, or after illness, injury, deconditioning, or aging changes have occurred.

The baseline of all functional capacity evaluations is the ability to identify human

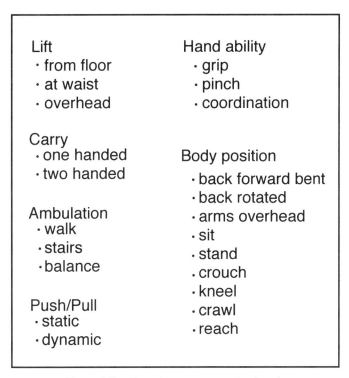

Figure 5.5. The primary components of work.

movement patterns. Because safety and productivity are enhanced through these processes, not only is activity documented, but the method of performing the activity also becomes critically important (Isernhagen, 1988; Johnson, 1995; Miller, 1991).

Functional testing is most often utilized in two areas of the WINMAP system: (1) For the new employee who must enter a job and be able to perform it safely and competently, and (2) for an injured worker who is being evaluated for return to work with possible impairment or deconditioning.

Because individual human performance underlies functional testing, all functional capacity evaluations, whether prework or after illness/injury, should be preceded by a history and a neuromusculoskeletal examination to determine physical attributes that may hinder performance and any contraindications to physical testing itself.

Once the specifics of functional testing are performed, the information gained through the musculoskeletal exam and history is correlated with the results. Therefore, as in the previous example, limitations in overhead lifting could be explained through rotator cuff weakness. Lifting with low-level limitations could be explained by the presence of knee degeneration or quadricep weakness.

Putting the physical cause and the functional result together in a qualitative/quantitative report will not only allow the functional ability of the worker to be matched to the work, but it also presents options for reasonable accommodation, work modification, or worker conditioning. All three types of remediation can be used individually or together to promote the matching of the work with the worker. Employees, medical providers, safety personnel, and workers benefit from this explicit explanation and opportunity for remediation. Outcomes can also be derived from measuring any work–worker mismatch prior to testing and intervention and competency (work) level after intervention.

IDENTIFYING AND INTEGRATING WINMAP CONTINUUM COMPONENTS

The occupational health professional planning to implement the WINMAP continuum has two ethical and professional responsibilities. The first is to be an expert in service provision. All of the continuum components require specialized knowledge and expertise. Professional competence must be displayed, and evaluations, interventions, and recommendations must conform to scientific objectivity and legal parameters. No one profession brings knowledge of all aspects of implementation to the system. Therefore, each professional must undertake individual training and education and participate in team collaboration in order to assure that the system can withstand a rigorous evaluation of its medical objectivity and legal credibility.

Second, the service provided must accomplish the goals stated in the written agreement. The financial agreement for reaching those goals should also be honored. Unfortunately, many employers remember the battle scars (disgruntled employees, lawsuits, wasted dollars) of previous work-injury managers/consultants. The occupational health professionals, specifically, and the professions, collectively, must be able to demonstrate effectiveness.

The following nine components form the definition and policies for WINMAP.

Prevention

1. Functional Job Analysis

Definition: Quantification and measurement of the active components of the job, including movements, functions, forces, actions, and postures, required to produce desired job outcome. This analysis becomes the basis for ergonomics, education, and pre-work screening.

Aspects
- Objective measurement
- Employer involvement
- Employee input and validation
- Professional interpretation

Methods
- Videotapes
- Questionnaires
- On-site measurement
- Validation process

Avoid
- Quantification only: Qualitative description analysis must be included as well. The job analysis process performed by a professional affords a rich opportunity to identify

potential for ergonomic changes, educational needs, and fitness/conditioning/screening needs for the workforce. This cannot be done when only numerical measurements are obtained.

- Paperwork input only: Questionnaires of either employees or supervisors are opinions only. Legal objectivity requires measurement and validation.
- Video analysis only: Videotapes do not produce forces, work climate, and other qualitative information. They are an excellent base and review mechanism but do not offer objective measurement.

Process

- Establish goals, process, outcomes, and method with the employer.
- Use only trained professionals with background in functional analysis, ergonomics, measurement, and the legal validation process.
- Review the job before going on-site (e.g., video, questionnaire, old job description).
- Evaluate and measure the job with assistance of a worker who performs the job.
- Validate job description through discussion and interactive dialogue.

Outcome

- Written description of job specifically addressing the functional aspects
- Bonding of management, workers, and occupational health providers as a result of measurement and the validation process
- The baseline of other occupational health components
- ADA compliance

2. Ergonomics

Definition: A design, development, or modification process, biomechanically and physiologically based, that provides maximum worker safety and productivity through matching the demands of the job to the worker's abilities.

Aspects

- Based on minimization of physiological, neuromusculoskeletal, and psychological demands identified in functional job analysis
- Best when it is an interactive process involving workers who perform the job
- Can be generalized to groups but can also be individualized
- Continual process as workers, work, worksite, and productivity requirements change

Methods

- Kinesiological evaluation of work movements
- Quantification/evaluation of specific forces and stressors
- Analysis of process of producing the "product"
- Application of engineering, physiologic, neuromusculoskeletal, and psychological principles to reduce stressors and increase productivity

Avoid

- Using prepackaged, heavily marketed ergonomic saviors
- Making ergonomic changes without involving the worker
- Considering only one solution instead of options
- Putting ergonomic changes in place without evaluating their effect on morale, safety, productivity, profitability

Process

- Utilize a functional job description.
- Determine the options for ergonomic changes to work and worksite (including tools).
- Determine physical/functional changes to reduce stressors.
- Confer with employer and pertinent worker groups (union, safety director, etc.) to discuss potential ergonomic changes.
- Delineate each ergonomic change possibility by description, cost, and outcome.
- Measure the effects on safety and productivity after ergonomic intervention.

Outcome

- Worksite, work methods, and work tools that maximize safety, and productivity, of work for the worker
- A base for further dynamic ergonomic problem solving
- Integration as a solution with prework screening, return to work, or ADA application

3. Fitness Conditioning

Definition: A program of exercise and work simulation that is designed to improve workers' neuromusculoskeletal and cardiopulmonary abilities. The conditioning program is specific to a job or group of jobs.

Aspects

- Target goals set at the beginning of program
- Progress toward meeting outcome goals measured at end of program
- Work ability measured after placement on the job to determine effectiveness of conditioning program
- Exercise targeted toward muscle groups or systems that are used in work
- Work simulation design to increase technique, safety, and method, as well as ability
- Program used at any time there is a mismatch between work and worker, such as preplacement after leave of absence, postinjury or illness, or with aging process

Methods

- Professional design and monitoring of activity
- Specific time frame for accomplishment of goals
- Conditioning done on-site or off-site
- If done off-site for injured worker, follow American Physical Therapy Association guidelines on work conditioning

Avoid

- Absence of a preplacement conditioning program for physically demanding jobs
- Making the program director responsible for the progress of the workers rather than the workers themselves
- Nonprofessionally supervised generic exercise programs

Process

- Evaluate the physical capacity level of the worker as compared with job demands.
- Design a general program of strengthening and conditioning and aerobic improvement to bring the body to a higher level of competence.
- Design a specific program targeted toward improvement of specific job-related skills.
- Provide supervision and encouragement during the process.

- Provide the worker with ongoing information on his or her progress toward goals.
- See that the worker takes self-responsibility for his or her own improvement.
- Conduct outcome matching of the worker's ability and job entrance requirements.
- Undertake outcome measurement of the worker's success on the job after conditioning.

Outcomes

- Decreased injuries to new hires
- Decreased lost time days when compared with no work conditioning program after injury
- Improved technique and productivity on beginning the job
- Increased worker resilience reducing occurrence of cumulative traumas
- Designed program to maintain physical status available to worker during course of employment
- Integrated with prework activity; after leaves of absence, illnesses, or injury; ADA application, transfer process, and aging

4. Prework Screening

Definition: The physical, functional testing of a job applicant, new hire, or transferring worker on the appropriate, validated essential functions of a specific job.

Aspects

- Based on validated functional job description (ensures job-relatedness) performed by a professional
    nonmedical in preoffer stage
    medical background in postoffer stage
- Safety as a criteria for passing
- Same screen given to all people testing for a specific job

Method

- Functional tests
- Standardized or actual work materials
- Kinesiophysical evaluation that identifies safety concerns
- Nondiscriminatory attitude and test items
- Utilization of accommodation guidelines for disabled
- Outcome measurement of effectiveness of screening

Avoid

- Nonfunctional testing to determine ability to do work
- Testing that favors strongest, gender-preferred age groups in ways that discriminate against those capable of doing the job with or without accommodation
- Making hiring decisions
- Providing medical/therapeutic advice
- Designing or providing tests that do not predict ability to do the job (*Note:* "Doing the job" is much more comprehensive than avoiding injury.)

Process

- Design a functional screen based on a functional job description.
- Validate the screen.

- Design specific test and scoring parameters.
- Integrate screening with physical and/or other evaluations.
- Test and record performance results.
- Provide employee with the performance test outcome.
- Identify potential direct threats and disability accommodations in conjunction with a physician and the employer.

Outcomes

- Reduced injury in new hires due to placement based on employee's functional ability
- Increased understanding of physical aspects of the job by potential new hires
- Improved associated activities, such as job transfer and return to work
- Effective ADA compliance in relation to "business necessity" and "job-relatedness"

5. Education for Injury Prevention

Definition: A process that provides an opportunity for the worker and supervisors to interact with the work environment to reduce the risk of sudden or cumulative trauma.

Aspects

- Interactivity of the learner and the lesson
- Empowerment of the worker to take self-responsibility for his or her health and safety and that of the work group
- Empowerment of the worker to actively change is or her work behaviors to ensure safety
- Extrapolation of the work education to home and recreational activities

Method

- Lecture, videotape, slides, reading material, or computer models
- Group or individual process
- Opportunity to be interactive, ask questions, clarify points, and make the general information specific to the job
- Learning opportunities reinforced with feedback
- Use of actual job slides, tools, or videotapes and/or educate at worksite

Avoid

- "Canned" programs of any media that do not emphasize interactivity with teaching material, allow for questions, and demonstrate personal application
- One-time only teaching sessions
- Teaching modules that do not promote self-responsibility
- Teaching methods that do not apply to the worker's own situation (which will lead to discarding material)
- Boring teacher or material

Process

- Teach and demonstrate.
- Interact with the worker.
- Evaluate the outcome of sessions immediately and over time.

Outcome

- Knowledgeable workers
- Interactive problem solving between workers and supervisors
- Potential or reduced injury at work and at home
- Interacts with ergonomics, conditioning, and return to work
- OSHA effectiveness

Injury Management

1. Immediate Active Therapy

Definition: Therapeutic care targeted to improve work function (increase mobility, strength, coordination, and tissue healing and decrease discomfort and inflammation). Self-treatment methods and education to prevent reinjury are provided within hours of report of problem.

Aspects

- Exercise, education, self-responsibility for positioning and work patterns
- Emphasis on function not pain
- Recognition of the person as a worker not a patient
- Functional testing of job demands
- Results in no or minimized lost work time

Method

- Active exercise to improve job-related function
- Appropriated (but limited) rest and palliative modalities
- Kinesiophysical functional testing to set goals of early return to work and problem-aggravation prevention
- Interact with employer and physician if necessary
- Education and empowerment to reduce the potential for further injury

Avoid

- Pain-focused treatment
- Inactivity or deconditioning of noninjured parts of the body
- Subjective return-to-work decisions
- Prolonged treatment or time off work (consult physician for "healing-time" guidelines and therapists for algorithms of care)

Process

- Build in a referral system for the early reporting process at the worksite.
- Provide access to therapy within 8–24 hours.
- Confer with a physician.
- Ensure that policies are in place and followed.
- Communicate with the employee to guarantee an immediate or early return to work.
- Recommend or provide job modifications when they are necessary.
- Provide functional testing prior to the worker's return to his or her job.
- Manage the return to work process until full duty or an agreed-on plateau is achieved.
- Conduct outcome studies on effectiveness, using cost, productivity, and lost work-time analyses.

Outcome

- Fewer lost time days
- Reduced impact of injury
- Decreased possibility of adversarial attitudes
- More self-responsible workers
- Reduced reinjury rates

2. Functional Capacity Evaluation (FCE)

Definition: Standardized testing of an injured or ill worker to determine ability to do a specific comprehensive set of work tasks that can be matched against real-world functional job descriptions.

Aspects

- Use of medical diagnostic information
- Safe functional testing
- Interaction with worker regarding abilities and limitations
- Job grid job-matching
- Emphasis on safe function not pain
- Interaction with employer

Method

- Kinesiophysical functional testing
- Movement testing, not static testing
- Nonadversarial attitude
- Complete understanding of test purpose and scoring method
- Education on ergonomic and safe movement patterns to be utilized during testing process
- Report format that is concise, clear, and easily readable by worker and employer

Avoid

- Psychophysical testing that puts pain or client in *charge* (discomfort patterns considered in the kinesiophysical approach but interact with rather than defy or overrule professional expertise)
- Comparing FCE results to a very generalized dictionary of occupational titles unless there is no other option
- Using nonfunctional tests or technology
- Negative labeling
- Using tests not designed for injured workers (e.g., those designed on "normals" or specific disease categories not prevalent in work injuries)
- Comparing results to "norms" (the ADA is clear that the worker must be compared to essential functions of the job)

Process

- Prepare referrer's order with history and medical records.
- Obtain functional job descriptions either before or after the FCE.
- Obtain client consent, work and medical history, and physical assessment.
- Administer the functional test.
- Compare FCE results with FJA (DOT not considered accurate for specific jobs).

- Make recommendations regarding the worker's ability to return to specific work and the options that would facilitate a return to specific work.
- Establish medical-legal credibility.
- Undertake outcome studies to measure the effectiveness of the return to work or case settlement.

Outcome

- Increased return to work rates
- Decreased disability costs
- Improved worker–work matching
- Expeditious physician work release
- Expeditious employer offer of return to work
- Improved worker self-understanding and empowerment
- Objective medical-legal information

3. Work Rehabilitation

Definition: Specific programming, on or off the job, utilizing rehabilitation methods (exercise, real or simulated activity, education and training) to bring an injured or ill worker up to or as close as possible to the level of the essential functions of the job.

Aspects

- Acceptance of a physical problem in the worker
- Focus of program is on improving function, not cure
- Measured improvement in functional goals
- Outcome orientation of return to work
- Integration with actual work when possible

Methods

- Standardized programs with individual tailoring
- The kinesiophysical method of ongoing progress
- Self-responsibility of client
- Progressive strength, endurance, and aerobic programs
- Actual work or work simulation
- Education in safety, body mechanics, and work techniques
- Functional job description as target goal

Avoid

- "Packaged" programs rather than individually designed programs
- Promises of cure or elimination of pain
- Ending a program in the clinic without going on-site to ensure return to work
- Taking care of client rather than facilitating self-responsibility

Process

- Determine work readiness state with an absence of medical contraindications to the program.
- Coordinate functional capacity testing with job matching to ensure that the program is necessary and set specific goals.

- Design and put in place a time-oriented program with the designated outcome, costs, and time lines projected.
- Integrate program with work until a full return to work is accomplished.
- Conduct outcome studies on cost effectiveness, return-to-work effectiveness, and impact on reinjury.

Outcome

- Physically improved workers at return to work
- Decreased disability costs and lost time
- Educated workers involved in preventing further injury

4. Modified Duty Determination/Permanent Accommodation

Definition: Providing a physical alteration in a work task, equipment, or method to facilitate a match between the current functional capacity of a worker and the demands of a regular job.

Aspects

- Cost-effective solutions that reduce lost work time
- Uses of the base of kinesiophysical functional testing and functional job demands to identify specific work capabilities and limitations
- Time-limited orientation that triggers reevaluation toward return to full duty when the person is ready
- Worker and team education in agreement with bringing a team member back with modifications

Method

- Ergonomic tools and/or modifications
- Job matching—functional testing with physical work demands

Avoid

- Promoting the "100% perfect to return to work" policy
- Creating groups of nonjobs as a "light-duty" dumping ground
- Keeping workers on modified duty forever (without reevaluation)
- Generating work team resentment at having to bring worker back on modified duty
- Creating modified duties that physically overstress other team members

Process

- Determine the person's functional ability to do specific work tasks.
- Match the functional ability against the demands of the worker's current job. If it is not a match, abilities are measured against demands of other available jobs. (If a 100% match, return to work is accomplished and no modification is needed.)
- If not a complete match, evaluate modifications that allow the worker to return to the job satisfactorily.
- Set a time for reevaluation of the match with the goal of return to full duty at his or her regular job as a goal.
- Undertake an outcome study to evaluate the modified duty cost-effectiveness, safety effectiveness, and impact on lost work time and disability.

Outcome

- Few lost work time days
- Improved productivity–dollars ratio
- Decreased likelihood of disability
- ADA compliance

THE WINMAP CONTINUUM AT WORK: FUNCTIONAL CAPACITY MATCHING OF WORK AND WORKER

Case Study 1

PROBLEM: New employees in the production department of a company have an increasingly high rate of injury in their first three months after hire. The employer is dismayed because many new employees are quickly hurt and placed on light duty. Separate jobs, not including the regular job, are created to keep employees at work. Those workers who go on light duty early in their employment have a tendency to stay on light duty for years. Current workers exhibit a resistance to accepting back workers who come back to their regular shifts after being on light duty. They are considered "complainers." This resistance reinforces the desire of workers to stay on light duty and not return to their regular jobs. What will the employer do?

Solution 1: Utilize WINMAP prevention components. The causes of the injuries should be investigated and the appropriate remediation designed, dependent on these causes. For example, workers may suffer back injuries, cumulative traumas, and the inability to finish full shifts due to lack of strength and conditioning on entrance to the job. To remedy, recommend the following possibilities:

a. Institute prework screening specific to the job for all new hires and jobs with high injury rates.
b. Institute a fitness conditioning program prior to placement to build up the strength and endurance level of new hires who have passed the initial screening. (Prework screening measures strength and coordination, but it is not as good at measuring endurance. Work conditioning builds the endurance portion.)
c. Revisit the education given during the preplacement period to identify whether the proper techniques and methods have been used by new hires.
d. Evaluate the effectiveness of the employer's "light-duty" program (see Solution 2)
e. Implement ergonomic changes. If one specific job is creating most of the problems for new hires, it is possible that the demands of the job have greater stressors than most new workers can handle. Making ergonomic changes to reduce the stressors—new tools, positions, work methods, or workplace design—would be appropriate.

Solution 2: Reevaluate return to work WINMAP components. Light duty may be popular as a way to bring people back to the worksite. In many cases, however, light duty is a "dumping ground"; people are brought back to work but not given respected work by either the company or the team. Because not being able to do the full job often carries a negative connotation, those who go on the "light-duty" program often find themselves in adversarial relationships with those who are doing "full work" for their pay.

Rather than support a light-duty program of relatively meaningless work, the occupational health consultant works with the team to design a more logical method of modified work, noting the following aspects:

a. The sooner the problem is reported the more likely it is that the person can stay on his or her regular job with only slight modifications. Changes may include a modified tool or work method, the temporary elimination of one of the work tasks, or additional help. These modifications should be temporary.
b. The adversarial relationship should be addressed. All workers should understand they could be offered the opportunity for brief modified work if an illness or injury occurs. This is a right of all those who are working, and, therefore, this right should not be seen as something that is given only to a select few.
c. All modified duty should be of a temporary nature. A restorative program should be implemented so that a target date is set for return to full duty. Having a target date allays the fears of co- workers that the person will be doing less than her or his full work for a long period of time.
d. Only if modification of the original job cannot be made through temporary modified duty, should another job be sought. In the event another job is utilized, it should not be considered "light duty." Elimination of a light-duty pool is the first step to having all workers respected for doing pertinent and valuable work.
e. A matrix of job demands developed through the process of job analyses and descriptions should now be utilized. If there is another job in the plant to which the person can be temporarily assigned, this assignment should be made. Reassignment allows productive work to continue even if the worker is doing a different job. Again, this reassignment should be seen as a temporary situation.
f. If the worker cannot physically return to his or her former full productive work, further accommodation should be made. At this time, ADA protection should be evaluated. However, whether or not the person falls under the ADA definition of disabled, the employer should seek a permanent accommodation for a valuable worker. Again, this permanent accommodation could be an assignment to a vacant job the worker can do, or it could be permanent modification of the original job.
g. If there is no legitimate job in the plant that the worker is able to do safely and productively, it may have to be acknowledged that the worker no longer meets the demand of any of the essential functions of any of the jobs in the plant. Therefore, the disability system rightfully can be brought in. This action will occur in a minority of cases, but it is important for morale and for productivity. If a worker truly is not able to do productive work at any job in a plant, the case should be resolved so that all parties can go on with their futures.

Case Study 2

PROBLEM: A worker with cerebral palsy demonstrates the following: Mild left hemiparesis, adequate ambulation, uses right side well, uses left upper and lower extremities as helper limbs, and exhibits a limp. The worker has always been able to do his job adequately. This worker dropped a bucket of nails in a work area, creating the possibilities that workers in the area could slip and that tires of the equipment used in that area could be punctured. The worker was written up as having caused a safety problem. The employer immediately called the worker in, took him off the job, and referred him to a physician for medical evaluation with the intention of determining whether the worker should receive a medical discharge. The employer justified his actions by stating that the accident created a dangerous condition for other workers. The physician was uncomfortable with medically disqualifying a current employee. The physician also considered the Americans with Disabilities Act and thought the worker was being treated discriminatorily. The WINMAP process was called into action.

The employer and occupational health consultant analyzed the problem, and there appeared to be two primary questions: (1) Was there discrimination toward the worker according to the terms of the Americans with Disabilities Act? (2) Is the worker capable of doing the job? (Has his condition worsened? Has aging made him weaker and not as able to control his body?)

Solution 1: In determining whether there is discrimination as defined by ADA, one must first identify whether the worker fell under the protection of ADA. Since the definition of *disability* indicates "a significant impairment in the ability to do … work" or the "perception of a disability," it is very likely that this worker would fall under the ADA protection. Not only was it known that the person had cerebral palsy and had obvious physical problems, but cerebral palsy may be a common diagnosis afforded ADA protection. In addition, the employer who pulled the worker off the job immediately had the "perception of disability," which also may place the worker under protection of ADA. Therefore, there is a strong likelihood that if this case went to court, the person would be classified as disabled.

Another test is to identify whether the action of the employer in pulling the worker off work immediately was different from the actions taken against others who had dropped buckets of nails. An examination of the records would indicate whether this type of safety accident had ever happened before and what the disposition of the situation was. If this accident had happened previously, and the worker who had the accident was only warned or reeducated, then it is clear that the worker with cerebral palsy had a much stronger action taken against him. This precedent strengthens the "perception of disability" action.

Solution 2: Determine a worker–work match. Is the worker physically capable of doing the job? A review of the records would also indicate whether in the past this person has had other safety violations that suggested physical deficiencies. For example, was this the first time he had dropped a bucket, or was this the tenth time? If this was the first, and the worker had successfully completed several years of employment, then it would be clear that by merely having done the job adequately in the past, the worker had the ability to do the essential functions of the job. The accident could then be identified as only that, an accident.

If, on the other hand, over a recent period of time, the worker had begun to have more accidents related to physical abilities, the suspicion that there may be a medical or functional problem in matching the work would be supported by this increase in physical difficulties.

It is important also to ascertain whether the work itself had changed. For example, if carrying the bucket of nails was a new job activity, then it is possible that the worker was now being asked to do something that was not formerly an essential function. This situation offers a good opportunity to look at ergonomic modifications or eliminate one task to ensure a successful performance. In this case, perhaps if the new activity were eliminated, the former job could then continue to be done productively and safely.

Solution 3: If a legitimate question exists regarding the current physical status of the worker under ADA, this could allow a medical evaluation to be made. A referral to a physician or therapist would be appropriate. However, without certain criteria present, employers must not require medical evaluations of workers who are currently doing their jobs. Unless there is a safety concern, productivity issue, or indication of a true medical problem, the employer cannot discriminate against the worker with cerebral palsy by requesting a medical evaluation. A worker who does not have a production or safety problem and concurrently has been performing the essential functions of the job is not required to take a medical evaluation. Under those circumstances, therefore, the physician was correct in wondering whether a medical evaluation was appropriate.

Solution 4: If medical testing is justified, then the physician and therapist become part of the team that continues to evaluate the functional capacity match between the work and the worker. Functional capacity testing can be done to identify abilities and limitations relating to work. Job-specific testing can then be added to the FCE to identify whether the person can do the essential functions of her or his job. Testing would provide information on the overall functional abilities of the worker, and more specifically, information on his ability to do his job. The physician and employer would not have to rely on subjective information or innuendos, but rather then would have objective functional capacity matching information for making further employment decisions.

In addition, this type of objective testing with job matching clarifies for the worker whether there is a mismatch. This clarification reduces the perception that there has been discrimination. If objective information indicates that there is a limitation, then the steps to remove that limitation can be initiated objectively and proactively. Taking these steps prevents the development of an adversarial relationship.

Solution 5: If the functional capacity job matching reveals deconditioning or an increase in a physical limitation, then the employer can bring the worker into a work-conditioning program to improve his physical ability to again perform the full demands of the job. If this cannot, then a job modification may be indicated.

If physical abilities match the job, then the worker merely had an "accident," and the safety team can assist the worker in preventing future accidents.

The following components were utilized to solve this problem:

- Functional job descriptions define the physical requirements of the job.
- Investigation into the parameters of the accident help determine if the worker's accident rates differ from others.
- The functional capacity evaluation identifies the worker's abilities.
- Functional job matching utilizes the functional job description and FCE results.
- A conditioning program can be utilized if weakness or treatable physical dysfunction causes a job mismatch.
- Ergonomics can be considered to modify a specific work area, allowing the person to do the full job.
- Educate the worker if safety procedures were not followed.

- Consultation in ADA protects the worker and employer, ensuring that no discrimination occurs.

Case Study 3

PROBLEM: A worker has been off work from his plant for nine months. The employer, in reviewing the disability records, determines that the worker will go on long-term disability in the near future if decisions are not made that allow him to return to work. The medical records indicated that seven months ago the physician noted that "the worker cannot lift more than five pounds." Given this restriction, there was nothing in the plant that the worker could do. Therefore, the worker stayed off work, and the employer did not create a "light-duty" position for him. At this juncture, the employer wonders if the person can return to work harnessed with this old medical restriction. The employer decides to call an occupational health consultant.

In analyzing this situation, the consultant reviewed the job descriptions at the plant. The employer was correct in believing that all jobs involved some type of materials handling. The "lightest" job available required a 15-pound lift. Other jobs required lifting up to 60 pounds. The employer concluded that with the medical restriction the person could not return to a current job.

The consultant considered performing a functional capacity evaluation with the worker to identify whether he has the safe ability to do the job. The physician's restrictions however, remained a problem.

Solution 1: The occupational health consultant must first consult the physician to determine whether the restriction given to the worker was to be temporary or permanent. In this case, the worker had a laminectomy with decompression at L4–L5. The physician was called and stated that the restriction was temporary. The worker had not been back to see that physician, and no other physician had called to inquire about lifting the restriction, so the original surgeon's restriction stood.

Solution 2: The occupational health consultant asked the physician to see the worker once again and remove the restriction if possible. The physician saw the worker, and the restriction was removed. The physician stated he had meant the original restriction only to cover the "healing time."

Solution 3: A functional capacity evaluation that used the kinesiophysical approach, in which safety is paramount, stability of the back is ensured, and full lifting capacity is identified, was ordered. In addition, the full FCE was ordered because of the possibility of deconditioning after a nine-month layoff from work. The specific job task components (developed earlier in a prework screen) were to be added after the FCE. Therefore, an FCE plus prework screen components were ordered.

Because of the deconditioning and the possibility of increasing low-back-pain symptoms, a two-day FCE was instituted to make sure that the testing would not make the person more symptomatic or unable to perform well.

The functional capacity evaluation was performed and showed that functionally the employee could do the minimum requirements of three jobs in the plant, including his former job. His lifting capacity was at 40 pounds, maximum. He had an ability to handle 20 pounds on an occasional basis.

Deconditioning was identified as a factor. The worker's heart rate remained high after exertion, and there was evidence of shortness of breath after lifting several items. In addition, on the second day he experienced muscle soreness. There was no change in ability or level of safety, but the muscle soreness indicated that the muscles were not in condition to handle much of the work.

Solution 4: A work conditioning program was implemented to improve the worker's endurance and technique and, if possible, even improve his lifting capacity.

Solution 5: Following the work conditioning program, retesting was performed and the worker returned work able to do his previous job safely. A determination of disability was not made. He returned to work at his previous job.

This problem was solved by using many components of the WINMAP system.

- Functional job descriptions were developed for the job analysis.
- Working with the physician to find any medical restrictions alleviated an adversarial relationship because the physician felt like part of the team.
- A full functional capacity evaluation was performed for this chronically off-work worker.
- Prework screen components were ordered after the FCE.
- A work conditioning program was able to target goals for the worker.
- Education was used to make sure that safety precautions were followed during the return-to-work process.

EVALUATION OF CASE STUDIES

Too many occupational health consultants will give employers "magic answers." These case studies demonstrated that solutions must be derived from analysis of the problem. Many WINMAP components were utilized in possible solutions to these problems. Without having all of the WINMAP options available, many of the solutions could not be accomplished. The employer who has all of the programs in place will have a much wider range of options.

CONCLUSION

Future Perspectives

The following sets summarize the points made in this chapter:

Set 1. Dynamics of Work and Worker

- Workers capabilities change with age, conditioning, illness, and injury.
- The physical demands of the job change and are changeable.
- Matching the worker and work for safety and productivity is a dynamic process.

Set 2. Outcomes of Mismatches

- When demands of the job override physical capacity of workers, production errors occur and/or the workers are subject to injury.
- Both are costly to employers and employees.

Set 3. Medical–Legal Responsibilities

- OSHA suggests matching the work to the worker.
- ADA requires nondiscrimination, using objective information regarding a worker's ability to perform a job.
- Workers' compensation facilitates decisions to allow the matching of the worker to the job.
- Legal action is increasing. Medical-legal knowledge and compliance are imperative.

Set 4. WINMAP Integrated Components

- There are at least five components to physical-injury prevention.
- There are at least four major components to injury management.
- These nine components are interdependent and interrelated. They form the continuum of care.

The occupational health professional utilizes comprehensiveness, dynamic action, and competence to facilitate positive outcomes from the basic drive of a worker to generate productive work and the fundamental need of business for cost-effective productivity.

The occupational health professional is in a unique position and has an obligation to proactively use a functional capacity matching continuum. Improving productivity, enhancing safety, and reducing costs are facilitated by the WINMAP process.

REFERENCES

Anderson, M. A. (1995). Ergonomics: Analyzing work from a physiological perspective. In S. Isernhagen (Ed.), *The comprehensive guide to work injury management* (pp. 3–39). Gaithersburg, MD: Aspen.

Baum, B. (1995). Working with the workers: The "buy in" to maintenance of wellness. In S. Isernhagen (Ed.), *The comprehensive guide to work injury management* (pp. 254–264). Gaithersburg, MD: Aspen.

Benz, L. N. (1995). Carpal tunnel syndrome measurement and surveillance management. In S. Isernhagen (Ed.), *The comprehensive guide to work injury management* (pp. 231–253). Gaithersburg, MD: Aspen.

Bullock, M. (1990). *Ergonomics*. London: Churchill-Livingstone.

Clifton, D. W. (1992). Risk management in work therapy. In S. Isernhagen (Ed.), *Orthopaedic physical therapy clinics of North America* (pp. 167–176). Philadelphia, PA: W. B. Saunders.

Darphin, L., Smith, R., & Green, E. (1992). Work conditioning and work hardening. In S. Isernhagen (Ed.), *Orthopaedic physical therapy clinics of North America* (pp. 105–124). Philadelphia, PA: W. B. Saunders.

EEOC. (1992a). *Americans with Disabilities Act: Handbook*. Washington, DC: U.S. Equal Employment Opportunities Commission.

EEOC. (1992b). *Americans with Disabilities Act: Technical Assistance Manual*. Washington, DC: U.S. Equal Employment Opportunity Commission.

Hart, D., Matheson, L., & Isernhagen, S. (1993a). Guidelines for functional capacity evaluation of people with medical conditions. *Journal of Orthopaedic Sports and Physical Therapy, 18*(6), 682–686.

Hart, D., Matheson, L., & Isernhagen, S. (1993b). Refining the practice of ergonomics. *Work, 3*(3), 69–72.

Himmelstein, J. S. (1988). Worker fitness and risk evaluation in context. In J. Himmelstein & G. Pransky (Eds.), *Worker fitness and risk evaluations* (pp. 169–176). Philadelphia, PA: Hanley & Belfus.

Isernhagen, S. (1988). "Functional capacity evaluation." In S. Isernhagen (Ed.), *Work injury: Management and prevention* (pp. 139–192). Gaithersburg, MD: Aspen.

Isernhagen, D. (1992a). The continuum of care. In S. Isernhagen (Ed.), *Orthopaedic physical therapy clinics of North America* (pp. 7–14). Philadelphia, PA: W. B. Saunders.

Isernhagen, D. (1992b). Ergonomic basics. In S. Isernhagen (Ed.), *Orthopaedic physical therapy clinics of North America* (pp. 23–36). Philadelphia, PA: W. B. Saunders.

Johnson, L. (1995). The kinesiophysical approach matches worker and employer needs. In S. Isernhagen (Ed.), *Comprehensive guide to work injury management* (pp. 399–409). Gaithersburg, MD: Aspen.

Nygard, C.-H., Suurnakki, T., & Ilmarinen, J. (1988). Effects of musculoskeletal work load and muscle strength on strain at work in women and men aged 44–58 years. *European Journal of Applied Physiology, 58*, 13–19.

Pheasant, S. (1991). *Ergonomics, work and health*. Gaithersburg, MD: Aspen.

Pope, M., Andersson, G., & Chaffin, D. (1991). The workplace. In M. Pope, G. Andersson, J. Frymoyer, & D. Chaffin (Eds.), *Occupational low back pain* (pp. 131–177). St. Louis, MO: Mosby.

Rodgers, S. H. (1988). Matching worker and worksite–ergonomic considerations. In S. Isernhagen (Ed.), *Work injury: Management and prevention* (pp. 65–79). Rockville, MD: Aspen.

II

PREVENTION OF WORK INJURY

6

Education and Training

Robin L. Saunders and Mark R. Stultz

ATTEMPTS TO PREVENT MUSCULOSKELETAL INJURY

Cumulative trauma disorders have gotten the nation's attention. Medical practitioners and executives in business and industry have long been aware of the escalating problem. Cumulative trauma injuries negatively affect the economy and individuals' lives. In many cases, workers' compensation insurance premiums are a significant budget item, affecting a company's profitability or ability to survive. Nearly everyone can identify a friend or relative whose life has been dramatically affected by a musculoskeletal injury.

To address these concerns in business and industry, several preventive strategies have evolved, including ergonomic evaluation and design of the workplace, employee selection and screening, proactive injury management, and education and training for the workforce. Ergonomic redesign is a seemingly obvious choice as the primary preventive strategy. After all, if the workplace is optimally designed, education should not be necessary. The workplace design would never encourage poor work practices. Work heights would be conducive to proper sitting, standing, and material-handling postures. The size, shape, and weight of materials handled would be appropriate for every worker. Indeed, common sense tells us that ergonomic design should be the primary preventive strategy. However, an awareness of ergonomics has not solved all workplace problems. In some work settings, redesigning existing equipment is cost-prohibitive. In many occupations, poor ergonomic conditions are a given, and even the most creative ergonomist would be hard-pressed to find a solution. It is for these reasons that employers have sought additional solutions, among them, education of their employees.

Education of the workforce has been a key component of the preventive strategy for many companies. Cumulative trauma and back injury prevention videos and booklets are easy to find. Companies and individuals skilled in motivation and education make a

Robin L. Saunders • The Saunders Group, 4250 Norex Drive, Chaska, Minnesota 55318. **Mark R. Stultz** • Medtronic Neurological, Advanced Pain Therapies, 800 53rd Avenue N.E., Minneapolis, Minnesota 55421.

Sourcebook of Occupational Rehabilitation, edited by Phyllis M. King. Plenum Press, New York, 1998.

living teaching employees how to change personal habits and work practices to better their chances of escaping injury. However, in some circles injury prevention education has come under attack. In any discussion about workforce education, there are fierce advocates and critics, each citing literature that supports his or her unique viewpoint.

The education of individuals currently experiencing pain is also controversial. The literature has not convincingly shown that education alone speeds recovery or prevents reinjury. In fact, a review of the literature reveals that there is a general lack of agreement about proper timing, content, audience, and even the methods of measuring the success of injury prevention education in industry and in clinical environments.

Preventive Education Variables

Most of the available literature concentrates on back injury prevention and education. It is difficult to analyze the success of back injury prevention education programs because of the vast differences among the various programs described in the literature. The main variables encountered when examining the literature include (a) the audience receiving the education, (b) the number of components in the education, (c) the philosophy/method taught, (d) the education and experiences of the trainer, and (e) the varied measures used to determine effectiveness.

The audiences varied from pain-free individuals to individuals who had recently suffered an acute episode of low back pain to chronic pain suffers. The goals of education for each population were somewhat different. For the pain-free individual, the primary goal was to educate her or him to prevent an episode of pain. Most of the articles written about this population had to do with back injury prevention programs in industry. For the individual currently experiencing pain, the goal was to reduce the severity of pain, speed recovery, and minimize the disability resulting from the episode. For the person with chronic pain, the goal became management of pain, improvement of function, and return to gainful employment with minimal risk of further injury. Most of the research on back injury prevention programs for individuals currently experiencing pain was performed in a clinical environment, with a variety of additional interventions taking place. These programs, usually termed *back schools* in the literature, often consisted of education and exercise.

There were a wide variety of components present in the education sessions described. The most common program elements included discussions about anatomy and physiology, the effects of exercise, proper posture, optimum material handling techniques, basic ergonomic principles, modification of activities of daily living, pathophysiology and the mechanics of injury, and basic acute care of injuries. However, there was no clear consensus on which components were most important because each program described a different use of them. Some programs stressed certain components more than others or omitted various components. And, as pointed out earlier, for individuals currently experiencing pain, the educational sessions occurred in a clinical environment while a variety of other interventions simultaneously took place. These conditions made it difficult to determine the specific effect of the education variable. Compounding the difficulties of program comparison was the fact that vastly different philosophies and methods were taught. For example, some of the articles stressed a lifting method using a posterior pelvic tilt to minimize lordosis, while other articles stressed either a straight back lifting position or a lordotic lifting position.

The education of the trainers as described in the literature varied as well. Some trainers were physical or occupational therapists; others were ergonomists and nurses. Each profession tended to have its particular biases. Additionally, the specific experiences of the trainers in particular industries or job practices tended to make them more or less suited to teach a particular group of trainees. The presentation styles and skills of individuals varied. A more evangelical style compared with a didactic style could make a difference, depending on the content of the message and the audience to whom it was being delivered. In fact, Snook stated, "the back schools which have enjoyed the greatest success have done so largely because their evangelistic 'deans' have the ability to sell their concepts to participants and motivate them to use the methods taught" (Snook & White, 1984, p. 234).

Finally, the variables assessed to show program efficacy varied considerably. For example, two studies looked at intra-abdominal pressure recordings to assess the effects of preventive education (Scholey, 1983; Stubbs, Buckle, Hudson, & Rivers, 1983), while another looked at the extent to which mechanical lifting devices were used (Linton & Kamwendo, 1987). Relatively few of the studies looked at actual injury or reinjury rates, which should be the definitive variable to assess when determining whether back education is effective.

Because of the differing variables contained in the literature, the following review of articles attesting to the effectiveness or ineffectiveness of education must be viewed with a critical eye. When considering those articles that claim education is not worthwhile, as well as those that tout the benefits of educating the workforce or providing a back school for patients, one must carefully consider the audience, components and philosophies taught, education and experiences of the trainer, and measures used to determine effectiveness. Otherwise, inappropriate generalizations could be made.

THE EFFECTIVENESS OF EDUCATION

In an analysis of health maintenance organization (HMO) clients, Berwick concluded that back schools had no clinical effect in reducing pain levels or increasing the functional status of participants experiencing an acute episode of low back pain when compared with patients in a control group who received "usual care" (Berwick, Budman, & Feldstein, 1989). Several studies have claimed that back schools that instruct participants exclusively on material handling practices had little or no effect (Dehlin, Hedenrud & Horal, 1976; Scholey, 1983; Snook, 1988a; Stubbs et al., 1983). However, Berwick's study was unusual in that it showed a lack of effectiveness in multiple-component back school education. The method described included anatomy, physiology, and exercise training.

One of the earliest studies of back-school effectiveness looked at low-back-injured auto workers at a Volvo plant in Sweden (Bergquist-Ullman & Larsson, 1977). Workers who participated in an educational program were compared to a placebo group who received an inconsequential dosage of an electrotherapeutic modality. The workers who participated in the program had a 30% reduction in the time required to return to work and a near 50% decrease in the amount of time required for recovery (14.8 days for the back-school group and 28.7 days for the placebo group).

Another series of articles detailed the short- and long-term effects of inpatient and outpatient back schools in Sweden (Harkapaa, Mellin, Jarvikoski, & Hurri, 1989; Harkapaa et al., 1990; Mellin, Hurri, Harkapaa, & Jarvikowski, 1989; Mellin et al., 1990). These authors found that back school participants initially had statistically significant improvements in pain and disability reports and compliance with treatment. Inpatient results were better than outpatient results. The inpatient back school group also improved in physical measurements. After one and one-half years, improvements had faded. Results suggested that repeated intervention was necessary for a more than temporary effect. The back school described included exercise and education as well as passive treatment.

A study looking at a flexion-oriented exercise/education approach (LeClaire, Esdaile, Suissa, Rossignol, Proulx, & Dupuis, 1996) showed that patients receiving physiotherapy and back school improved in knowledge and exercise performance when compared with a control group receiving physiotherapy only. However, there were no differences between groups in return-to-work time or the number or duration of recurrences.

Other authors cited the positive results of a clinical back school in their controlled trial (Moffett, Chase, Portek, & Ennis, 1986). They compared a back school and exercise group with an exercise only group. Patients in both groups improved at 6 weeks, but back school participants continued to improve at 16 weeks, while the exercise only group reverted to their original level of disability.

One study (Stankovic & Johnell, 1990) compared the McKenzie method of treatment to a "mini back school," and found that McKenzie treatment was superior in five of seven variables studied. However, their mini back school did not teach or encourage exercise. Most other back schools reporting success included exercise as a significant component.

In a meta-analysis of the literature, one author found that clinical back schools were most effective when combined with comprehensive rehabilitation programs (DiFabio, 1995). Back schools tended to be effective for treatment of pain, physical impairment, and education/compliance. The articles reviewed did not demonstrate effectiveness in work/vocational and disability outcomes.

In another critical review of 16 randomized clinical trials, poor quality of the research methods was found (Koes, van Tulder, van der Windt, & Bouter, 1994). Out of a possible 100 points for quality of research methods, only two articles scored more than 50 points. The studies reporting positive results of clinical back schools tended to have higher scores. Reported benefits of back schools were usually of short duration only.

One study (Schenk, Doran, & Stachura, 1996) supported the use of "live" back schools for influencing lifting posture and conveying information. The authors were critical of video presentations because of the poor success found in their study. However, they admitted that the nonprofessional quality of the videotape they used may have influenced the outcome.

There were several reports of the effectiveness of education in industry. PPG Industries reportedly had a 70%–90% reduction in injury costs and incidence rates two years after preventive education implementation (Johnson, 1991, in Snook, 1988b). A 67% reduction in back injury liability and a 70% decrease in lost workdays were seen after introduction of a back injury prevention program at Lockheed Missiles and Space Company (Tomer, Olson, & Lepore, 1984). Two years after education was initiated, Southern Pacific Transportation Company saw a 22% decrease in low back injury rates and a 43% decrease in lost work days with 39,000 employees (Snook & White, 1984).

A 90% reduction in back injury claims, a 50% reduction in lost workdays, and a massive reduction in workers' compensation costs (from $200,000 to $20,000 per year) had been reported at American Biltrite (Fitzler & Berger, 1983). In a study of eight different industries, a 40% decrease in lost work days was seen with an associated reduction in medical insurance premiums (Melton, 1983). There was, however, an increase noted in the reporting of low back pain.

In another study, municipal employees participated in a mandatory, intensive six-week education and exercise program (Brown, Sirles, Hilyer, & Thomas, 1992). The protocol involved supervised strength and flexibility exercises 20 minutes per day, five days per week, and educational sessions 30 minutes long, four days per week. The results were compared to a randomly selected control group. Participants in the program had half as many reinjuries as nonparticipants during the six-month period following intervention. Because exercise and education occurred simultaneously and with fairly equal intensity, it is difficult to assess the effect of the education alone.

Several studies showing a poor effect of education interventions used questionable assessment. For example, two separate studies (Scholey, 1983; Stubbs, Buckle, Hudson, & Rivers, 1983) used intra-abdominal pressure recordings in their evaluation of behavior change and compliance to taught principles. Scholey's study contained only four subjects and acknowledged that limited time was allowed for education. No studies exist that conclusively relate reduced intra-abdominal pressure levels to a reduction in incidence and severity of low back injury. Therefore, both the assessment method and the conclusions drawn in these two studies should be viewed with suspicion.

In other studies that claimed educational interventions were ineffective, flaws existed. In one study (Snook, Campanelli, & Hart, 1978), the authors acknowledged that no attempts were made to evaluate the quality or type of procedures used to train employees in safe lifting habits. Other studies pointed out that the type of lifting procedure used is of extreme importance (Anderson & Chaffin, 1986; Chaffin, Gallay, Wooley, & Kuciemba, 1986; Hart, Stobbe, & Jaraedi, 1987; Park & Chaffin, 1974). And even though one study concluded that a relationship exists between the incidence of low back injury and the lifting technique used (Dehlin, Hedenrud, & Horal, 1976), a questionable metric was used to assess effectiveness. Rather than look at injury rates (the definitive variable), the authors looked at the frequency of leisure activity pursuit and the extent to which mechanical lifting devices were used. Even studies that claimed positive educational effects used questionable study methods. In one study, for example, written test scores rather than direct observation were used to predict adherence to biomechanical principles taught (Wollenberg, 1989).

THE CONTROVERSY SURROUNDING TECHNIQUE

There has been considerable controversy regarding effective exercise techniques and lifting practices. The main controversy revolves around the "flexed versus extended" philosophy. One philosophy, made popular by Williams, assumes that low back pain is primarily due to tightness of the lumbar extensors and weakness of the abdominal musculature (Williams, 1982). It also assumes that a posteriorly tilted pelvis is the desired posture. Proponents of this philosophy advocate abdominal strengthening and knees-to-chest stretching, which involve a flexed lumbar posture, and a lifting method that utilizes a posterior pelvic tilt.

McKenzie (McKenzie, 1981) advocated a different philosophy. This approach encourages the use of passive lumbar extension to effect a change in the intervertebral disc. Additionally, it encourages an anteriorly tilted pelvis with a slight lumbar lordosis. The basic premise is that the nucleus of the disc tends to migrate posteriorly with repeated flexion of the spine (Harris & McNab, 1954). Also, the posterior aspect of the annulus tends to fatigue and fissure because of the stress that flexion induces to the posterior elements (Hickey & Hukins, 1980; Park, 1976). One adhering to the McKenzie philosophy might argue that back schools that teach flexion exercises and the posterior pelvic tilt lifting posture are compounding rather than preventing lower back problems. Indeed, a study assessing the results of McKenzie's protocols showed that they were twice as effective in relieving low back pain as was a treatment involving a flexed lumbar position (DiMaggio & Mooney, 1987).

In the back school articles reviewed, there are actually two types of lifting positions advocated: the posterior pelvic tilt lift described earlier, and a lift using a straight back-bent knee approach. None of the back schools reviewed instructed participants in lordotic (anteriorly tilted pelvis) lifting. The use of the posterior pelvic tilt lift is infrequently advocated (Mattmiller, 1980; Morrison, Chase, Young, & Roberts, 1988). Arguments against this lift include the probable negative effects on the disc discussed earlier. Additionally, researchers point to our knowledge of length-tension relationship in muscles when they theorize that the erector spinae are at a disadvantage with the lumbar spine flexed (Hart et al., 1987). Because they are less able to quickly develop the force required to counter a sudden increase in load, a bigger burden may be placed on the posterior ligamentous structures and the annulus in a sudden slip or fall.

There is a less obvious distinction between the straight back-bent knee lift and the lordotic lift. The literature does not do a good job of comparing the actual injury rates resulting from the use of the two techniques. Instead, biomechanical modeling is used to theorize that one method is better than another. However, a careful review of the literature suggests that a lordotic lifting position may be best. Hart found that 80% of the painful lifting postures he studied involved lumbar kyphosis (Hart et al., 1987). Furthermore, researchers have observed that most injured workers naturally assume a lordotic posture when lifting, presumably for protection and comfort (Snook & White, 1984).

THE POWER POSITION

Based on published studies (Anderson & Chaffin, 1986; Hart et al., 1987) and the theoretical models proposed by McKenzie (1981), a lordotic lift with the weight held close the to body is highly recommended. The weight can be held closest to the body when a lordotic lift is combined with a straddled stance. Also advocated is the lordotic position when performing non-material-handling activities, such as reaching and bending and recreational activities (Figure 6.1).

To effectively teach this concept, the Saunders Group has adopted the term *power position*, described to participants in the following way:

> Stand in an upright posture with your feet in a diagonal position at least shoulder width apart. Bend your knees a little and then bend forward at the hips by pushing your rear backward, while keeping your head and chest up. Keeping your head and chest up ensures a neutral curve in the spine. Remember to keep the object lifted close to your body, and don't jerk or twist.
>
> If you are lifting something from the floor, the correct position is a lot like the three-point stance of a football lineman. Bend the knees a little, the hips a lot, stick your rear out, and keep your head and shoulders up. This is the "power position" for an athlete, and it works just as well as the factory. Even something as awkward as reaching into the trunk of your car can be done safely if you use the "power" position.

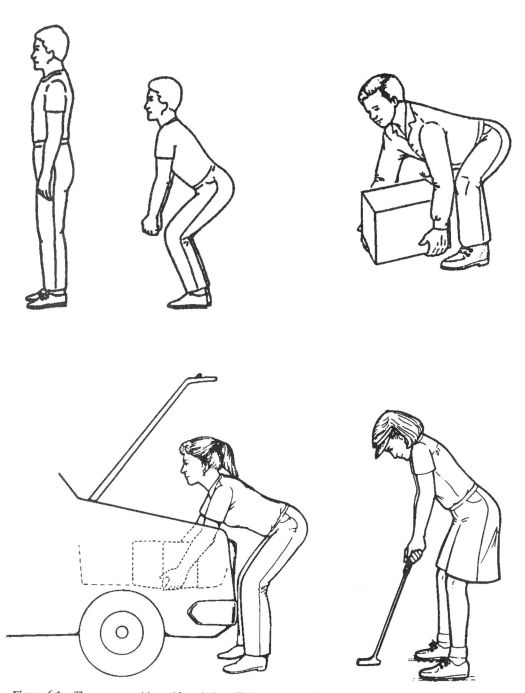

Figure 6.1. The power position with variations. Trainees are taught to use the power position in any lifting, reaching, or recreational activity involving forward bending. From H. D. Saunders (1992). *For Your Back* (pp. 29, 32). Chaska, MN: The Saunders Group.

The power position puts less stress on the legs because the knees don't bend quite so far. Less energy consumption is required, and muscles don't fatigue as readily. Less compression on the knee joints results. Awkward and cumbersome weights can be lifted more safely because the object can be held closer to the spine.

SUGGESTED COMPONENTS IN PREVENTIVE EDUCATION

There is more to back injury prevention education than exercise and lifting techniques. A comprehensive back school (Saunders, 1992) combines the following elements. First, a frank discussion about the current confusion and misperceptions about back injury management must occur. The instructor should emphasize that even among medical practitioners, disagreement about effective treatment is the norm. The back school participants must be convinced that the problem is serious enough to demand their full attention if they are to change their behavior. They will not be convinced if they feel that back injury treatment is "the doctor's problem." An attitude of self-responsibility in back injury prevention starts with the knowledge that an injury is not always easy to cure and severe disability can result.

Some clinicians even advocate detailing the risks of noncompliance, including lost income, inability to participate in athletics or hobbies, permanent or partial disability, chronic pain, sexual dysfunction, impaired bowel and bladder control, and many other morbid effects (Schwartz, 1989).

Anatomy and physiology principles must be taught, but the information cannot be either boring or overly detailed. For participants to buy into a lordotic position philosophy, they need to understand enough about anatomy to understand the reason for the recommended techniques. Only anatomy and physiology that is relevant to a desired behavior change should be taught. Otherwise, the participant will not be able to prioritize the information learned. For example, it is only important to know that the interior of the disc is not innervated to convince the participants that repetitive poor posture can cause damage even if pain is not felt.

Next, the work and lifestyle practices that cause injury should be explored in detail. It is important to give examples relevant to the audience's actual work practices and experiences. If a "generic" program that contains many irrelevant examples is presented, the participants will assume the information does not apply to them. A program presented at work that incorporates a video or slides of employees performing actual work tasks not only has extreme relevance, but also keeps the audience's attention and gives the instructor credibility. It is essential to emphasize that back injuries result from a cumulative set of factors, not from a one-time slip, twist, lift, or fall. Back injuries should be equated with a gradual-onset disease process like heart disease. Heart disease results from an accumulation of a long list of risk factors, including high blood pressure, obesity, smoking, poor diet, and lack of exercise. Likewise, back problems result from an accumulation of such risk factors as poor posture, faulty body mechanics, stressful work and lifestyle activities, lack of exercise, and a decline in general flexibility and fitness. To treat back problems, one must address the risk factors rather than concentrate on quick fixes that only relieve symptoms (Figure 6.2).

Common treatments for back injury should be discussed. However, a major point that should be made is that most passive treatments (rest, physical therapy modalities, medications, and manipulations) only treat the symptoms of a problem and not the fac-

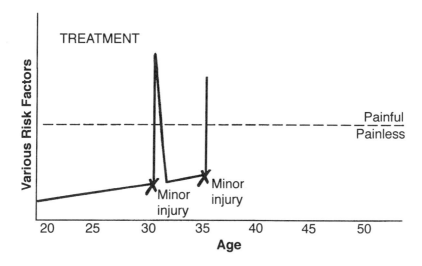

Figure 6.2. Back pain versus risk factors. The two lists below represent risk factors for back problems. The problems can be slowly worsening with time, but the individual does not yet have pain. A minor incident causes pain, and the pain is relieved with treatment. However, if the treatment does not address the risk factors, the back problem is still present and may continue to worsen, eventually leading to a major disorder. *Source:* H. D. & R. L. Saunders (1993). *Evaluation, Treatment and Prevention of Musculoskeletal Disorders: I. The Spine.* Chaska, MN: The Saunders Group.

tors that actually cause back injury. To truly treat back injuries, it is important to address the causes.

No back injury education program would be complete without a thorough discussion of ergonomic design and body mechanics. Although lifting should be stressed, other work and home risk factors, such as reaching too far, slumped sitting or standing postures, repetitive movements without changing positions frequently, and twisting should be addressed. In this discussion, it is absolutely essential that the instructor include examples that are relevant to the participant's actual activities. The program loses all credibility if the instructor gives advice that is impractical or impossible to implement on the actual job site or in the participant's home. Also, it should be acknowledged that it is not always possible to use optimum techniques or make the job or home site ergonomically ideal. In these instances, the participant will have to rely on other preventive strategies.

Exercise also should be discussed. At a minimum, participants should be encouraged to stay aerobically fit; at least one important study (Cady, Bischoff, O'Connell, Thomas,

& Allan, 1979) shows a correlation between aerobic fitness and a healthy back. Additionally, specific exercises can be taught. It is most beneficial to do an individualized flexibility and strength screening, including instruction in the exercises that would either correct inadequacies or counteract stressful positions assumed at work or home. The fewer exercises taught, the better. Individuals will be more motivated to comply with an exercise program that is individualized, simple to perform, easy to remember, and doesn't consume a lot of time. The content and scope of the educational session should vary, depending on the audience. Participants in a clinical environment who are currently experiencing pain will have different perspectives than industrial workers attending an on-the-job, mandatory preventive class. In general, injured participants are easier to educate because they have an interest in improvement. Noninjured participants are more difficult to motivate, and it is particularly important to make sessions relevant and the suggested actions easy to implement.

EDUCATION VERSUS TRAINING

A company puts it workers through a back injury prevention class. Everyone is taught the basics of body mechanics. These basics are demonstrated and practiced in the class. Literally ten minutes after the course is over, a tour through the shop area reveals that not a single person has improved their body mechanics on the job! What happened?

This scenario has probably occurred countless times in industry, and it is the reason back education programs have a mixed reputation. A central question in the whole process of education and training is, "Does increased awareness result in a change in performance?" In other words, is it enough to simply raise a person's awareness level and expect a change in their behavior? If that is true, then

- why do some people still drink and drive?
- why do some people still smoke cigarettes?
- why do some people still use poor body mechanics?

A look at the literature shows that educational efforts have often been ineffective. Noncompliance with preventive treatment regimens has been estimated as high as 67% (Wollenberg, 1989). One article reported the poor application of principles taught in the workplace (St. Vincent, Tellier, & Lortie, 1989). Of six principles taught, simultaneous application by workers occurred in only 1% of the cases. Even when the principles were assessed independently, the compliance rate was only 11%–33%.

Many programs fail because they only raise awareness levels; they stop short of providing what is really needed to facilitate performance change. Although the terms *education* and *training* are often used interchangeably, there are distinct differences. The dictionary has this to say (*Merriam-Webster's Collegiate Dictionary*, 1993): "[*Education* is] knowledge and development resulting from an educational process"; "[*training* is] preparing for a test of skill." In other words, education provides the foundation of knowledge, while training develops the skills necessary to integrate learning with new behavior.

Matthew B. Miles described six steps in the learning process (Miles, 1981):

1. Dissatisfaction, recognition of a problem
2. Selection of new behaviors

3. Practicing new behaviors
4. Getting evidence on results
5. Generalizing, applying, and integrating the behaviors
6. Finding new dissatisfactions and problems

Step One   Dissatisfaction, Recognition of a Problem

If people don't believe there is a problem in the first place, why should they change their behavior? They must recognize their dissatisfaction and be willing to do something about it. Injury prevention programs should emphasize problems with particular relevance to the population addressed. Getting upper-management's attention, for example, requires an emphasis on the cost of injury. Workers, on the other hand, will be motivated by a hard look at injury rates, disability percentages, and statistics on job loss, pain, and suffering.

Step Two   Selection of New Behaviors

The person must become aware of and be willing to try out changes that will make an improvement. The motivation can come at three levels:

1. Compliance — "I do because someone with power says so."
2. Identification — "I do because I want to be like you."
3. Internalization — "I do because it accomplishes something of value to me."

Of the three, only internalization works effectively. Therefore, injury prevention classes must convincingly show a benefit to the participant. The presumed benefits of a behavior change, such as increased productivity and less fatigue, should be dramatic and immediate. Longer term, less obvious benefits, such as a decreased injury rate, are less meaningful.

Step Three   Practicing New Behaviors

Affording many opportunities to practice the new behaviors is the next step. The practice should take place both within the "safety" of the course and in the "real" environment. The behavior practiced must be done with reasonable correctness. Therefore, injury prevention sessions should include ample time for the practice of desired techniques in a real environment, and the student–instructor ratio should be small enough to allow one-on-one feedback to participants.

Step Four   Getting Evidence on the Results

Because many results of an improvement in back care are not immediately evident, it is essential that individuals receive feedback on new behavior. The feedback must be specific, nonpunitive, and immediate. Such feedback requires that supervisors and upper management get actively involved in the training process. In other words, the program cannot be presented to workers alone; there should also be a change in management practices. Positive results should be publicized, and management should foster an atmosphere in which ergonomic improvement and safe work practices are prioritized.

Step Five   Generalizing, Applying, and Integrating the New Behaviors

Once individuals accept that the new behaviors are successful, they must integrate them into the general context of activity. In other words, the successful new behavior must become the accepted and comfortable "normal behavior." The goal is to create a work environment in which new work stations are automatically designed with an ergonomic thought process, and new work procedures are developed with safe worker practices in mind. Ideally, workers will integrate safe practices into their home and recreational environments.

Step Six   Process Continuation

New dissatisfactions are found and the process continues!

OVERCOMING PASSIVITY—ONE APPROACH IN INDUSTRY

When teaching musculoskeletal injury prevention classes to noninjured workers, we have found that many participants adopt a passive attitude. It is very easy for a participant to feel, "This stuff doesn't apply to me, because my job is different." Or, "Why should I change my behavior—a safe work environment is the company's responsibility." Or, "My situation is so terrible, there is nothing I can do." To combat these attitudes, the instructor must emphasize that an attack on back injuries consist of the following elements in order of priority: making ergonomic change, learning to do the job the best way, reversing stressful positions, and maintaining good physical condition.

Ergonomic Change

With management's approval, the instructor should openly point out the ergonomic hazards of the participant's job. (The instructor should also work with management to improve ergonomic hazards. Implementation of recommendations will depend on the feasibility of the recommended changes.) If ergonomic challenges are ignored, the instructor risks losing credibility with the audience and having them think that he or she is on management's side. This situation is particularly harmful when there is adversity between employees and management to begin with. Many simple things can be done to improve the worksite: Hold a discussion of basic "layman's" ergonomics, or stress individual accountability for suggesting changes to management, for example. With good training and empowerment, workers can make simple, commonsense changes to their own work stations.

If the instructor has been asked by management to ignore ergonomics and simply teach body mechanics, he or she should be wary. If management has already implemented good ergonomic principles, the instructor should point these out in the class. If management has not addressed existing ergonomic hazards and has no plans to do so, the class will surely be a waste of time. Management must be open to addressing ergonomics in order for any educational effort to succeed.

Learn to Do the Job the Best Way

When ergonomic changes are not possible or feasible, one should take responsibility to do the job the best way possible. In this situation, education and training in body mechanics and proper posturing is important. Training in real job situations is essential. Teaching how to properly lift a box while standing in a roomful of nurses can border on absurdity. The instructor's credibility is key. At a minimum, the instructor should try the recommended techniques in actual job situations to determine whether the job tasks can be done as taught. Videotape or slides of workers performing tasks correctly and incorrectly should be shown, and workers should be asked to propose alternate approaches to tasks using the principles taught. An interactive teaching style works quite effectively when the instructor has credibility with the class.

Reverse Stressful Positions

When appropriate, the instructor must acknowledge that it is not only impossible to improve ergonomic conditions, but it is also impossible to do a job a better way. Visualize ironworkers tying rod while straddling joists 50 feet off the ground. There are some jobs that are inherently hard on our bodies. It is impractical to either change the job or improve workers' technique. In such instances, workers can be trained to frequently reverse stressful positions by taking breaks, stretching, or rotating jobs. In the case of the ironworker who performs prolonged and repetitive bending, standing lumbar extension performed frequently during the day can help maintain extension flexibility and reverse the stressful position of flexion.

Maintain Good Physical Condition

Occasionally, the instructor will encounter particularly recalcitrant individuals who will claim that their employers will not allow ergonomic changes, that they cannot perform their jobs with any improved techniques, and that they do not have enough time to perform frequent stretch breaks. In such cases, instructors should stress the maintenance of good physical condition. Studies show that general fitness plays a big part in the prevention of back injuries (Cady et al., 1979).

Presenting these multiple strategies gives workers options that are within their control and lends credibility to the presentation. Better yet, an overall training strategy that incorporates "prioritization of principles" prevents individuals from arguing that there is nothing that can be done to improve their situations.

OVERCOMING PASSIVITY—ONE APPROACH IN THE CLINIC

In chronic pain patients, passivity is usually caused by patients' frustrations with the conflicting information they have received from medical professionals. Also, they tend to feel that treatment for their condition is the physician's/therapist's responsibility—not theirs. Educational efforts must focus on self-responsibility and empowerment to allow patients to manage their conditions. Empowerment begins with the knowledge that back problems are a cumulative effect of several risk factors, many of which they can control.

Patients feel overwhelmed and cannot imagine beginning activity again, until they are "cured." One should attempt to convince them that activity is part of the treatment not the end result. Actively addressing risk factors, such as poor ergonomic conditions, faulty body mechanics, lack of strength and flexibility, and poor posture, is done through exercise, ergonomic correction at home, and an examination of the lifestyle practices that contribute to back pain.

EDUCATION AND TRAINING ARE NOT ENOUGH—A FOUR-STAGE PROCESS

In industry, musculoskeletal injury prevention is a process not an activity. There are several necessary components in this process. To educate and train the workforce alone assumes that musculoskeletal injury is caused solely by worker practices. This assumption is simply not true. A review of the literature shows that many factors, ranging from ergonomic to psychological, influence the incidence and severity of injuries. Attempting to manage back injury problems with a "back care presentation" is like putting a Band-Aid on a gushing wound. A successful preventive strategy has to coordinate an attack on many fronts.

Based on experience and perusal of the literature, the authors suggest the following training process:

- *Stage One: Development.* The development stage consists of four parts: (a) gaining management support, (b) developing a specific plan to address ergonomics and worker behavior, (c) developing a training strategy that involves both management and nonmanagement employees, and (d) identifying measures to evaluate effectiveness.
- *Stage Two: Implementation.* Implementation of the strategy involves conducting a preintervention employee survey, ergonomic evaluation and redesign, and management and employee training, collecting postintervention data, and analyzing that data to determine effectiveness.
- *Stage Three: Process Modification.* Process modification involves examining the data obtained and processes used. It determines the results of the efforts thus far and briefs the appropriate management about them. At this point, modification of the plan occurs. The team must identify lessons learned and then modify the process as needed.
- *Stage Four: Process Continuation.* Assuming that implementation was demonstrated to be effective, and that there is corporate-level buy-in to continue, a plan is developed to ensure the continual prioritization of the ergonomic and training interventions.

This training strategy is heavily influenced by ergonomics. Management and workers are trained to look for ergonomic hazards and implement fixes. The fixes are often inexpensive and involve common-sense adaptations to the existing environment. Additionally, workers are trained to change their behaviors, including the way they use tools and handle materials. However, technique changes are only successful when they are part of an overall plan to improve the work environment. Anything less would be hypocritical and short-sighted—and would not be effective.

Gaining management support for the educational effort is vital to the success of the program. Management should be educated about ergonomics and ergonomic goals as well as the potential cost/benefit of the company's participation in the effort. Management support must come at three distinct levels, otherwise there will not be the necessary buy-in. These three levels are corporate, occupational medicine, and individual site.

Support at the corporate level is necessary because commitment cannot occur at the other management levels without it. Financial resources are only one issue. Upper management must foster an environment in which safety is clearly a priority. This change often involves rethinking the way middle-management personnel are compensated or rewarded for their jobs. For example, monetary bonuses may need to be based on safety statistics as well as productivity.

Support from the company's occupational medicine team is also essential. This is true whether or not the medical staff are employees or on contract. Physicians must support the principles taught to management, including the necessity of early return to work plans and treatment that focuses on restoring function and addressing the causes of cumulative trauma rather than on only relieving symptoms. The participation of occupational health nurses in case management is a key to successful implementation of these efforts.

Support from middle management at the sites involved is also critical. Supervisors and site managers must understand the principles being taught so that they can positively reinforce changes in worker behavior and actively solicit worker involvement in ergonomic change. With the active support of management, the occupational rehabilitation provider becomes more than simply a "trainer." The provider assists management in developing data-analysis models, ergonomic implementation processes, and follow-up programs. He helps to appoint an ergonomics/education team and assists in empowering the team to effect true change in both work design and attitude toward job functions. In large corporations with multiple sites, success may be achieved with a "train-the-trainer" approach, where ergonomics/education teams are taught to actually implement all stages of the process independently at their sites. This type of approach is necessary in larger corporations because it is impractical and costly for consultants to evaluate, train and follow up with thousands of workers. The largest and most successful example of this intervention is with the U.S. Navy, where the Saunders' model has been implemented at over 30 different Naval Command Stations. Some command stations have reported up to a 50% reduction in reportable back injuries. NAV AIR total savings were estimated at $250,000,000.

THE USE OF VIDEO PROGRAMS

The popularity of injury prevention programs has led several companies to develop and market video and slide/tape training packages to health care professionals and corporations. Back care booklets and consumer-oriented videotapes can also be found in book and video stores. Can these educational efforts succeed? As noted earlier, Schenk and colleagues' study (1996) were critical of video back schools in industry. Presentation of a videotape to workers or patients without any other intervention or follow-through is ineffective.

Success has also been achieved by having patients in the clinic watch video presentations as an adjunct to one-on-one education with their therapists. Learning occurs through repetition. Some individuals learn better by listening, while others learn better using visual aids. Patients should be educated individually first. Then, videos and booklets may be used to support and enhance the message.

When giving injury presentations to workers, it is important to capture their attention. Professionally produced videos or slides help increase the professionalism of a presentation and assist the learning process. It is not beneficial to show a video to workers unless a facilitator who can lead a discussion and demonstrate techniques is present. The facilitator must have credibility with the audience. This requires that the facilitator be familiar with the job site and adequately trained to answer medical questions. The facilitator need not be a medical professional to be credible, but she or he must have sufficient training in medical facts to explain relevant concepts accurately. A favored method of training is to use professionally produced slides and videos in combination with slides and videos of jobs being performed by employees. In this way, the presentation is "customized" for each company. Video training packages may be used in refresher courses and for new employee training. It is recommended that large corporations use an in-house facilitator to develop a streamlined train-the-trainer process.

SUMMARY

In summary, the literature is mixed regarding the success of preventive training programs, both in clinical and industrial environments. A perusal of the literature reveals that, in general, study design is poor, and there is no consensus on the method, number of components involved, audience, trainer, and measures used to determine effectiveness. Some trends can be observed, however. Training programs that incorporate multiple components, including exercise, tend to be most effective in the clinic. The successful industrial programs described in the literature also tended to have multiple interventions, using employee education as just one component of an overall prevention strategy.

Indeed, common sense would tell us that successful preventive strategies attack the many causes of musculoskeletal disorders rather than focusing on a single cause. Because it is well accepted that cumulative trauma injuries are a result of many factors, including poor ergonomic conditions, faulty worker practices, psychosocial factors, and physical fitness, it follows that sensible efforts at prevention would attempt to address these factors through ergonomic change, worker and management training, and exercise. Unfortunately, this real-world strategy is not easy to study, which explains the anecdotal/descriptive nature of many of the articles available.

Education and training have a place in musculoskeletal injury prevention. The authors of this chapter have had good results with a multicomponent process that involves ergonomic change, worker and management training, and aggressive data analysis and follow-up. Worker training focuses on education about basic ergonomic principles and empowerment to effect changes in the work environment. Material-handling instruction is based on a technique called the power position, which is a lordotic lumbar spine position, incorporating a wide base of support with the weight held close to the body.

When teaching patients in the clinic, the focus should be on symptom/activity improvement and prevention of future episodes. The principles taught are similar to the authors' industrial worker training, emphasizing the components most relevant to workers' current situations. The stress is on self-responsibility for improvement and prevention of future episodes. Return of function and pain relief were achieved when self-responsibility was coupled with an exercise rehabilitation approach.

Education alone is not a panacea. However, education can be effective in the prevention of musculoskeletal disorders, especially when used in conjunction with other sensible prevention strategies.

ACKNOWLEDGMENT. The authors wish to acknowledge Mark A. Anderson, M. A., P. T., for his ideas on education versus training and his involvement with our education/ergonomics process.

REFERENCES

Anderson, C. K., & Chaffin, D. B. (1986). A biomechanical evaluation of five lifting techniques. *Applied Ergonomics, 17*(1), 2–8.

Bergquist-Ullman, M., & Larsson, U. (1977). Acute low back pain in industry: A controlled prospective study with specific reference to therapy and confounding factors. *Acta Orthopaedica Scandinavica, 170*, 1–117.

Berwick, D., Budman, S., & Feldstein, M. (1989). No clinical effect of back schools in an HMO: A randomized prospective trial. *Spine, 14*(3), 338–344.

Brown, K. C., Sirles, A. T., Hilyer, J. C., & Thomas, M. J. (1992). Cost effectiveness of a back school intervention for municipal employees. *Spine, 17*(10), 1224–1228.

Cady, L. D., Bischoff, D. P., O'Connell, E. R., Thomas, P. C., & Allan, J. H. (1979). Strength and fitness and subsequent injuries in firefighters. *Journal of Occupational Medicine, 21*(4), 269–272.

Chaffin, D., Gallay, L. S., Wooley, C., & Kuciemba, S. R. (1986). An evaluation of the effect of a training program on worker lifting postures. *International Journal of Industrial Ergonomics, 1*, 127–136.

Dehlin, O., Hedenrud, B., & Horal, J. (1976). Back symptoms in nursing aides in a geriatric hospital. *Scandinavian Journal of Rehabilitation Medicine, 8*, 47–53.

DiFabio, R. (1995). Efficacy of comprehensive rehabilitation programs and back school for patients with low back pain: A Meta-analysis. *Physical Therapy, 75*(10), 865–878.

DiMaggio, A., & Mooney, V. (1987). Conservative care for low back pain: What works? *Musculoskeletal Medicine, 4*(12), 63–74.

Fitzler, S. L., & Berger, R. A. (1983). Chelsea back program: One year later. *Occupational Health and Safety, 52*(7), 52–54.

Harkapaa, K., Mellin, G., Jarvikoski, A., & Hurri, H. (1989). A controlled study on the outcome of inpatient and outpatient treatment of low back pain: Part I. Pain, disability, compliance, and reported treatment benefits three months after treatment. *Scandinavian Journal of Rehabilitation Medicine, 21*, 81–89.

Harkapaa, K., Mellin, G., Jarvikoski, A., & Hurri, H. (1990). A controlled study on the outcome of inpatient and outpatient treatment of low back pain: Part III. Long-term follow-up of pain, disability, and compliance. *Scandinavian Journal of Rehabilitation Medicine, 22*, 181–188.

Harris, R. L., & McNab, I. (1954). Structural changes in the lumbar intervertebral discs. *Journal of Bone & Joint Surgery, 36B*(2), 304–322.

Hart, D. L., Stobbe, T., & Jaraedi, M. (1987). Effect of lumbar posture on lifting. *Spine, 12*(2), 138–145.

Hickey, D. S., & Hukins, D. (1980). Relation between the structure of the annulus fibrosus and the function and failure of the intervertebral disc. *Spine, 5*(2), 106–116.

Koes, B. W., van Tulder, M. W., van der Windt, D. A. W. M., & Bouter, L. M. (1994). The efficacy of back schools: A review of randomized clinical trials. *Journal of Clinical Epidemiology, 47*(8), 851–862.

LeClaire, R., Esdaile, J. M., Suissa, S., Rossignol, M., Proulx, R., & Dupuis, M. (1996). Back school in a first episode of compensated acute low back pain: A clinical trial to assess efficacy and prevent relapse. *Archives of Physical Medicine Rehabilitation, 77*, 673–679.

Linton, S. J., & Kamwendo, K. (1987). Low back schools: A critical review. *Physical Therapy, 67*(9), 1375–1383.

Mattmiller, A. W. (1980). The California back school. *Physiotherapy, 66*(4), 118–122.

McKenzie, R. A. (1981). *The lumbar spine: Mechanical diagnosis and therapy.* New Zealand: Spinal Publications.

Mellin, G., Hurri, H., Harkapaa, K., & Jarvikowski, A. (1989). A controlled study on the outcome of inpatient and outpatient treatment of low back pain: Part II. Effects on physical measurements three months after treatment. *Scandinavian Journal of Rehabilitation Medicine, 21,* 91-95.

Mellin, G., Hurri, H., Harkapaa, K., & Jarvikowski, A. (1990). Controlled study on the outcome of inpatient and outpatient treatment of low back pain. Part IV. Long-term effects on physical measurements. *Scandinavian Journal of Rehabilitation Medicine, 22,* 189-194.

Melton, B. (1983). Back injury prevention means education. *Occupational Health and Safety, 52*(7), 20-23.

Merriam-Webster's collegiate dictionary (10th ed.). (1993). Springfield, MA: Merriam-Webster.

Miles, M. (1981). *Learning to work in groups* (p. 341). New York: Teacher College Press.

Moffett, J. A., Chase, S. M., Portek, I., & Ennis, J. R. (1986). A controlled, prospective study to evaluate the effectiveness of a back school in the relief of chronic low back pain. *Spine, 11*(2), 120-122.

Morrisson, G., Chase, W., Young, V., & Roberts, W. (1988). Back pain: Treatment and prevention in a community hospital. *Archives of Physical Medicine and Rehabilitation, 69*(8), 605-608.

Park, K. S., & Chaffin, D. B. (1974). A biomechanical evaluation of two methods of manual load lifting. *AIIE Transactions, 6,* 2105-2113.

Park, W. M. (1976). Radiological investigation of the intervertebral disc. In M. I. V. Jayson (Ed.), *The lumbar spine and back pain* (pp. 185-230). London: Pitman Publishing Limited.

Saunders, H. D. (1992). *The back care program.* Minneapolis, MN: The Saunders Group.

Schenk, R. J., Doran, R. L., & Stachura, J. J. (1996). Learning effects of a back education program. *Spine, 21*(19), 2183-2189.

Scholey, M. (1983). Back stress: The effects of training nurses to lift patients in a clinical situation. *International Journal of Nursing Studies, 20*(1), 1-13.

Schwartz, R. K. (1989). Cognition and learning in industrial accident injury prevention: An occupational therapy perspective. *Occupational Therapy in Heath Care, 6*(1), 61-85.

Snook, S. H. (1988a). Approaches to the control of back pain in industry: Job design, job placement and education/training. *State of the Art Reviews in Occupational Medicine, 3*(1), 45-59.

Snook, S. H. (1988b). *The control of low back disability: The role of management* (pp. 97-101). San Francisco: American Industrial Hygiene Association.

Snook, S. H., Campanelli, R., & Hart, J. (1978). A study of three preventive approaches to low back injury. *Journal of Occupational Medicine, 20*(7), 478-481.

Snook, S. H., & White, A. H. (1984). Education and training. In M. H. Pope, J. Frymoyer, & G. Anderson (Eds.), *Occupational low back pain* (pp. 233-244). Philadelphia, PA: Praeger Scientific.

St. Vincent, M. Tellier, C., & Lortie, M. (1989). Training in handling: An evaluative study. *Ergonomics, 32*(2), 191-210.

Stankovic, R., & Johnell, O. (1990). Conservative treatment of acute low back pain. A prospective randomized trial: McKenzie method of treatment versus patient education in "mini back school." *Spine, 15*(2), 120-123.

Stubbs, D. A., Buckle, P. W., Hudson, M. P., & Rivers, P. M. (1983). Back pain in the nursing profession: The effectiveness of training. *Ergonomics, 26*(8), 767-779.

Tomer, G. M., Olson, C., & Lepore, B. (1984, January). Back injury prevention training makes dollars and sense. *National Safety News,* pp. 36-39.

Williams, P. (1982). *Low back and neck pain.* Springfield, IL: Charles C Thomas.

Wollenberg, S. P. (1989). A comparison of body mechanic usage in employees participating in three back injury programs. *International Journal of Nursing, 26*(1), 43-52.

7

Wellness and Fitness Programs

Jeffrey Rothman

Within the last decade, society has clearly begun to recognize the importance of a lifestyle as a vehicle moving the individual toward or away from behavior that is beneficial to health. The process of the individual's taking responsibility for realizing his or her maximum health potential is referred to as *wellness*. Wellness takes into consideration the multidimensionality and interrelationships of a person's existence and being. Physical fitness, proper nutrition and diet, positive self-image and social relationships, and the ability to take responsibility for self-care are interwoven and integral to maximizing the potential to live life to its fullest. This chapter will discuss the interrelationship of wellness and fitness in occupational rehabilitation and present the elements of a program for occupational fitness.

WELLNESS AS A DYNAMIC PROCESS

Wellness is a dynamic process. It is never static. You don't simply stay well or get well. There are many degrees of wellness. For example, an individual may not exhibit physical symptoms of illness but may have unmanaged emotional and stress-related behaviors that lower the body's resistance to disease. Health is a dynamic process, running along a continuum—from optimal health to death. At one end of the continuum is optimal health. At the opposite end is low-level wellness, leading to death—the complete loss of function. Movement toward premature death is characterized by progressively worsening states of health, while movement toward wellness is in the direction of continually improving health (see Figure 7.1).

This continuum of health (sometimes referred to as an illness–wellness continuum) also illustrates the importance of self-responsibility in maintaining one's health. Self-responsibility include awareness, health screening, education, and growth. Looking at

Jeffrey Rothman • Director of Physical Therapy, College of Staten Island, City University of New York, Staten Island, New York 10314.

Sourcebook of Occupational Rehabilitation, edited by Phyllis M. King. Plenum Press, New York, 1998.

Figure 7-1. Health and wellness continuum.

how one is conducting his or her life makes the individual aware of potential risk factors. Health screening provides specific information from appropriate health professionals about the presence and degree of severity of risk factors for illness or disease. Education explores alternatives ways to modify risk factors and provides the information necessary to make informed choices about health care. Growth allows the individual to take action on health care options. The key point is that the individual has control over the direction and pathway she or he chooses to travel on the health continuum. These processes allow the individual to assume self-responsibility for his or her lifestyle behaviors (see Figure 7.2).

THE MULTIDIMENSIONALITY OF HEALTH

The five basic dimensions of health—or definitions of healthy functions—that are often referred to in the literature (Dintiman & Greenberg, 1986) are as follows

Physical health—ability to carry out daily tasks with sufficient energy and strength, with ample reserve available for circumstances that may arise
Emotional health—ability to express and control emotions appropriately
Social health—ability to interact well with others and the environment and have positive interpersonal relationships
Mental health—ability to learn, including cognitive capabilities
Spiritual health—belief in some unifying force, such as a Supreme Being, nature, or scientific laws.

The degree of health that one achieves depends on how one functions in each of these dimensions. We do have control over some factors. Lifestyle choices, diet, environment, and genetics all play an important role and help determine how much control we have over our health. Wellness implies that the way in which we care for our bodies has a significant influence on our total health. Lifestyle behaviors—the daily choices we make about our lives—have been singled out as the most important influences on our health. Recent research indicates that almost 85% of all illness and injury is the result of life-

High-Level Wellness

Awareness   Health Screening   Education   Growth   →   Optimum Health

Figure 7-2. Self-responsibility for one's health.

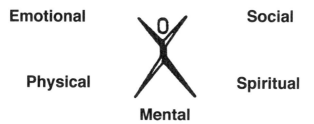

Figure 7-3. The multiple dimensions of health.

style choices (Jamieson, 1997). Healthy lifestyle behaviors and self-responsibility for health are the keys to a high level of wellness (see Figure 7.3).

HEALTH PROMOTION AND PREVENTION

Health promotion is the movement toward optimal health and high-level wellness. Activities that maintain or improve one's level of health are health promotional. Health promotion is a broad concept and can encompass any of the major dimensions of health, such as improving emotional health by fostering interpersonal relationships. The health promotion activity can also be specific, such as exercising three times per week for 30 minutes per session to promote physical fitness.

Prevention is defined as taking steps to avert the development of disease or illness. Prevention can also limit the progression of a disease along its course. There are three levels of prevention: primary, secondary, and tertiary.

Primary prevention includes the general and specific health promoting activities that protect the individual from disease and illness. The populations involved are generally healthy and do not exhibit any symptoms of disease, but they may be susceptible to the development of disease. Health-promotion activities include immunizations, lifestyle behavior modifications, smoking cessation, and nutritional counseling.

Secondary prevention involves early diagnosis and treatment to stop or limit disease and avert the sequelae of a disease or illness. Screening activities play an important role at this level. They may be administered to detect such diseases or disorders as hypertension, high cholesterol levels, malignancies, osteoporosis, and acquired immune deficiency syndrome (AIDS).

Tertiary prevention occurs after a disability or condition is irreversible. It is important in limiting the degree of disability or handicap. The goal of tertiary prevention is to limit the disability and enable the individual to utilize whatever residual function he or she has available to maximize the ability to function in society.

HEALTH CARE PROFESSIONALS' ROLES IN HEALTH PROMOTION AND PREVENTION

Only recently has the long-standing disease treatment orientation of conventional medicine been challenged. Medical professionals have begun to realize that a different philosophy is needed to promote better health and prevent disease in our society. The disease treatment approach is very expensive; health care costs now exceed 15% of the gross national product (Clinton, 1993). These escalating costs for health care, limited access to the health care system, and increasing illness and disease in segments of our society have mandated the need for health care reform. Preventive practice and the promotion of optimal levels of health can contribute significantly to improving the quality of health care and decreasing its costs. For the past two decades, researchers have found that prevention and wellness programs, both community- and those at work-site-based can improve health and prevent injury (Farquhar et al., 1990; Gebhardt & Crump, 1990; Harris, Caspersen, DeFriese, & Estes, 1989; Kellett, Kellett, & Nordholm, 1991; Pelletier, 1993; Thompson, 1994; Viru & Smirnova, 1995).

Professional organizations, managed care systems, and private and state insurance companies have emphasized the importance of prevention. It is the health care profes-sional's responsibility as well to take an active role in promoting health and wellness. The health care practitioner must be able to model and reflect the attitudes and healthy lifestyle behaviors that she or he wishes to convey to patients. Health care practitioners must assess their own health status nd lifestyle behaviors and formulate strategies for personal health. Active participation in evaluating and modifying one's personal lifestyle behaviors helps provide a foundation for a lifelong commitment to a high level of well-ness. This practice contributes to the practitioner's professional career and augments the decision-making process, playing a role in the development of health promotion strate-gies with and for clients. The adage "practice what you preach" applies to the health practitioner as a model for health and wellness.

To augment their "model of health," the health practitioner must document and research the effectiveness of health promotion and prevention programs. Research is necessary to provide the validity and reliability of these programs. Health care reform will support those programs that provide an economic return and cost savings for the delivery of health care services.

FITNESS

The past decade has witnessed a surge of interest in exercise and fitness. There has been a proliferation of health clubs and exercise videotapes, with noted health experts and celebrities expounding on the importance of exercising and fitness to maintain or improve health. Research on the benefits of exercise clearly demonstrate a positive relationship between regular exercise and reduced stress, improved muscle strength and endurance, decreased risk for coronary heart disease, increased efficiency of the cardio-pulmonary system, and decreased risk for low back injuries (Blair, 1985; Blair, Kohl, & Paffenbarger, 1989; Haskell, Montoye, & Orenstein, 1985; Jackson, 1994; Kellett et al., 1991; Paffenbarger & Hale, 1975; Paffenbarger, Hyde, Wing, & Chung-Cheng, 1986).

The importance of fitness in the workplace has not been examined as thoroughly. However, large and small companies have begun to open on-site health promotion and prevention centers. The purpose of these centers is to improve the health and well-being of employees by facilitating proper lifestyle behaviors. Decreased absenteeism, reduced health care costs, protection from lower back problems and musculoskeletal injuries, and improved productivity are among the benefits of exercise, nutritional counseling, and stress management and health-promotion programs in the workplace.

Before we describe occupational rehabilitation fitness programs, it is necessary to discuss the general guidelines for fitness and exercise. *Fitness*, in its broadest sense, is an ongoing state of health, whereby the body has the capacity to meet the physical demands and rigors of modern life and perform at an optimal level with relatively little strain and without injury. A person who is physically fit is able to perform his or her duties and responsibilities at work and participate in play and personal activities and obligations. The fit individual also has the capacity to meet the physical demands of unusual situations such as hiking across heavy terrain or climbing steep stairs. The economic and personal benefits of being physically fit can be measured by fewer sick days from work, decreased injury to the lower back, and reduced medical expenses.

CLASSIFICATIONS OF FITNESS

There are two major classifications of fitness: performance-related fitness and health-related fitness. Performance-related fitness is concerned with measures of strength, speed, flexibility, and agility and is often considered in association with specific athletic events. Health-related fitness concerns physical conditioning related more to health and occupational rehabilitation. (Health-related fitness is more pertinent to our discussion of occupational rehabilitation and will be discussed in greater detail than performance-related fitness.)

Performance-Related Fitness

Performance-related fitness measures levels of strength, skill, power, endurance, and agility in recreational sports and specific athletics. Although these are important aspects of fitness, in actuality they are not directly related to health and wellness. The nonathletic individual and typical occupational worker have little need of the strength and skill to throw a football 40 yards to a specific target. The ability to run fast for an extended period of time and to change direction of movement quickly can be invaluable assets for a professional baseball player or weekend athlete but are not as valuable to the typical worker as it relates to a level of wellness.

Health-Related Fitness

Health-related fitness comprises four components of health and wellness: cardiopulmonary fitness, body composition, strength and endurance, and flexibility. Cardiopulmonary fitness, also referred to as aerobic fitness, is the body's ability to provide sufficient oxygen and nutrients to all vital organs and muscles during continuous rhythmical exercises for extended periods of time, using the cardiopulmonary system. Levels of inefficient cardiopulmonary fitness can result in coronary heart disease and a decreased capacity to perform physical activities. A heart in excellent condition and an effective pulmonary system can function at a high level of fitness. Proper aerobic training and conditioning can strengthen the cardiopulmonary system and increase its ability to transport oxygen throughout the body. Studies have shown that individuals who have suffered a heart attack or were predisposed to coronary heart disease benefit significantly from exercise (Blair et al., 1989; Garcia-Palmieri, Costas, & Cruz-Vidal, 1982; Ornish, 1990;

Paffenbarger, et al., 1986; Rippe, Blair, & Freedson, 1987). Effective cardiopulmonary exercise programs can prevent coronary heart disease by improving cardiovascular and metabolic fitness.

According to Bazley (1992), cardiovascular fitness is improved through exercise by

- increasing collateral circulation
- slowing heart rate at rest and during a specific workout
- improving peripheral circulation
- lowering blood pressure
- increasing stroke volume
- enlarging coronary vessels
- increasing cardiac output
- increasing physical work capacity
- improving aerobic capacity (Vo_2max)

Bazley added that exercise can improve metabolic fitness by

- lowering blood concentrations of low-density lipoprotein cholesterol (LDL-C)
- lowering concentrations of very low-density lipoprotein cholesterol (VLDL-C)
- reducing levels of serum triglycerides
- increasing levels of high-density lipoprotein cholesterol (HDL-C)
- decreasing fibrinolytic activity at rest via reduced circulating catecholamines
- increasing insulin sensitivity
- increasing blood volume
- reducing blood glucose levels

In addition to affecting coronary heart disease, research has shown that a regular program of cardiorespiratory or aerobic fitness can help prevent and control hypertension, noninsulin-dependent diabetes mellitus, osteoporosis, obesity, depression and anxiety, and colon cancer (Harris et al.,1989; Thompson, 1994).

Cardiopulmonary Fitness

The body's capacity to consume oxygen at a maximum rate, referred to as Vo_2max, is the primary measurement in evaluating cardiopulmonary endurance. There are several methods that can be used to estimate cardiopulmonary fitness. Direct measurements of oxygen uptake through the use of sophisticated equipment is the most accurate, but it is expensive and requires substantial time and technical expertise. There are a number of other tests that can estimate cardiopulmonary fitness indirectly by determining the heart-rate response to specific exercises. Although these tests are not exact measurements, they do provide more than an adequate approximation of aerobic fitness. These tests can also provide baseline information by which to measure improved fitness over time. They can easily be administered at a work site and require minimal equipment and space. Two of the many tests available will briefly be described. (The reader is referred to other sources of information for more complete, detailed references on these assessment instruments and how they are administered) (Altug, Hoffman, & Martin, 1993; American College of Sports Medicine, 1991).

The Step Test. The individual is asked to step up and down on a bench (of a specific size) at a fixed rate for five minutes. Heart rate is taken five minutes before the test and five minutes after the test. Based on the postexercise heart rate, age, sex, and body weight, a fitness score assessing the level of fitness from superior to very poor is determined.

Bicycle Ergometer. On a stationary bicycle, the subject pedals at a preset RPM (revolutions per minute) and at a specified workload for five minutes. Heart rate is measured during the last minute. Tables based on the age of the subject, sex, workload, and heart rate determine the subject's level of fitness.

Body Composition

Body composition is the relative proportion of body fat to lean body tissue. Most experts agree that the proportion of body fat to fat free weight is a better determinant of an individual's fitness level than ordinary body weight. An excessive proportion of body fat puts an individual at greater risk for health problems, such as cardiovascular disease and diabetes. Body composition can provide the information needed to assess weight loss and design exercise programs. The recommended percentage of body fat is based on the sex of the individual, age, and level of fitness. It is suggested that for the adult male, the percentage of body fat should be between 12% and 17%, while females should be between 17% and 22%. Based on the fact that approximately 50% of the body's fat is stored just below the skin, the skin fold test for determination of body fat is often used.

Although the skin fold method is subject to error (3%–4%), it is inexpensive and easy to learn and administer when compared with other methods. With the use of skin fold calipers, measurements are taken at preselected anatomical sites. Using formulas and tables, an individual's percentage of body fat is determined. The individual's current fat weight, lean body weight, and desired body weight can also be calculated by use of a formula and equation through this method. (For a more detailed description of this method, the reader is referred to other sources) (Althoff, Svoboda, & Girdano, 1992; Altug, Hoffman, & Martin, 1993; McGlynn, 1990).

Strength and Endurance

The basic foundation for physical exercise is the muscle system. Muscle strength is the force required by a muscle or group of muscles to perform a movement. Muscle endurance is the ability of the muscle to maintain a contraction over a period of time. When performing any activity, muscle strength and muscle endurance determine the level of performance in that activity. It is important to emphasize that the muscular system does not work independently of other body systems. Muscles are dependent on the heart, pulmonary systems, and blood vessels to provide sufficient energy and waste product elimination in order to perform work effectively. Therefore, proper conditioning is necessary for all bodily systems to maintain a maximal level of fitness.

The strength and endurance of the body's major muscles play an important role in many aspects of health. For example, proper body mechanics involving use of the leg muscles instead of the back muscles can help ensure a safe lifting performance and moving of objects at work or home. Adequate strength in the muscles of the lower back and especially the abdominals are cited as important for the prevention of injuries to the low back (Cady, Bishoff, O'Connell, & Allan, 1979; Doolittle, Spurlin, Kaiyala, & Sovern, 1988; Jackson, 1994; Kellett et al., 1991). The capacity to perform physical activities for a given period of time without undue strain and stress is a direct result of adequate muscle strength and endurance. Muscles that are weak and cannot sustain a contraction for the time needed to complete an activity are at greater risk for injury.

The strength and endurance of a muscle can be determined by using a variety of methods and instruments. A brief description of the most common methods used to assess muscle strength and muscle endurance follows.

Isometric Static Strength. Isometric static strength can be measured by using special devices referred to as dynamometers or tensiometers. The handheld dynamometer is often used to measure grip strength. Similar devices measure the strength of back and leg muscles. These instruments are easy to administer and record. However, static strength is limited because it only measures strength at one joint angle and not through full range of motion. Muscle endurance can be measured by having the individual maintain the contraction over time.

Dynamic Isotonic Strength. Muscle strength and muscle endurance are assessed through the use of free weights, weight stacks (such as the universal gym equipment), or computerized exercise machines. Isotonic exercises are performed against resistance while the load remains constant; the resistance varies depending on the angle of the joint. Muscle strength can be measured separately from that of endurance by having the individual lift the weight for one or a number of repetitions against a preset speed. Recommended standards for the dynamic strength of different muscle groups are available. Dynamic muscle strength can provide an objective strength measure provided that the individual properly performs the activity without building up momentum when lifting the weights. It is important to closely monitor the individual while performing this method of assessment to prevent injury. There are also computerized muscle testing machines available to assess isotonic muscle strength and endurance.

Isokinetic Strength. Isokinetic strength assessment measures the muscle's ability to contract maximally at a constant speed over a full range of motion against a variable resistance. Muscular endurance can be measured as the muscle contracts against a preset speed for a given time period. An *isokinetic contraction* is defined as equal motion or equal speed. The isokinetic machine is set to provide only one speed of movement, regardless of how hard one pushes. An isokinetic contraction utilizes the present resistance. This resistance is directly related to the applied force; as one pushes, the isokinetic device resists in proportion to the force used. Isokinetic measurement provides objective documentation to assist in determining muscle strength or weakness. However, isokinetic machines are expensive, bulky, and are usually only available in rehabilitation centers.

Flexibility

Flexibility is the range and extent of movement of a joint. Muscles should be flexible to allow the full range of motion required for activities of daily living at home and work and during recreation. All activities require different degrees of flexibility—reaching for an object, painting, stacking supplies, or climbing stairs. Lengthening of muscles is necessary to allow for efficient and safe movement. A shortened muscle can be a result of inactivity, improper exercising, arthritic joint changes, or muscle weakness. Injury and damage to a muscle can result when an inflexible joint is placed in a lengthened position. It is important to note that flexibility varies from individual to individual and may result from lifestyle behaviors or occupational activities.

Joint flexibility depends on the integrity of the joint capsule, connective tissue, ligaments, tendon, and muscle. Any limitations of these structures can result in decreased flexibility. Flexibility of the lower spine and hip are particularly important because they relate to low back problems. Decreased range of motion of the lower spine and hip can limit or decrease the muscle strength of the lower back and abdominals, making the back more susceptible to injury.

Assessment of flexibility should be performed carefully by trained professionals because improper stretching can result in tearing of the joint capsule. There are several approaches to stretching, including static stretching, passive stretching, active stretching, and ballistic stretching. For static stretching, the procedure is to place the joint slowly in a position of stretch whereby the muscle is lengthened. Static stretching involves exercises through which a stretch is held in a fixed position for a short period. Passive or manual stretching occurs when the professional applies an external force. In active stretching, the individual provides the stretch. Ballistic stretching involves rapid bouncing and jerky movements. This type of stretching is not recommended because it may result in injury.

In summary, the components of health-related fitness—cardiorespiratory fitness, body composition, muscle strength and endurance, and flexibility—are important to achieving a high level of wellness. These components can be used to improve the body's response to exercise, decrease an excessive percentage of body fat, strengthen major muscle groups to prevent injury, improve the capacity of muscle to work over a period of time, and increase joint flexibility for physical activities. An individual who is "fit" is better able to function at home and at work.

FITNESS IN OCCUPATIONAL REHABILITATION

The principles of wellness and health-related fitness previously discussed should be applied when designing and implementing occupational fitness programs. An effective employer recognizes the multidimensionality of each individual. The physical aspects of health are positively or adversely affected by emotional or social interactions. How an individual interacts with her or his supervisor and other employees will be influenced by how well that individual is able to meet and perform the physical demands of the job. It is in the best interest of management to consider health promotion and injury prevention and make them part of the work environment. The delivery of health care services in the workplace can facilitate optimal employee health. To do so, it is necessary to identify potential health problems before they exist, the primary level of prevention. Many organizations already provide significant employee assistance programs, such as stress management, nutritional guidance, smoking cessation, psychosocial counseling, and fitness programs. The benefits of these programs as they relate to health care costs, productivity, and morale are enormous and have only recently begun to be examined.

The components of health-related fitness provide the basic framework necessary to implement an effective fitness program. Although there is a paucity of research in this area, it is important to describe briefly some of the benefits of fitness programs that have been reported in the literature: reduced absenteeism, decreased health care costs, improved health status of employees, and injury prevention.

Reduced Absenteeism and Decreased Health Care Costs

A regular program of exercise and fitness correlates with reduced absenteeism. For example, the relation between exercise and absenteeism due to illness and injury was assessed in 21,924 male workers in manufacturing companies in Japan (Muto & Sakurai, 1993). Exercisers I (those engaging in exercise less than once a week), Exercisers II (once or twice a week), and Exercisers III (more than three times a week) had significantly lower incidences of absence from work than nonexercisers. The proportion of cases of absence in Exercisers I, II, and III was 10%, 10%, and 14% lower, respectively, than that of nonexercisers. The number of days absent among Exercisers I, II, and III was 48%, 43%, and 26% lower, respectively, than among nonexercisers. Other studies similarly found that fitness programs in industries resulted in reduced absenteeism (Bey & Jones, 1986; Wood, Olmstead, & Craig, 1989). Wood and colleagues (1989) studied the Tri-Healthalon Program at General Mills and compared absenteeism with the cost for the program. The program included an employee fitness program. The authors reported a return on investment of $3.10 the first year and $3.90 in subsequent years for every dollar spent on the program. There was also a 23% increase in the number of employees who exercised three times per week. In a study of Johnson & Johnson's "Live for Life" program, Bly and Jones (1986) found that the increase in the mean annual in-patient cost of insurance was reduced significantly because of decreased hospital stays. The annual cost increase for the fitness group was $43 as compared with $76 for the group that did not participate in the fitness program.

Improvement in Health Status

Exercise and fitness programs are a preventive intervention for chronic disease processes and improve the individual's health status. Employers must recognize that a healthy employee has the potential to be a productive member of the organization for a significant number of years of service. The savings in health care costs are also significant if major chronic diseases are prevented. A regular program of physical exercise has been found to prevent such chronic diseases as coronary heart disease (Paffenbarger & Hale, 1975), hypertension (Bjorntorp, 1982), non-insulin-dependent diabetes mellitus (Kriska, Blair, & Pereira, 1994), osteoporosis (Alois, Cohn, & Ostuni, 1978), and colon cancer (Paffenbarger, 1984; Powell, Caspersen, Koplan, & Ford, 1989).

There have been a number of long-term studies on the benefits of corporate wellness programs. Bjurstrom (1978) studied 600 employees who received a comprehensive health and physical activity program over a five-year period. The study showed a significant reduction in the risk of coronary heart disease, amelioration of a wide range of health problems, and a large reduction in employee absenteeism. Shephard (1983) studied 534 men and women who participated in a fitness program for one year. The author noted a significant reduction in medical reimbursement costs and a 50% reduction in employee hospitalizations.

Injury Prevention

A major factor motivating companies to initiate fitness programs is the reduction of work-related injuries and the concomitant workers' compensation costs. Musculoskeletal injuries account for a majority of these injuries, with a high proportion involving the low back. Fitness levels and exercise training appear to be related to injury (Jackson, 1994). For instance, high levels of aerobic fitness, strength, and flexibility were shown to be inversely related to the workers' compensation costs of firefighters (Cady et al., 1979; Cady, Thomas, & Karwasky, 1985) and lineworkers (Doolittle, 1988).

The important Cady study (Cady et al., 1979) found a relationship between the incidence of back injuries and levels of fitness among firefighters. He reported the injury rates for the least fit to be 7.1%, the middle fit to be 3.2%, and the most fit to be 0.8%. Back injuries among those firefighters who were fit were less costly than those of firefighters who were not fit. A study of electrical lineworkers found similar results (Battie, Bigos, & Fisher, 1989). Based on these studies, it would appear that fitness programs help reduce musculoskeletal injuries. Several other studies have shown that strength is related to injury rates, and that a worker is more likely to sustain a musculoskeletal injury when a job's lifting requirements approach or exceed the worker's strength capacity (Chaffin, Herrin, & Keyserling, 1978; Keyserling, 1986).

Based on a review of the literature and the author's experience, an effective program to prevent injuries to the musculoskeletal system needs to encompass the following components:

Job analysis: Analyze the physical job requirements including duties, behaviors, and worker outcomes.

Education and training: Train workers on safety precautions, such as lifting techniques, body mechanics, and postures for sitting, reaching, and standing.

Exercise and fitness programs: Initiate muscle strengthening exercises and fitness programs to strengthen those muscles that are needed to perform the job safely, and help improve and maintain the health status of the individual.

Strengthening exercises to condition the muscles that will be used to perform the job activity and endurance training exercises that will allow the individual to withstand the particular physical stresses on the job are crucial to injury prevention. An example of how these components can be implemented is as follows: An individual works on a loading dock. He or she performs activities that require lifting, pushing, and pulling objects (based on the job analysis). At times, he or she must be able to move quickly along the dock as the merchandise arrives. To prevent injuries, the subject should be trained in proper lifting techniques (education and training); regularly perform exercises to strengthen the abdominals, quadriceps, and lower spine; and perform aerobic exercises, such as walking or running.

ELEMENTS OF A FITNESS PROGRAM

Based on the previous discussion of the components of health-related fitness and the review of the benefits of fitness programs in industry, important elements in designing and implementing an effective fitness program for employees can be identified. It is necessary to note that the extent of a fitness program depends on the financial resources that a company is able to commit to it. Larger companies collaborate with managed care systems to provide health fitness programs as a vehicle to curtail medical costs. Smaller companies may be able to join with similar-sized companies in offering such programs. Analysis of a company's injury and compensation costs may lend support for health fitness programs. This analysis reviews the company's injury statistics, rate of absenteeism from injury, and medical claims that are related to the occupation and job description. Consultants with experience in designing a fitness program can help to ensure that sufficient space is available for the program and that the equipment to be purchased is appropriate for that facility. A survey of the workplace—especially an ergonomic assessment—can also gather information on the type of exercise and fitness program that should be considered. The following sections describe those elements recommended for consideration when planning a fitness program for a company or industry.

Health Survey and Physical Activities Readiness Questionnaire

Employees should complete a health survey that provides information on lifestyle behaviors, levels of exercise and physical activity, nutritional and dietary habits, stress, and general health. Any physical or health problem, such as injuries to the musculoskeletal system, are thus identified. The Physical Activities Readiness Questionnaire (Harris et al., 1989) is a simple and reliable preexercise screening tool that can be used to determine if the individual can begin the exercise program or should return to his or her referring physician before beginning the program.

Medical Screening and Assessment

Ideally, medical screening and assessment should be performed on-site at the company's medical facility. The screening usually includes a maximal stress test and full exam, including blood analysis. The tests are usually performed by a cardiologist and registered nurse. If the facility does not provide a medical facility for the screening, employees should be referred to a physician before beginning the fitness program. The physician should have experience in identifying potential health risks for exercise. It is up to the physician to determine whether a cardiovascular stress test is necessary. This determination is often based on the age of the individual, family history, blood chemistry results, and physical examination.

Cardiovascular Assessment

Assessment of the body's capacity to utilize oxygen at a maximum rate will provide information on the individual's cardiovascular fitness level. (Several indirect methods—the steptest and the bicycle ergometer—were described previously in this chapter.)

Body Composition

The relative proportion of body fat to lean body tissue, referred to as body composition, provides information needed to assess weight loss and design a fitness program. (The use of skin fold calipers to measure body composition as an assessment tool was described earlier.)

Muscle Strength and Endurance

Evaluation of muscle strength and endurance helps to develop a proper conditioning program. (Isometric, isotonic, and isokinetic strength parameters are the assessment methods described earlier in this chapter.)

Flexibility

An assessment of a joint's range of motion for efficient and safe movement is important to the prevention of injury or damage to that joint. Flexibility can be measured by static, active, or passive stretch of the joint by a trained professional. (A brief description of these methods appears earlier in this chapter.)

Consultation by Trained Professionals

Consultants should be involved early in the planning process. They may include physical therapists, athletic trainers, exercise physiologists, and nutritionists.

Nutritional Guidance

Proper nutritional guidance is an integral component of a fitness program. A nutritionist or dietician should be included among those whose expertise is necessary to effectively implement a program.

Health Education Program

An ongoing regular session of educational programs on topics related to personal wellness should be offered to the participants. Topics may include stress management, smoking cessation, and exercise.

Comprehensive Fitness Program

A comprehensive fitness program with up-to-date exercise equipment and a variety of fitness classes are crucial to maintaining participants' interests. Classes on yoga, tai chi, low impact aerobics, and cross-training are some examples. The equipment in the center should be maintained and replaced as newer exercise devices become available.

Individuality in Programming

The exercise and fitness program should be individualized and meet the goals and expectations of the individual. Following the initial assessment, a regular progress assessment should be performed, and the exercise program should be modified, depending on its results. A written assessment of each employee should be kept on file.

A MODEL PROGRAM

Many corporations have initiated exercise and fitness programs with significant results. Successful model programs exist. The following is a brief description of one such program.

At its corporate headquarters in midtown Manhattan, Pfizer Incorporated, a research-based health-care company, offers a state-of-the-art health and fitness center to its 2,500 employees. Pfizer knows the importance of keeping healthy. It has designed the facility and offers services that improve the health of its employees by reducing their risk of

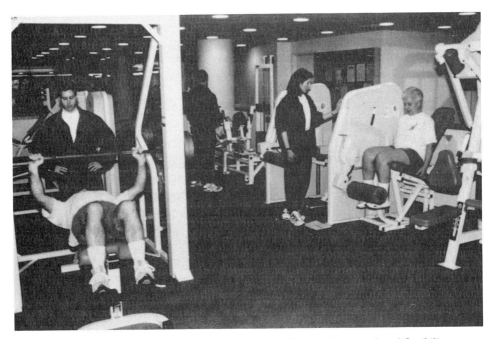

The facility offers a wide range of equipment to develop muscle strength and flexibility.

cardiovascular disease and other lifestyle-related illnesses. Staffed by exercise physiologists, a physical therapist, certified athletic trainers, and a health promotion specialist, Pfizer has designed their facility to offer a comprehensive wellness program, including fitness health promotion, orthopedic care, cardiac rehabilitation, and ergonomics.

Pfizer's Programs for Integrating Total Health (PFIT) is one of the many fitness programs Pfizer has established worldwide. "Focusing on employee wellness makes good business sense," said Pfizer Chair and CEO William C. Steere Jr., someone who exercises regularly at the headquarters' facility. "When you're under stress, it's hard to focus on exercise, but I always feel better when I do."

Every employee is eligible to join PFIT, which is subsidized by Pfizer and requires minimal monthly payments from employees. Each new member is required to undergo a series of medical assessments: a maximal stress test, body fat analysis, and a full physical exam, including blood analysis. Tests are performed at Pfizer's on-site medical facility by a registered nurse and internist/cardiologist. These assessments are used as a tool to determine cardiovascular risk factors and the current fitness levels of prospective members. The results are evaluated by the medical and fitness staffs. After reviewing the tests, a fitness staff member gives the new participant an exercise orientation. During the orientation, the staff member and the participant discuss the results of the medical and nutritional assessment, identify cardiovascular risk factors, and develop a personalized exercise program that is based on these results and the individual's goals. Members are assessed annually or biannually, depending on age and medical history.

PFIT is equipped with treadmills, computerized bicycles, recumbent bikes, cross-country skiers, stairclimbers, and rowing machines. Each piece of cardiovascular equipment has a heart rate monitor. The treadmills and recumbent bikes each have a color

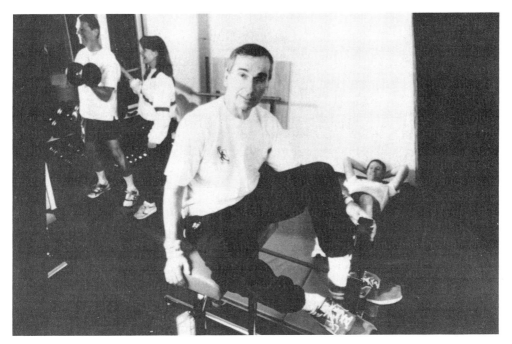

"Focusing on employee wellness makes good business sense," says Pfizer Chair and CEO William C. Steers, Jr.

television and videocassette recorder. There is a combination of Nautilus and Cybex weight equipment and free weights available for members who want to strengthen and tone muscles. The health and fitness staff offers one-on-one training to all members. A comprehensive group exercise program includes low-impact aerobics, beginning and advanced step classes, body conditioning, stretching, and box aerobics. Specialty classes, such as ballroom dance, country line dancing, yoga, and tai chi, are also rotated into the schedule.

Pfizer also makes it convenient for employees to exercise by providing each member with a locker and full exercise attire, including T-shirt, shorts, and socks. The locker rooms are equipped with a steam room, several showers, fresh towels, and other amenities. Participation in the health and fitness programs has steadily increased to a current daily participation of 250 employees.

The physical therapy program employs a licensed physical therapist and certified athletic trainer. If an employee is in need of physical therapy, he or she provides Pfizer with a prescription for therapy, and the physical therapy is provided on-site. Each employee receives an initial evaluation that includes a medical history, subjective and objective information, assessment, short- and long-term goals, and a treatment plan. Progress notes are kept and sent to physicians on request. All the necessary modalities and equipment are provided to ensure the success of the physical therapy program. The physical therapist and certified athletic trainer currently treat approximately 30–35 different employees each week.

An annual health promotion calendar is designed to offer all employees (members and nonmembers) monthly program options, which include screenings, lectures, seminars, and intervention programs. Some examples of the intervention programs include

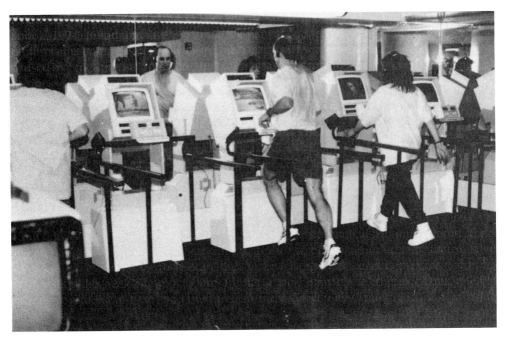

PFIT is equipped with treadmills and stairclimbers, which provide an excellent way to improve cardiovascular fitness.

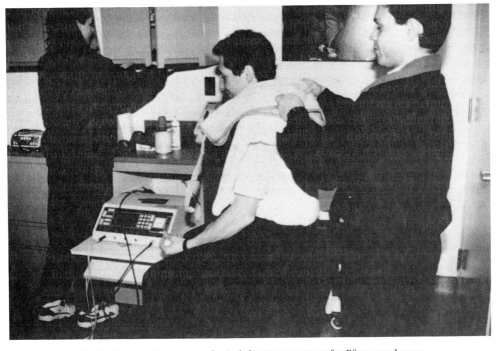

The facility provides on-site physical therapy treatment for Pfizer employees.

high blood pressure and cholesterol intervention, smoking cessation, diabetes control, stress management, nutrition education, and cancer screenings.

Pfizer is proud to offer the PFIT as a valuable tool in retaining its employees. The center is an attractive benefit for potential new employees. The goals and objectives of the center are consistent with Pfizer's commitment to health and excellence. The facility is an integral part of the company's goal to be "Part of the Cure."

ACKNOWLEDGMENT. Matthew Donofrio, M.S., A.T.C., Assistant Manager of the Pfizer Program for Integrating Total Health (PFIT), helped to provide the information on the exercise and fitness programs at Pfizer.

REFERENCES

Alois, J. F., Cohn, S. H., & Ostuni, J. A. (1978). Prevention of involutional bone loss by exercise. *Annals of Internal Medicine, 89,* 356–358.

Althoff, S. A., Svoboda, M., & Girdano, D. A. (1992). *Choices in health and fitness.* Phoenix: Gorsuch Scarisbrick.

Altug, Z., Hoffman, J. L., & Martin, J. (1993). *Manual of clinical exercise testing, prescription and rehabilitation.* Norwalk: Appleton & Lange.

American College of Sports Medicine. (1991). *Guidelines for exercise testing and prescription.* Philadelphia, PA: Lea & Febiger.

Battie, M. C., Bigos, S. J., & Fisher, L. S. D. (1989). A prospective study of the role of cardiovascular risk factors and fitness in industrial back complaints. *Spine, 14,* 141–149.

Bazley, R. D. (1992). Promoting health through exercise. In J. Rothman & R. E. Levine (Eds.), *Prevention practice: Strategies for physical therapists and occupational therapists* (pp. 36–59). Philadelphia, PA, W. B. Saunders.

Bjorntorp, P. (1982). Hypertension and exercise. *Hypertension, 4,* 56–59.

Bjurstrom, L. A. (1978). A program of heart disease prevention for public employees. *Journal of Occupational Medicine, 20,* 521–531.

Blair, S. N. (1985). Physical activity leads to fitness and pays off. *Physician Sports Medicine, 13,* 153–157.

Blair, S. N., Kohl, H. W., & Pfaffenbarger, R. S. (1989). Physical fitness and all-cause mortality: A prospective study of healthy men and women. *Journal of the American Medical Association, 262,* 2395–2401.

Bly, J., & Jones, R. (1986). Impact of worksite health promotion on health care costs and utilization. *Journal of the American Medical Association, 256,* 3240–3253.

Cady, L. D., Bishoff, E. R., O'Connell, P. C., & Allan, J. H. (1979). Back injuries in firefighters. *Journal of Occupational Medicine, 21,* 269–272.

Cady, L. D., Thomas, P. C., & Karwasky, R. J. (1985). Program for increasing health and fitness of firefighters. *Journal of Occupational Medicine, 27,* 110–114.

Chaffin, D. B., Herrin, G. D., & Keyserling, W. M. (1978). Pre-employment strength testing: An updated position. *Journal of Occupational Medicine, 20,* 403–408.

Clinton, W. J. (1993). *Health security: The president's report to the American people.* Washington, DC: White House.

Dintiman, G., & Greenberg, J. S. (1986). *Health through discovery.* New York: Random House.

Doolittle, T. L., Spurlin, O., Kaiyala, K., & Sovern, D. (1988). Physical demands of lineworkers. *Proceedings of the Human Factors Society, 32,* 632–636.

Farquhar, J. W., Fortmann, S. P., Flora, J. A., Taylor, C. B., Haskell, W. L., Williams, P. T., Maccoby, N., & Wood, P. T. (1990). Effects of community-wide education on cardiovascular disease risk factors. *Journal of the American Medical Association, 264,* 359–366.

Garcia-Palmieri, M. R., Costas, R., & Cruz-Vidal, M. (1982). Increased physical activity: A protective response against heart attacks in Puerto Rico. *American Journal of Cardiology, 50,* 749–755.

Gebhardt, D. L., & Crump, C. (1990). Employee fitness and wellness programs in the workplace. *American Psychology, 45,* 262–272.

Harris, S. S., Caspersen, C. J., DeFriese, G. H., & Estes, E. H. (1989). Physical activity counseling for healthy adults as a primary preventive intervention in the clinical setting. *Journal of the American Medical Association, 261,* 3590–3598.

Haskell, W. L., Montoye, H. J., Orenstein, D. (1985). Physical activity and exercise to achieve health-related physical fitness components. *Public Health Report, 100,* 202–212.

Jackson, A. (1994). Pre-employment physical evaluation. *Exercise and Sports Sciences Reviews, 22,* 53–90.

Jamieson, J. E. (1997, March/April). Health care: A misnomer? *Alternative Therapies in Clinical Practice,* 57–59.

Kellett, K. M., Kellett, D. A., Nordholm, L. A. (1991). Effects of an exercise program on sick leave due to back pain. *Physical Therapy, 71,* 283–293.

Keyserling, W. (1986). Postural analysis of the trunk and shoulders in simulated real time. *Ergonomics, 29,* 569–583.

Kriska, A. M., Blair, S. N., & Pereira, M. A. (1994). The potential role of physical activity in the prevention of non-insulin diabetes mellitus: The epidemiological evidence. *Exercises and Sports Sciences Reviews, 22,* 121–144.

McGlynn, G. (1990). *Dynamics of fitness: A practical approach.* Dubuque, IA: Wm. C. Brown.

Muto, T., & Sakurai, H. (1993). Relation between exercise and absenteeism due to illness and injury in manufacturing companies in Japan. *Journal of Occupational Medicine, 35,* 995–999.

Ornish, D. (1990). Can lifestyle changes reverse coronary heart disease? *Lancet, 336,* 129–133.

Paffenbarger, R. S., & Hale, W. E. (1975). Work activity and coronary heart mortality. *New England Journal of Medicine, 292,* 545–550.

Paffenbarger, R. S., Hyde, R. T., Wing, A. L., & Chung-Cheng, H. (1986). Physical activity, all-cause mortality and longevity of college alumni. *New England Journal of Medicine, 314,* 605–613.

Paffenberger, R. S., Hyde, R. T., Wing, A. L., & Steinmetz, C. H. (1984). A natural history of athleticism and cardiovascular health. *Journal of the American Medical Association, 252*(4), 491–495.

Pelletier, K. R. (1993). A review and analysis of the health and cost-effectiveness outcome studies of comprehensive health promotion and disease prevention programs at the work site: 1991–1993 update. *American Journal of Health Promotion, 8,* 50–61.

Powell, K. E., Caspersen, C. J., Koplan, J. P., & Ford, E. S. (1989). Physical activity and chronic diseases. *American Journal of Clinical Nutrition, 49,* 999–1006.

Rippe, J. M., Blair, S. N., & Freedson, P. S. (1987). The health benefits of exercise: Part 1. *Physician Sports Medicine, 15,* 115–132.

Shephard, R. J. (1983). Employee health and fitness: the state of the art. *Preventive Medicine, 12,* 644–650.

Thompson, W. G. (1994). Exercise and health: Fact or hype? *Southern Medical Journal, 87,* 567–574.

Viru, A., & Smirnova, T. (1995). Health promotion and exercise testing. *Physician Sports Medicine, 19,* 123–136.

Wood, E. A., Olmstead, G., & Craig, J. (1989). An evaluation of lifestyle risk factors and absenteeism after two years in a worksite health promotion program. *American Journal of Health Promotion, 58,* 128–133.

8

Ergonomics

Donald S. Bloswick, Tim Villnave, and Brad Joseph

HISTORY

For thousands of years, humans have been concerned with tools and devices that might make work and life easier. Christensen (1987) noted that the importance of a "good fit" between humans and tools was probably realized early in the development of the species. Australopithecus Prometheus selected pebble tools and made scoops from antelope bones to make tasks easier to perform. Sketches of early farm tools show that they were designed to match the size and shape of the human body well.

Probably the first formal discussion of the relationship between physical effort and musculoskeletal maladies was presented by the Italian physician Bernardino Ramazinni, who noted in 1713:

> The maladies that afflict the clerks aforesaid arise from three causes: First, constant sitting; secondly, the incessant movement of the hand and always in the same direction; thirdly, the strain on the mind from the effort not to disfigure the books by errors or cause loss to their employers when they add, subtract, or do other sums in arithmetic.... In a word, they lack the benefits of moderate exercise, for even if they wanted to take exercise, they have no time for it; they are working for wages and must stick to their writing all day long. Furthermore, incessant driving of the pen over paper causes intense fatigue of the hand and the whole arm because of the continuous and almost tonic strain on the muscles and tendons, which in the course of time results in failure of power in the right hand. (Herington & Morse, 1995)

What might be called contemporary ergonomics began soon after World War II. Kroemer (1988) noted that a group of physical, biological, and psychological professionals from the United Kingdom met in 1950 to address issues associated with the interaction between humans and machines in military systems. This group created the

Donald S. Bloswick and Tim Villnave • Department of Mechanical Engineering, University of Utah, Salt Lake City, Utah, 84112.   **Brad Joseph** • Ford Motor Company, 1500 Century Drive, Dearborn, Michigan, 48210.

Sourcebook of Occupational Rehabilitation, edited by Phyllis M. King. Plenum Press, New York, 1998.

work *ergonomics.* At about the same time, engineering and behavioral professionals in the United States were discussing similar concerns. The study of these issues became known as "human factors" or "human factors engineering." Gradually the distinction between ergonomics and human factors changed from one based on geography to one based on content area. As noted by Budnick (1994), those concentrating on the physical aspects of work and human abilities (work physiology, occupational biomechanics, anthropometry) became known as ergonomists or industrial ergonomists. Behavioral scientists, concerned more with the psychological aspects of the relationship between humans and their environment (sensation/perception, the decision-making process, organizational design), were called human factors professionals or human factors engineers. These are not clear-cut distinctions, however, and there is considerable overlap between the professions.

DEFINITION

Ergonomics is a term derived from the Greek words *ergon,* meaning "work" and *nomos,* meaning "law" (*Webster's New Twentieth Century Dictionary*, 1979). Ergonomics therefore relates to the laws of work. The laws noted here are the natural or physical laws of work as opposed to human-made regulations or rules. Ergonomics is often defined as the study of the natural laws of work, in particular, the relationship between the worker and the work environment. A more contemporary definition might be the one developed and used by the UAW Ford Ergonomics Process:

> Ergonomics means fitting jobs to people. Ergonomics examines the interaction be-
> tween the worker and the work environment. It uses the knowledge from many
> different sciences to help us understand the effects of the job on the worker. (UAW-
> Ford National Joint Committee on Health and Safety, 1988, p. 7)

The Board of Certification in Professional Ergonomics (1996) has defined ergonomics as

> a body of knowledge about human abilities, human limitations, and other human
> characteristics that are relevant to design. Ergonomic design is the application of this
> body of knowledge to the design of tools, machines, systems, tasks, jobs, and environ-
> ments for safe, comfortable, and effective human use.

Reflecting its mission to protect worker safety and health, the Occupational Safety and Health Administration (ErgoWeb, 1995) has defined ergonomics as

> the field of study that seeks to fit the job to the person, rather than the person to the
> job. This is achieved by evaluation and design of workplaces, environments, jobs,
> tasks, equipment, and processes in relationship to human capabilities and interactions
> in the workplace.

Ergonomics is concerned with the problems and processes involved in designing systems for effective human use and in creating environments that are suitable for living and working. It recognizes that work methods, equipment, facilities, and tool design all influence the worker's motivation, fatigue, likelihood of sustaining an occupational injury or illness, and productivity.

General issues that must be considered in the design of the workplace and the fitting of the workplace to the worker include the following:

1. Forces required to perform the task
2. Postures involved in the task
3. Energy required to perform the task
4. Frequency of performance of the task and rest between exertions
5. Environmental conditions

The ergonomist deals with the relationship between the worker and the work environment to optimize the fit between the worker and the job. A poor fit can cause unnecessary stress to the operator and may adversely affect the worker through job-related injuries or illnesses, or it can adversely affect the product through reduced quantity, quality, or efficiency of production. This fit may be pictured as an overlap between the capabilities of the individual and the requirements of the task (shown in Figure 8.1).

When task requirements match the capabilities of the individual, job-related stresses are at a minimum. When task requirements exceed or do not match the capabilities of the individual, job-related stresses increase. This fit can be enhanced by increasing the capabilities of the individual through physical conditioning or training, or by decreasing physical task requirements through task analysis and redesign.

A proper fit between the worker and the workplace can accomplish the following:

1. Reduce occupational injury and illness
2. Reduce workers' compensation, sickness, and accident costs
3. Reduce medical visits
4. Reduce absenteeism
5. Improve productivity
6. Improve quality and reduce scrap material
7. Improve worker comfort on the job

Notice that Items 1 through 6 directly relate to the profitability of the enterprise. Even Item 7 actually relates to profitability because worker comfort will affect Items 1 through 6. It is important to realize that the implementation of ergonomics programs is cost-effective and pays off in the long run.

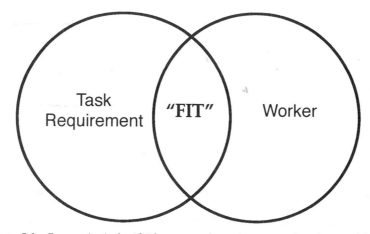

Figure 8-1. Ergonomics is the "fit" between task requirements and worker capabilities.

INDUSTRIAL RISK FACTORS

Based on a sample of 250,000 private industry establishments, the United States Bureau of Labor Statistics found that in 1994, 27.4% (612,828) of nonfatal occupational injuries in private industry that involved days away from work were due to overexertion (National Safety Council, 1996). The Liberty Mutual Insurance Company (Webster & Snook, 1994) found that in 1989, low back pain accounted for 16% of all claims, and 33% of all claims compensation. In 1996, Joe Dear, OSHA administrator, noted that injuries caused by repetitive motion were the nation's fastest growing hazard, costing the nation's businesses about $20 billion each year ("Ergonomics: Reich 'Anxious to Move' on Ergonomics," 1996). The indirect costs of cumulative trauma disorders (CTDs) have been estimated to be five times that amount, or $100 billion per year (OSHA, 1996).

Task Risk Factors

Force

The forces acting on the body result from resistance to body movement. These forces are often generated by gravity (lifting or lowering a load), but they may also result from gravity and friction (pushing or pulling a load), mechanical friction or interference (assembling parts), holding or activating hand tools, or any other activity that involves external forces acting on the body. High force has been associated with risk of injury at the shoulder/neck (Berg, Sanden, Torell, & Jarvholm, 1988), the low back (Herrin, Jariedi, & Anderson, 1986) and the forearm/wrist/hand (Silverstein, Fine, & Armstrong, 1987).

Posture

Posture describes the position of the body. Body posture combines with the forces noted earlier to generate external or resultant moments about the joints. These moments are defined as force multiplied by the distance the force acts from the joint. For example, a ten-pound load generates a higher moment at the shoulder when held out in front of the body than when held at the side, close to the body. The muscles in the body must generate force to create opposing or reactive moments about each joint. This action results in stress on the muscles, tendons, and connective tissue. Awkward postures tend to increase the moments resulting from a given external force and increase the required muscle forces. Awkward postures also reduce the ability of the body to generate muscle force and reactive moments. Hence, awkward postures tend to increase the moment on the body and decrease the body's ability to generate a reactive moment, resulting in biomechanical stress. Awkward posture is associated with an increased risk for injury (Armstrong, Fine, & Silverstein, 1985; Fine, Punnett, & Keyserling, 1987; Punnett, Fine, & Keyserling, 1987).

Specific postures have been associated with injury. (What follows is a list of examples.) At the wrist:

1. Flexion and extension positions were associated with carpal tunnel syndrome (de Krom, Kester, Knipschild, & Spaans, 1990).
2. Ulnar deviation of greater than 20° was associated with increased pain and pathological findings (Hünting, Laübli, & Grandjean, 1981).

At the shoulder:

1. Abduction or flexion of greater than 60° maintained for more than one hour per day was associated with acute shoulder and neck pain (Bjelle, Hagberg, & Michaelsson, 1981).
2. Hand positioning at or above shoulder height was associated with tendinitis and various shoulder pathologies (Herberts, Kadefors, Hogfors, & Sigholm, 1984).

At the cervical spine:

1. A position of 30° of flexion took 300 minutes to produce severe pain symptoms, while a position of 60° of flexion took 120 minutes to produce severe pain symptoms (Chaffin, 1973).
2. Extension with arm elevation was associated with neck/shoulder pain/stiffness, shoulder muscle tenderness, and pain in neck motion (Sakakibara, Miyao, Kondo, & Yamada, 1995).

At the low back:

1. Trunk sagittal angle was associated with occupationally related low back disorder (Marras et al., 1995).

Posture issues can be created by work methods (bending and twisting to pick up a box or bending the wrist to assemble a part) or workplace dimensions (extended reach to obtain a part from a bin at a high location or kneeling in the storage bay of an airplane while handling luggage because of confined space).

Repetition

Repetition is the time quantification of a similar exertion performed during a task. A warehouse worker may lift three boxes per minute from the floor to a countertop; an assembly worker may make 20 units per hour. Repetitive motion has been associated with injury (Armstrong, Foulke, Joseph, & Goldstein, 1982; Hagberg, 1981) and worker discomfort (Ulin, Ways, Armstrong, & Snook, 1990). Generally, the greater the number of repetitions, the greater the degree of risk. However, there is no specific repetition threshold value (cycles/unit of time, movements/unit of time) associated with injury.

Velocity/Acceleration

Angular velocity/angular acceleration is the speed of body part motion and the rate of change of speed of body part motion, respectively. Marras and Schoenmarklin (1991, 1993) found a mean wrist flexion/extension acceleration of 490 deg/s/s in low-risk jobs, while acceleration of 820 deg/s/s in high-risk jobs. Marras and colleagues (1995) associated trunk lateral velocity and trunk-twisting velocity with medium-risk and high-risk, occupationally related low back disorder.

Duration

Duration is the time quantification of exposure to a risk factor. It can be measured as the minutes or hours per day a worker is exposed to a risk. Duration can also be viewed as the years of exposure to a risk factor or a job characterized by a risk factor. In general, the greater the duration of exposure to a risk factor, the greater the degree of risk. Duration limits for biomechanical risk factors have not been established. However, duration has been associated with injury for particular tasks that involve interaction of risk factors, such as video display terminal (VDT) work (Kamwendo, Linton, & Mortiz, 1991), and checkout work done by grocery clerks (Margolis & Krause, 1987; National Institute for Occupational Safety and Health, 1991).

Recovery Time

Recovery time is the time quantification of rest, performance of low-stress activity, or performance of an activity that allows a strained body area to rest. Short work pauses have reduced perceived discomfort (Hagberg & Sundelin, 1986), and rest periods between exertions have reduced performance decrement (Caldwell, 1970). The recovery time needed to reduce the risk of injury increases as the duration of risk factor increases. Specific minimum recovery times for risk factors have not been established.

Environmental Risk Factors

Vibration

Segmental. Vibration applied to the hand can cause a vascular insufficiency of the hands/fingers (Raynaud's phenomenon or vibration white finger). Also, it can interfere with sensory receptor feedback, leading to increased handgrip force to hold the tool. Furthermore, a strong association has been reported between carpal tunnel syndrome and segmental vibration (Silverstein et al., 1987; Wieslander, Norback, Gothe, & Jublin, 1989).

Whole Body. Exposure of the whole body to vibration (usually through the feet/ buttocks while riding in a vehicle) has some support as a risk contributing to injury. Boshuizen, Bongers, and Hulshof (1990) found the prevalence of reported back pain to be approximately 10% higher in tractor drivers than in workers not exposed to vibration; the prevalence of back pain increased with the vibration dose. Dupuis and Zerlett (1987) reported that operators of earth-moving machines with at least ten years exposure to whole-body vibration showed lumbar spine morphological changes earlier and more frequently than did nonexposed people.

Workplace epidemiological studies have shown a relationship between whole body vibration with musculoskeletal and peripheral nervous system disorders (Seidel & Heide, 1986), and low back pain, early degenerative changes to the lumbar spine, and herniated lumbar disc (Hulshof & van Zanten, 1987).

Heat

Heat stress is the total heat load that the body must accommodate. The body is subject to heat produced externally (environment temperature) and generated internally (human metabolism). Excessive heat can cause heatstroke, a condition that can be life threatening or result in irreversible damage. Less serious conditions associated with excessive heat include heat exhaustion, heat cramps, and heat-related disorders (e.g., dehydration, electrolyte imbalance, loss of physical/mental work capacity). The 1985

Statistical Abstracts of the United States (105th ed.) estimated that there were 5 to 10 million workers in industries where heat stress was a potential health hazard (U.S. Department of Commerce, 1985). Heat stress is associated with reduced work time, reduced performance, increased error rates, severe illness, and fatalities (Schneider, Johanning, Bélard, & Engholm, 1995).

Cold

Cold stress is the exposure of the body to cold that lowers the body's deep core temperature. Cold can result in frostbite when an unprotected extremity is exposed to temperatures below freezing (Schneider, Johanning, Bélard, & Engholm, 1995). Cold temperatures can also reduce dexterity and increase generated grip force through tactile desensitization. Cold can indirectly contribute to injury/illness. When gloves are used to protect from low temperatures, a reduction in grip strength occurs. Some authors have suggested that as a result of reduced grip strength the muscle force generated for a given task must increase, increasing the risk for musculoskeletal injury (Hagberg et al., 1995). Gloves may also increase grip strength, decreasing the coefficient of friction between the glove and the tool.

Lighting

With industrialization, the trend in lighting has been to provide higher lighting levels. In certain work settings, such as the office, where problems with glare and eye symptoms have been associated with levels above 1000 lux (Grandjean, 1988), this has proven hazardous. Barreiros and Carnide (1991) found differences in visual functions over the course of a workday among VDT operators and other office workers who worked in badly lit environments. For VDT workers, eye fatigue is sometimes associated with glare and poor office lighting.

Noise

Noise is unwanted sound. In the industrial setting, it may be continuous or intermittent and present in various ways (bang of a rifle, load dropped on the floor, clatter of a pneumatic wrench, whirl of an electric motor). Exposure to noise can lead to temporary and permanent deafness, tinnitus, paracusis, or speech misperception. The louder the noise and the greater its duration, the greater the risk to hearing.

Also, noise well below thresholds that cause hearing loss may interfere with the ability of some people to concentrate. An estimated 8 million civilian workers in the United States are exposed to potentially damaging levels of noise (Davis & Hamernik, 1995). Exposure to aircraft noise was associated with a high-frequency loss prevalence of 41.9% among 112 airport employees (Chen, Chiang, & Chen, 1992).

ERGONOMICS PROGRAMS

OSHA Publication 3123

In 1991, OSHA published OSHA 3123, *Ergonomics Program Management Guidelines for Meatpacking Plants* (Occupational Safety and Health Association, 1991). This document was intended to be OSHA's "first step" in assisting the meatpacking industry in the development of a comprehensive health and safety program with ergonomics as an integral part. Although these guidelines were prepared for meatpacking plants, they also can be used as the foundation for an overall ergonomics program in nearly any facility. These guidelines suggested that ergonomics programs include the following:

1. Worksite analysis
2. Hazard prevention and controls
   Engineering controls
   Work practice controls
   Personal protective equipment
   Administrative controls
3. Medical management
4. Training and education
   General training
   Job-specific training
   Training for supervisors
   Training for managers
   Training for engineers and maintenance personnel

Worksite Analysis

Worksite analysis is concerned with the identification of existing or potential ergonomic hazards. One component of this process involves a review of injury/illness records to locate departments, work areas, or positions where the rate or cost of ergonomic-related disorders are high or are increasing. This review may include an OSHA 200 log and medical, safety, and insurance records. The OSHA incidence rate is presented in terms of ergonomic-related disorders per 200,000 work hours (100 full-time equivalent employees for one year). This can be represented by the following equation:

$$\text{Incidence rate} = \frac{\text{no. of ergonomic-related cases} \times 200{,}000}{\text{no. of hours worked in the department}}$$

The incidence rate should be analyzed to determine the overall ergonomic-related incidence and to see if specific types of ergonomic disorders are concentrated in specific departments or if trends exist.

A second component of this process involves an analysis of the workplace to determine the existence of ergonomic hazards. This includes an analysis of the job, workstation, or process that contributes to the risk of developing an ergonomic-related disorder. This analysis frequently focuses on risk factors for upper extremity cumulative trauma disorders (UECTD) and back disorders.

Hazard Prevention and Control

Once ergonomic hazards have been identified, it is important to implement controls to reduce risks. The preferred method of reducing risks is to implement engineering controls, such as the redesign of workstations, work methods, and tools.

Medical Management

A medical management program for ergonomic-related disorders should include health care providers who understand the prevention, early recognition, evaluation, treatment, and rehabilitation of ergonomic-related disorders. The program also should include periodic workplace walk-throughs, surveys of symptoms in the work population, and monitoring of OSHA forms or other records for trends in ergonomic-related disorders. A health surveillance program should include evaluation and implementation of a conditioning period for new or transferred workers, a periodic health survey of all workers exposed to ergonomic stresses, and a compilation of a list of light duty jobs. Employees should be encouraged to report early symptoms of ergonomic-related disorders. Standard protocols for the evaluation and treatment of ergonomic-related disorders should be developed by health care providers.

Training and Education

It is essential that all employees be informed about ergonomic hazards and abatement methods at a level consistent with their needs and abilities to use the information. Training and education should be provided to employees, supervisors, managers, engineers, maintenance personnel, and health care providers. Employees should receive general training on the types and risk factors for ergonomic disorders and appropriate abatement measures. Supervisors should receive the same training as employees, plus additional training to enable them to recognize and correct hazardous work practices and reinforce employee training. Manager training should provide a basic understanding of the ergonomics of production processes and the overall cost-effectiveness of ergonomic hazard abatement measures. Plant engineers and maintenance personnel should be trained to prevent ergonomic hazards through proper workplace, tool, and process design and abate these hazards when discovered.

The UAW–Ford Ergonomics Process

For the past several years a cooperative agreement between the UAW (United Auto Workers) and Ford Motor Company, with assistance from the University of Michigan Center for Ergonomics, has facilitated the development of what is probably the most comprehensive corporate ergonomics program in the United States. The establishment of plant ergonomics committees has been a part of the UAW–Ford contract since 1987. The stated goal of the program is "to make significant reductions in workplace injuries and illnesses through the application of sound ergonomic principles in the work environment in every manufacturing and assembly facility at Ford Motor Company" (UAW–Ford National Joint Committee on Health and Safety, 1988).

The UAW–Ford Ergonomics Process has three major components: (1) process start-up, (2) job improvement cycle, and (3) long-term development.

Process Start-Up

The initiation of the ergonomics process involves the following:

1. Securing leadership commitment
2. Selection of members of the plant local ergonomics committee (L.E.C.)

3. Training of the L.E.C.
4. Development of a plant mission statement
5. Development of the teamwork process

The L.E.C. consists of management and employee representatives. Ex officio Chairpersons are the plant manager and employer (union) leader. The exact composition of the L.E.C. is not specified. L.E.C.s that have been found to be effective generally include management representatives from manufacturing engineering, medical, manufacturing supervisors, and plant safety. Employee representatives (equal in number to management) are drawn from skilled trades and production employees. Two functioning chairpersons are selected, one each from management and engineering representatives.

Job Improvement Cycle

The Job Improvement Cycle includes (a) identification of priority jobs, (b) evaluation of job stresses, (c) development of solutions, (d) implementation of solutions, (e) project documentation, and (f) project follow-up
(This is a closed loop process as shown in Figure 8-2.)

Identification of Priority Jobs. Priority job identification is based on a determination of the types and frequencies of ergonomic-related disorders in the plant. This determination can be accomplished using existing injury and illness records, such as the OSHA 200 log; through surveys of workers; or through job analyses. Consideration may also be given to the cost or complexity of a solution, the seriousness of the injuries, and the number of people who will benefit.

Evaluation of Job Stresses. This evaluation can be based on the judgment of the L.E.C., information from the operator, or ergonomic analytical tools, such as the Revised NIOSH Work Lifting Equation, compressive force calculations, or various ergonomic checklists.

Development of Solutions. Solutions may be accomplished by brainstorming within the L.E.C., soliciting ideas from supervisors and operators, working with vendors, seeking assistance from Ford corporate staff or other personnel outside the L.E.C., and consulting with experts outside the corporation.

Implementation of Solutions. Implementing solutions requires the organization of resources to effect the appropriate changes. This process may involve the development of proposals for funding; working with vendors, engineers, technicians, and skilled tradespeople to fabricate tools, equipment, and processes; training operators and super-

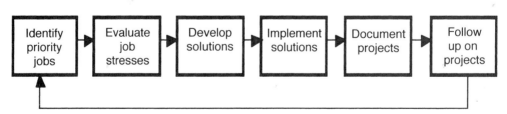

Figure 8-2. The Job Improvement Cycle of the UAW–Ford Ergonomics Process.

visors on how to use new methods and equipment; and monitoring the progress of the project.

Project Documentation. Documentation involves tracking ongoing projects to insure systematic completion and verifying the problem, solution, and cost savings for each completed project. The documentation of completed projects is essential to serve as the basis for continued ergonomic program development and as a resource base for personnel who identify new ergonomic-related problems.

Project Follow-up. Follow-up is necessary to determine the long-term effects of the ergonomics effort. Follow-up information should also be recorded in the project documentation noted previously.

Long-Term Development

Long-term development includes (a) specialized training for members of the L.E.C. and other personnel, such as engineers and medical staff; (b) communication of the importance of ergonomics to all plant personnel; and (c) continued review and improvement.

The results of the UAW–Ford Ergonomics Process appear to be positive. In one Ford plant the implementation of an ergonomics program is given much of the credit for a drop in lost workdays from 3,134 in 1990 to 1,355 in 1991 (Brandon, 1992).

Results of Ergonomics Programs

In one auto parts manufacturing plant, the implementation of ergonomics controls, such as load reduction and the installation of material lift assist devices, is credited with much of the 67% decline in the injury rate in a one-year period (Bureau of National Affairs, 1988a). Two Goodyear facilities reported nearly an 80% decrease in time lost to injuries during the two years after implementation of an overall ergonomics program (Geras, Pepper, & Rodgers, 1989). Beech Aircraft estimates a cost savings of approximately $200,000 per year from a reduction in UECTDs as a result of an early intervention/medical surveillance program ("Early Intervention Reduces Injuries," 1992).

In 1990, Siemens found that 43 of the 100 employees at its home office in Auburn Hills, Michigan, were complaining of pain in shoulders, backs, elbows, and fingers. Approximately $3,600 was invested in back cushions, lumbar supports, keyboard/mouse wrist rests, and document holders. The employees were trained in stretching and encouraged to take frequent short breaks. After the implementation of the program, Siemens has not had a CTD-related complaint in two years ("'Communication' drives process," 1997).

In the early 1990s, Silicon Graphics attributed 70% of its medical costs to upper limb disorders. A training program was initiated in 1992, and a self-directed ergonomics resource center was established. Silicon Graphics hired an ergonomics consultant in 1995. That same year, the company realized a 41% drop in reportable upper limb disorders, followed by a further 50% drop in reportable CTD cases in 1996 ("Silicon Graphics Melds," 1997).

In its helicopter assembly plant, Sikorsky noted a 75% drop in lost workday incident and severity rates, and a 25% drop in OSHA recordable incidents after the implementation of ergonomics training, work teams, and engineering controls (Thaler, 1996). In one AT&T facility, an investment of $373,000 in equipment, equipment modification, and ergonomic chairs resulted in an 80% decrease in its $400,000 workers' compensation costs ("AT&T Uses Cost-Conscious Program," 1995). In John Deere's Dubuque Works, a comprehensive ergonomics program reduced repetitive motion injuries by 60% and nearly eliminated back injuries (Jegerlehner, 1995). In Hawaii, Pepsico was cited by Hawaii OSHA for not providing a safe workplace for delivery drivers. An ergonomics program, which included training, exercise, task and equipment analysis/redesign, and the hiring of a consultant reduced back injury reports from 15 cases in 1991 to 4 in 1992 (Fehrenbacher & Wick, 1995).

Newport News Shipbuilding's welding department, with a total employment of about 1,800 workers, was averaging between two and four wrist injuries per month. After an in-depth training program covering tool selection, work methods, and scaffold placement, they experienced only six wrist injuries in over one year. A lifting training program in the maintenance department reduced the frequency of back injuries from one per month to zero. In 1996, they reported a total reduction in the ergonomic case rate of 30% and the lost time ergonomic case rate of 55%. The company saved $1.4 million in workers' compensation costs ("Training a 'limbsaver'," 1997).

Ergonomics programs are also frequently associated with productivity increases. A back program and ergonomic job analysis program at Fleming Companies Incorporated resulted in a 50% drop in back injury incidents, a decrease in workers' compensation costs, and an increase in productivity (Bureau of National Affairs, 1988b). An ergonomics intervention effort at Ethicon, a Johnson & Johnson company, had inconclusive results from an ergonomic standpoint but increased productivity by over 10% (Longmate & Hayes, 1990). In another Johnson & Johnson facility, ergonomic task and equipment changes reduced the physical stress in many jobs so that they could be done by a larger percentage of the workforce. This also increased productivity (Longmate, 1995).

At Red Wing Shoes, the implementation of an ergonomics program, which included training, conditioning, stretching, adjustable chairs, equipment modification, and the hiring of an ergonomist, reduced workers' compensation costs from $4.4 million in 1990 to about $1.3 million in 1995. It also reduced manufacturing time ("Red Wing Shoes'," 1995). At General Seating, ergonomics training, job rotation, and task and workstation redesign reduced lost workdays by 70% and increased productivity ("Problem-Solving by Committee," 1995).

It should be noted that in many cases there is also an increase in ergonomic-related cases reported on the OSHA 200 log during the first year or so after the implementation of a comprehensive ergonomics program. One manufacturing plant of approximately 1,100 employees, 700 of whom were involved in direct labor, had 10 UECTD cases costing approximately $100,000 in 1990. After the implementation of an ergonomics program and an aggressive medical management program, the cost of these injuries dropped to approximately $40,000 in 1991, but the *number* of cases increases to 45. This trend continued in 1992 (Bloswick, 1992). In another facility of approximately 4,500 workers, the implementation of an overall ergonomics program was a primary factor in the reduction of lost workdays associated with UECTDs. Lost workdays went from 613 in 1990 to 149 in 1991, with approximately 20 occurring during the first half of 1992. The actual *incidence* of ergonomic disorders remained relatively constant (Bloswick, 1992). This is not a sign of an ineffective program, rather, it is a sign of an environment within which workers are encouraged to report minor disorders early, when the disorders can be corrected with minor worksite modifications, before they become serious enough to require expensive medical intervention.

ERGONOMIC STANDARDS AND CERTIFICATION

Ergonomic Standards and Guidelines

The Occupational Safety and Health Act (OSHA)

At present OSHA does not have an ergonomics standard in place. In order to include the consideration of ergonomic hazards in normal workplace inspections, OSHA has turned to the provisions of Section 5(a) of the OSHA Act—the "general duty clause" (Ninety-First Congress, 1970)—which states the following:

1. [Each employer] shall furnish to each of his employees employment and a place of employment which are free from recognized hazards that are causing or are likely to cause death or serious physical harm to his employees.
2. [Each employer] shall comply with occupational safety and health standards promulgated under this Act (p. 4).

If an ergonomic hazard (or other hazard) exists, OSHA inspectors may issue a citation under Section 5(a) when the following criteria are met:

1. There is not an applicable OSHA standard.
2. The employer failed to keep the workplace free of a hazard to which employees were exposed.
3. The hazard is (or should have been) recognized by the employer.
4. The hazard is causing or was likely to cause death or other serious physical harm.
5. There is a feasible and useful method to correct the hazard.

The absence of specific ergonomic standards requires interpretation when using the general duty clause. For example: Would the hazard cause *serious* physical harm? Is the hazard recognized? Do *feasible* abatement methods exist? For purposes of citations, *serious physical harm* is defined as an impairment that makes part of the body functionally useless or substantially reduces the body's efficiency on or off the job. Such impairment may be permanent or temporary, chronic or acute.

In 1995, OSHA published the *Draft Proposed Ergonomics Protection Standard* (ErgoWeb, 1995) but never adopted it as official policy. There was substantial opposition to the proposed standard. Several private companies and trade groups joined together with the Republican Congressional leadership to end development of the standard, using funding riders that prevented OSHA from working on, proposing, or promulgating an ergonomics standard. In 1998, ergonomics is listed as a priority for OSHA.

American National Standards Institute (ANSI)

ANSI is a private, nonprofit organization founded in 1918. It is composed of 1,400 members, including the National Fire Protection Association, the American Society for Testing and Materials, professional groups, and private companies. ANSI itself does not write standards. The organization participates in standard development by assembling qualified groups and facilitating a consensus opinion to produce a voluntary American National Standard (American National Standards Institute, 1996). ANSI also assumes a clearinghouse role for standard development by sanctioning standards already written by organization members. By 1996, 11,500 American National Standards had been developed/sanctioned.

There are three ANSI ergonomic-related standards:

ANSI B-11: Ergonomic Guidelines for the Design, Installation, and Use of Machine Tools (American National Standards Institute, 1993)
ANSI/HFS 100-1988: American National Standard for Human Factors Engineering of Visual Display Terminals Workstations (Human Factors Society, 1988)
ANSI Z-365: Control of Work-Related Cumulative Trauma Disorders—Draft (American National Standards Institute, 1998)

International Organization for Standards (ISO)

The ISO, established in 1947, is a nongovernmental, worldwide federation of national standards bodies from over 100 countries. ANSI is the representative from the United States. The organization strives to promote standardization in the world to facilitate the international exchange of goods and services and a freer interaction within the intellectual, scientific, technologic, and economic communities (International Organization for Standardization, 1996).

Standards are written by technical committees, subcommittees and working groups composed of qualified representatives from industry, professional groups, and governmental agencies. Standards are written for many fields, except electrical and electronic engineering (these areas are managed by the International Electrotechnical Commission). The standards are developed through consensus (all interests are taken into account), intended to be applicable industry-wide, and are voluntarily enforced. ISO has developed 28 ergonomic standards and has 69 in preparation (Dul, de Vlaming, & Munnik, 1996).

Ergonomics Certification

Board of Certification in Professional Ergonomics (BCPE)

The Board of Certification in Professional Ergonomics (BCPE) was established in 1990 as a nonprofit corporation (Board of Certification in Professional Ergonomics, 1996). It provides procedures for examining and certifying qualified practitioners of ergonomics. A qualified applicant may be certified as either a Certified Professional Ergonomist (CPE) or a Certified Human Factors Professional (CHFP). The BCPE certifies *practitioners* of ergonomics, defined as individuals who have the following qualifications:

1. Superior knowledge of available ergonomics information
2. Command of the methodologies used by ergonomists and the ability to apply that knowledge to the design of a product, system, job, or environment
3. The ability to apply this knowledge to the analysis, design, testing, and evaluation of products, systems, and environments

To be certified, applicants must meet all of the following requirements:

1. Master's degree or equivalent in one of the correlative fields of ergonomics, such as biomechanics, human factors, ergonomics, industrial engineering, industrial hygiene, kinesiology, psychology, or systems engineering
2. Four years of demonstrable experience in ergonomics practice

3. Evidence of experience in applying ergonomics to "design" (submission of a work product to the BCPE)
4. A passing score on the BCPE examination

The BCPE is also investigating the creation of a new level of ergonomics certification, Certified Ergonomics Technologist (CET), that will encourage certification for health care providers ("Ergonomics Certification," 1996). This CET certificate will have requirements in the same areas as the CPE but with less depth of knowledge and experience requirement.

For more information contact:

Board of Certification in Professional Ergonomics
P.O. Box 2811
Bellingham, WA 98227-2811
USA
Phone: (360) 671-7601
Fax: (360) 671-7681
E-Mail: BCPEHQ@aol.com
Internet: http://tucker.mech.utah.edu/Pub/BCPE/home./html

Oxford Research Institute (ORI)

The Oxford Research Institute (ORI) has established a process for certification in industrial ergonomics or human factors engineering that uses a controlled peer review process formally instituted in 1993. A qualified applicant may be certified as a Certified Industrial Ergonomist (CIE) or a Certified Human Factors Engineering Professional (CHFEP). Specialty certification may be requested in a number of different areas.

To be certified, applicants must provide evidence of the following:

1. Resume that details B.S. plus six years, M.A. plus five years, or Ph.D. plus four years of experience in a related field of employment
2. Specialized training or formal education in fields related to ergonomics or human factors engineering
3. Duplicate copies of two or three work samples, such as books, articles, technical reports, inventions, patents, awards, honors, demonstrations, videotapes, or other media, showing the applicant to be the principle author
4. Two letters of recommendation from sponsors who are familiar with the applicant's work in the specialty field
5. A passing score on the certification examination not presently a requirement, but may be implemented (As of February 1998 and "for the next several months" this requirement will be waived for applicants who are "practicing ergonomists.")

For more information contact:

Oxford Research Institute
10153 Vantage Point Court
New Market, MD 21774
USA
Phone: (301) 865-4506

Roy Matheson and Associates (RMA)

Roy Matheson and Associates (RMA) provides certification as a Certified Ergonomic Evaluator Specialist (CEES). Applicants must be certified in a related safety, health, or engineering field and complete two 15–20 page papers on worksite evaluations. One evaluation must deal with a situation involving the risk of back injury; the other, where there is a risk of an upper extremity cumulative trauma disorder (UECTD). Applicants must also submit recommendations from three people who have received ergonomic evaluations from the applicant and proof of 25 workstation assessments.

For more information contact:

Roy Matheson and Associates
P.O. Box 492
Keene, NH 03431
USA
Phone: (800) 443-7690
Fax: (603) 358-0116
E-mail: info@roymatheson.com
Internet: http://www.roymatheson.com

Board of Certified Safety Professionals (BCSP)

The Board of Certified Safety Professionals (BCSP) was organized in 1969 as a peer certification board to certify practitioners in the safety profession. A qualified applicant may be certified as a Certified Safety Professional (CSP). Beginning in the latter half of 1997, individuals who hold the CSP designation may, by examination, seek specialty designation in ergonomics.

For more information contact:

Board of Certified Safety Professionals
208 Burwash Avenue
Savoy, IL 61874
USA
Phone: (217) 359-9263
Fax: (217) 359-0055
E-mail: bcsp@bscp.com
Internet: http://www.bcsp.com

Professional Organization in Ergonomics

Several international organizations exist which public journals, arrange conferences, and facilitate professional development.

For more information, contact

The Human Factors and Ergonomics Society (HFES)
P. O. Box 1369
Santa Monica, CA 90406-1369
USA
Phone: (310) 394-1811

Fax: (310) 394-2410
E-mail: 70732-2420@compuserve.com
Internet: http://www.hfes.org

The International Ergonomics Association (IEA)
Secretary General
Prof. ir. Pieter Rookmaaker
Netherlands Railways
SE ARBO/Ergonomics
P.O. Box 2286
3500 GG Utrecht
The Netherlands
Phone: (area/country codes) +31-30-354455
Fax: +31-30-2399456
E-mail: seaergo@knoware.nl
Internet: http://www.louisville.edu/speed/ergonomics

The Ergonomics Society
Devonshire House
Devonshire Square
Loughborough LE11 3DW
United Kingdom
Phone: (area/country codes) +44 1509 234904
Fax: +44 1509 234904
E-mail: ergosoc@ergonomics.org.uk
Internet: http://www.ergonomics.org.uk/

In addition to the above organizations, several professional societies have established technical interest groups related to ergonomics and include ergonomic issues at their regional and national conferences. Probably the largest of these are the Institute of Industrial Engineers (IIE), American Industrial Hygiene Association (AIHA), and American Society of Safety Engineers (ASSE). (Information on periodicals relating to ergonomics is listed in the appendix.)

APPENDIX

Ergonomics Related Journals

Applied Ergonomics
Elsevier Science
660 White Plains Road
Tarrytown, NY 10591-5153
Phone: (914) 524-9200
Fax: (914) 333-2444
$120.00 (personal)

Ergonomics
Taylor & Francis
1900 Frost Road
Suite 101
Bristol, PA 19007
Phone: (215) 785-5800
Fax: (215) 785-5515
$297.00

Ergonomics in Design
Human Factors and Ergonomics Society
P.O. Box 1369
Santa Monica, CA 90406-1369
Phone: (310) 394-1811
$33.00

Human Factors
Humans Factors and Ergonomics Society
1124 Montana Avenue
Suite B
Santa Monica, CA 90403
Phone: (310) 394-1811
$135.00

International Journal of Human Factors in Manufacturing
John Wiley & Sons
605 Third Avenue
New York, NY 10158-0012
Phone: (212) 850-6645
Fax: (212) 850-6021
E-mail: subinfo@jwiley.com
$98.00

International Journal of Industrial Ergonomics
Elsevier Science
P.O. Box 211
1000 AE Amsterdam
The Netherlands
Phone: (0-20-485) 36 42
Fax: (0-20-485) 35 98
E-mail: Fulfilment-F@Elsevier.NL
NY Office Phone: (212) 633-3750
$170.00

Journal of Occupational Safety and Ergonomics
Ablex Publishing
355 Chestnut
Norwood, NJ 07648
Phone: (201) 767-8450
Fax: (201) 767-6717
$50.00 (personal)

Occupational Ergonomics
Chapman & Hall
115 5th Avenue
New York, NY 10003
Phone: (212) 780-6233
Fax: (212) 260-1363

E-mail: fogarty@chaphall.com
$70.00 (personal)

Work
Elsevier Science Ireland
Customer Relations Manager
Bay 15K
Shannon Industrial Estate
Shannon, County Clare, Ireland
Phone: (+353-61) 471944
Fax: (+353-61) 472144
E-mail: Eirmailjournal@elsevier.ie
$137.60

Trade Publications

Material Handling Engineering
Penton Publishing
1100 Superior Avenue
Cleveland, OH 44144-2543
Phone: (216) 696-7000

Occupational Hazards
Penton Publishing
1100 Superior Avenue
Cleveland, OH 44144-2543
Phone: (216) 696-7000

Occupational Health & Safety
Stevens Publishing
222 Rosewood Drive
Danvers, MA 01923
Phone: (508) 750-8500

Professional Safety
ASSE
1800 E. Oakton Street
DesPlaines, IL 60018-2187
Phone: (847) 699-2929

Safety & Health
National Safety Council
1121 Spring Lake Drive
Itasca, IL 60143-3201
(630) 285-1121

Workplace Ergonomics
Medical Publications
Stevens Publishing
3630 I-35
Waco, TX 76706
(815) 734-1159

REFERENCES

American National Standards Institute. (1993). *Ergonomic guidelines for the design, installation, and use of machine tools* (ANSI B11 TR 1-1993). New York, NY: Author.

American National Standards Institute. (1995, April 17). *Control of work-related cumulative trauma disorders: Part 1. Upper extremities* (ANSI Z-365, 3rd working draft). New York, NY: Author.

American National Standards Institute. (1996). *ANSI online: American National Standards Institute home world wide web page* [On-line]. Available: http://www.ansi.org

Armstrong, T. J., Foulke, J., Joseph, B., & Goldstein, S. (1982). Investigation of cumulative trauma disorders in a poultry processing plant. *American Industrial Hygiene Association Journal, 43*, 103–116.

Armstrong, T. J., Fine, L. J., & Silverstein, B. A. (1985). *Occupational risk factors of cumulative trauma disorders of the hand and wrist: A final report* (Contract No. 200-82-2507). Cincinnati, OH: National Institute for Occupational Safety and Health.

AT&T uses cost-conscious program to fight CTDs. (1995). In M. Gauf, *Ergonomics that work: Case studies of companies cutting costs through ergonomics* (pp. 53–62). Haverford, PA: CTD News.

Barreiros, L., & Carnide, F. (1991). Luminous environmental influence on visual fatigue in VDT operators: Designing for everyone. In Y. Queinnec & F. Daniellou (Eds.), *Proceedings of the Eleventh Congress of the International Ergonomics Association* (pp. 719–721). London: Taylor & Francis.

Berg, M., Sanden, A., Torell, G., & Jarvholm, B. (1988). Persistence of musculoskeletal symptoms: A longitudinal study. *Ergonomics, 31*(9), 1281–1285.

Bjelle, A., Hagberg, M., & Michaelsson, G. (1981). Occupational and individual factors in acute shoulder-neck disorders among industrial workers. *British Journal of Industrial Medicine, 38*, 356–363.

Bloswick, D. S. (1992). *Technical reports file*. Salt Lake City, UT: University of Utah, Department of Mechanical Engineering.

Board of Certification in Professional Ergonomics. (1996). *Board of Certification in Professional Ergonomics home world wide web page* [On-line]. Available: http://bcpe.org.html.

Boshuizen, H. C., Bongers, P. M., & Hulshof, C. T. J. (1990). Self-reported back pain in tractor drivers exposed to whole-body vibration. *International Archives of Occupational and Environmental Health, 62*, 109–115.

Brandon, K. (1992, June). Ergonomics at UAW-Ford. *Occupational Health and Safety, 61*(6), 44–54.

Budnick, P. M. (1994). Ergonomics. In G. L. Key (Ed.), *Industrial therapy* (pp. 75–84). St. Louis, MO: Mosby.

Bureau of National Affairs. (1988a). Costs, rewards of redesign. In *Back injuries: Costs, causes, cases and prevention—A BNA special report* (pp. 49–50). Washington, DC: Author.

Bureau of National Affairs. (1988b). Warehousing and distribution: Fleming Cos. Inc. In *Back injuries: Costs, causes, cases and prevention—A BNA Special Report* (pp. 80–82). Washington, DC: Author.

Caldwell, L. S. (1970). Decrement and recovery with repetitive maximal muscular exertions. *Human Factors, 12*, 547–552.

Chaffin, D. B. (1973). Localized muscle fatigue: Definition and measurement. *Journal of Occupational Medicine, 15*, 346–354.

Chen, T., Chiang, H., & Chen, S. (1992). Effects of aircraft noise on hearing and auditory pathway function of airport employees. *Journal of Occupational Medicine, 34*(6), 613–619.

Christensen, J. M. (1987). The human factors profession. In G. Salvendy (Ed.), *Handbook of human factors* (pp. 4–16). New York: John Wiley.

"Communication" drives process at Siemens. (1997, January). *CTD News, 6*(1), 5–6.

Davis, R. I., & Hamernik, R. P. (1995). Noise and hearing impairment. In B. S. Levy & D. H. Wegman (Eds.), *Occupational health: Recognizing and preventing work-related disease* (pp. 321–336). Boston: Little, Brown.

de Krom, M. C. T. F. M., Kester, A. D. M., Knipschild, P. G., & Spaans, F. (1990). Risk factors for carpal tunnel syndrome. *American Journal of Epidemiology, 132*(6), 1102–1110.

Dul, J., de Vlaming, P. M., & Munnik, M. J. (1996, March). A review of ISO and CEN standards on ergonomics. *International Journal of Industrial Ergonomics, 17*(3), 291–297.

Dupuis, H., & Zerlett, G. (1987). Whole-body vibration and disorders of the spine. *International Archives of Occupational and Environmental Health, 59*, 323–336.

Early intervention reduces injuries at Beech aircraft, company hygienist says. (1992, June 10). *Occupational Safety and Health Reporter, 22*(2), 61–62.

Ergonomics certification program now under development will enhance professional status of providers in practicing prevention. (1996, December). *Work Injury Management, 5*(10), 3–4.

Ergonomics: Reich "anxious to move" on ergonomics, cost of illnesses demands action, Dear says. (1996, October 30). *Occupational Safety and Health Reporter, 26*(22), 668.

ErgoWeb (1995). *OSHA draft ergonomic protection standard: Summary of key provisions* [On-line]. Available: http://www.ergoweb.com:80/Pub/Info/Train/MODI/mod1def.html.

Fehrenbacher, D., & Wick, J. L. (1995). A successful back injury reduction program. In A. C. Bittner & P. C. Champney (Eds.), *Advances in industrial ergonomics and safety VII* (pp. 347–350). Bristol, PA: Taylor & Francis.

Fine, L. J., Punnett, L., & Keyserling, W. M. (1987). An epidemiological study of postural risk factors for shoulder disorders in industry. In P. Buckle (Ed.), *Musculoskeletal disorders at work* (pp. 108–109). Bristol, PA: Taylor & Francis.

Geras, D. T., Pepper, C. D., & Rodgers, S. H. (1989). An integrated ergonomics program at the Goodyear Tire and Rubber Company. In A. Mital (Ed.), *Advances in industrial ergonomics and safety I* (pp. 21–28). Bristol, PA: Taylor & Francis.

Grandjean, E. (1988). *Fitting the task to the man*. Bristol, PA: Taylor & Francis.

Hagberg, M. (1981). Electromyographic signs of shoulder muscular fatigue in two elevated arm positions. *American Journal of Physical Medicine, 60*(3), 111–121.

Hagberg, M., Silverstein, B., Wells, R., Smith, M. J., Hendrick, H. W., Carayon, P., & Perusse, M. (1995). Identification, measurement, and evaluation of risk. In I. Kuorinka & L. Forcier (Eds.), *Work-related musculoskeletal disorders: A reference book for prevention* (pp. 139–212). Bristol, PA: Taylor & Francis.

Hagberg, M., & Sundelin, G. (1986). Discomfort and load on the upper trapezius muscle when operating a word processor. *Ergonomics, 29,* 1637–1645.

Herberts, P., Kadefors, R., Hogfors, C., & Sigholm, G. (1984). Shoulder pain and heavy manual labor. *Clinical Orthopaedics and Related Research, 191,* 166–178.

Herington, T. N., & Morse, L. H. (1995). Cumulative trauma/repetitive motion injuries. In T. N. Herington & L. H. Morse (Eds.), *Occupational injuries: Evaluation, management, and prevention* (pp. 333–345). St. Louis, MO: Mosby

Herrin, G. D., Jariedi, M., & Anderson, C. K. (1986). Prediction of overexertion injuries using biomechanical and psychophysical models. *American Industrial Hygiene Association Journal, 47,* 322–330.

Hulshof, C., & van Zanten, B. V. (1987). Whole-body vibration and low back pain. *International Archives of Occupational and Environmental Health, 59,* 205–220.

Human Factors Society. (1988). *American national standard for human factors engineering of visual display terminal workstations* (ANSI/HFS Standard No. 100-1988). Santa Monica, CA: Author.

Hünting, W., Laübli, T., & Grandjean, E. (1981). Postural and visual loads at VDT workplace: 1. Constrained postures. *Ergonomics, 24*(12), 917–931.

International Organization for Standardization. (1996). *International organization for standardization home world wide web page: Introduction to ISO* [On-line]. Available: http://www.iso.ch/.

Jegerlehner, J. L. (1995). Workers' participation helps reduce cumulative trauma disorder injuries. In A. C. Bittner & P. C. Champney (Eds.), *Advances in industrial ergonomics and safety VII* (pp. 339–342). Bristol, PA: Taylor & Francis.

Kamwendo, K., Linton, S. J., & Mortiz, U. (1991). Neck and shoulder disorders in medical secretaries. *Scandinavian Journal of Rehabilitative Medicine, 23,* 127–133.

Kroemer, K. H. E. (1988). Ergonomics. In B. Plog (Ed.), *Fundamentals of industrial hygiene*, (pp. 283–334). Chicago, IL: National Safety Council.

Longmate, A. R. (1995). Ergonomic control measures in the health care industry. In A. Bhattacharya & J. D. McGlothlin (Eds.), *Occupational ergonomics: Theory and applications* (pp. 519–535). Bristol, PA: Taylor & Francis.

Longmate, A. R., & Hayes, T. J. (1990). Making a difference at Johnson & Johnson: Some ergonomic intervention case studies. *Industrial Management, 32*(2), 27–30.

Margolis, W., & Krause, J. F. (1987). The prevalence of carpal tunnel syndrome symptoms in female supermarket checkers. *Journal of Occupational Medicine, 29*(12), 953–956.

Marras, W. S., Lavender, S. A., Leurgans, S. E., Fathallah, F. A., Ferguson, S. A., Allread, W. G., & Rajulu, S. L. (1995). Biomechanical risk factors for occupationally related low back disorders. *Ergonomics, 38*(2), 377–410.

Marras, W. S., & Shoenmarklin, R. W. (1991). Quantification of wrist motion in highly repetitive, hand-intensive jobs, *National Institute for Occupational Safety and Health final report*. Cincinnati, OH: National Institute of Occupational Safety and Health.

Marras, W. S., & Schoenmarklin, R. W. (1993). Wrist motion in industry. *Ergonomics, 36,* 341–351.

National Institute for Occupational Safety and Health. (1991). *Shoprite supermarkets, New Jersey-New York* (HETA 88-344-2092). Washington, DC: U.S. Government Printing Office.

National Safety Council. (1996). *Accident facts*. New York: Author.

Ninety-First Congress, S. 2193. (1970, December 29). *Occupational Safety and Health Act of 1970* (Public Law 91-596). Washington, DC: U.S. Government Printing Office.

Occupational Safety and Health Administration (OSHA). (1991). *Ergonomics program management guidelines for meatpacking plants* (OSHA Publication No. 3123). Washington, DC: Author.

Occupational Safety and Health Administration (OSHA). (1996, December 10). *What are RSIs? Preventing repetitive stress injuries.* Washington, DC: U.S. Department of Labor.

Oxford Research Institute. (1996, October 28). *Oxford Report, 11*(3), 1–2.

Problem-solving by committee at General Seating. (1995). In M. Gauf, *Ergonomics that work: Case studies of companies cutting costs through ergonomics* (pp. 63–68). Haverford, PA: CTD News.

Punnett, L., Fine, L. J., & Keyserling, W. M. (1987). An epidemiological study of postural risk factors for back disorders in industry. In P. Buckle (Ed.), *Musculoskeletal disorders at work* (p. 74). Bristol, PA: Taylor & Francis.

Red Wing Shoes' early warning system. (1995). In M. Gauf, *Ergonomics that work: Case studies of companies cutting costs through ergonomics* (pp. 79–83). Haverford, PA: CTD News.

Sakakibara, H., Miyao, M., Kondo, T., & Yamada, S. (1995). Overhead work and shoulder-neck pain in orchard farmers harvesting pears and apples. *Ergonomics, 38*(4), 343–358.

Schneider, S., Johanning, E., Bélard, J.-L., & Engholm, G. (1995). *Occupational Medicine: State of the Art Reviews, 10*(2), 363–383.

Seidel, H., & Heide, R. (1986). Long-term effects of whole-body vibration: A critical survey of the literature. *International Archives of Occupational and Environmental Health, 58*, 1–26.

Silicon Graphics melds high- and low-tech. (1997, January). *CTD News, 6*(1), 7–8.

Silverstein, B. A., Fine, L. J., & Armstrong, T. J. (1987). Occupational factors and the carpal tunnel syndrome. *American Journal of Industrial Medicine, 11*, 343–358.

Thaler, J. (1996, March/April). The Sikorsky success story. *Workplace Ergonomics, 2*(2), 22–25.

Training a "limbsaver" at Newport news. (1997, January). *CTD News, 6*(1), 9–10.

UAW-Ford National Joint Committee on Health and Safety. (1988). *Fitting jobs to people: The UAW-Ford ergonomics process implementation guide.* Ann Arbor: University of Michigan.

Ulin, S. S., Ways, C. M., Armstrong, T. J., & Snook, S. H. (1990). Perceived exertion and discomfort versus work height with a pistol-shaped screw driver. *American Industrial Hygiene Association Journal, 51*(11), 588–594.

U.S. Department of Commerce, Bureau of the Census. (1985). *Statistical abstracts of the U.S.* (105th ed.). Washington, DC: National U.S. Government Printing Office.

Webster, E. D., & Snook, S. H. (1994). The cost of 1989 workers' compensation low back pain claims. *Spine, 19*(10), 1111–1116.

Webster's New Twentieth Century Dictionary (2nd ed.). (1979). San Francisco, CA: William Collins.

Wieslander, G., Norback, D., Gothe, C. J., & Jublin, L. (1989). Carpal tunnel syndrome (CTS) and exposure to vibration, repetitive wrist movements, and heavy manual work: A case-referent study. *British Journal of Industrial Medicine, 46*, 43–47.

9

Preemployment and Preplacement Testing

Lisa L. Perry

Preemployment and preplacement testing is used by employers to determine an individual's suitability for a specific job. This practice has become widespread in the last decade. Preemployment testing was first used in civil sector hiring (in police and fire departments), where adequate strength and agility were considered critical to ensure public safety. Preemployment and preplacement testing has recently gained popularity as an injury prevention strategy, and as a tool to help employers make nondiscriminatory hiring decisions.

Occupational and physical therapists utilize their expertise in work injury management, functional capacity testing, and ergonomics to offer preemployment and preplacement testing as a component of occupational rehabilitation and prevention services. To meet the growing demand of the industry, equipment and evaluation manufacturers have developed a wide variety of products. The result is a confusing blend of available testing methodologies of questionable validity for hiring purposes.

Legal issues need to be considered in the hiring process as well. It is critical to evaluate the facts about preemployment and preplacement testing and challenge unsupported assumptions in the process. This chapter will review what is known about testing so that we can build a test model that makes sense and can be upheld in the justice system. It will focus on strength testing because this is the most common application in occupational rehabilitation and prevention programs. Specifically, the following four key issues will be explored:

- The distinction between preemployment and preplacement testing
- The current uses for preemployment tests and the efficacy of these uses

Lisa L. Perry • Anthem Blue Cross and Blue Shield, 8845 Governor's Hill Drive, Suite 150, Cincinnati, Ohio 45242.

Sourcebook of Occupational Rehabilitation, edited by Phyllis M. King. Plenum Press, New York, 1998.

- The available testing methods and the validity and reliability of these methodologies for preemployment purposes
- The legal issues that must be considered when providing tests for the hiring selection process

PREEMPLOYMENT AND PREPLACEMENT TESTING

The terms *preemployment testing* and *preplacement testing* are frequently used interchangeably in the literature and in practice. However, there is a distinction between them that can be made to help lessen the confusion over terminology. This distinction is based on where in the hiring process the tests are performed

Preemployment testing most commonly refers to tests done prior to making a hiring decision. These tests frequently contain measures of strength, endurance, and possibly aptitude in a particular work task. The results of these tests are then used to determine if an individual should be hired.

Preplacement tests are similar in structure to preemployment tests but are commonly used after a conditional offer of employment has been made. In this situation, the test results are used to ensure that an appropriate match has been made between the worker and the job, most frequently from the perspective of physical ability.

The decision as to whether a test should be done before or after a job offer has been made is based primarily on the legal ramifications of each scenario. (These issues will be discussed in more detail in the legal section in this chapter.) Because the basic structure of these tests is similar, the term preemployment test will be used to refer to both preemployment and preplacement tests throughout the remainder of the chapter.

TESTING ASSUMPTIONS

Employers typically use strength testing in the hiring selection process for several reasons. Most notably, testing is performed to (a) reduce injuries in the workplace, (b) ensure public safety, and (c) objectively evaluate job functions.

This section describes the three common uses for preemployment strength testing to determine if they are justifiable and build a basis for our strength-testing model.

Injury Prevention

The Premise: It seems to make sense that if we match the strongest, most able individual to a job, we lessen the risk of a workplace injury. Most people instinctively feel vulnerable when they perform activities that they perceive to be beyond their limits. To validate this assumption, it is helpful to look at the research associated with the epidemiology of injuries in industry, such as low back pain.

Findings: Several investigators have explored the factors that correlate with workplace injury. Surprisingly, despite popular belief, these authors have found little correlation between injury and associated costs and the physical factors that one would commonly assume to be associated with injury. For example, in a 15-year retrospective study of 3,958 employees (Bigos, Spengler, Martin, Zeh, Fisher, & Nachemson, 1986a; Bigos et al., 1986b), researchers found little relationship between the incidence of low back pain and the type of job performed. Workers were found just as likely to be injured in jobs viewed as not being physically strenuous as those that were. They also found that although injuries caused by accidents (e.g., slips and falls) accounted for a small percentage of the total number of low back injuries, they accounted for a disproportionately high percentage of the costs. This finding was supported by Troup, Martin, and Lloyd (1981) in a study that showed a higher rate of postinjury absenteeism from injuries caused by accidents.

Perhaps the most compelling aspects of these studies was the significant correlation between the employees' most recent six-month performance appraisal and the cost of injury. A disproportionate number of injured employees, especially those associated with the highest case costs, had the lowest appraisal ratings. A significant correlation between psychosocial factors and injuries has also been supported by Troup, Foreman, Baxter, and Brown (1987) and Andersson (1981).

Cady, Bischoff, O'Connell, Thomas, and Allan (1979), studying a group of firefighters, found the most fit group to have the least frequent occurrence of injuries. However, the cost of injuries associated with the most fit group was substantially higher than that of the least fit group.

Snook, Campanelli, and Hart (1978) evaluated three preventative approaches to low back injuries used by industry: preplacement physicals, training, and job design. They found that all three methods of prevention were ineffective for controlling injuries.

Without clear evidence that measures of physical capacity are predictors for injury, it is difficult to justify the use of preemployment strength testing for the purpose of reducing injuries or injury costs at the work site. This conclusion is supported by the fact that other factors, including job type, accidental injury, and social factors, seem to be highly correlated with the cost and degree of disability of low back injury. The factors that make a worker successful in the job are complex. A unidimensional strength test does not appear sophisticated enough to critically determine which individuals will or will not injure themselves on the job, or to reduce the costs associated with workplace injuries.

Public Safety

The Premise: It is taken for granted that people entrusted to handle our safety will be able to meet the physical challenges of that job. We expect that when a firefighter responds to an emergency, he or she will be fully capable of maneuvering water hoses and climbing ladders and will have the physical endurance necessary to withstand the heat and intensity of the job. The use of preemployment tests to protect public safety has been an accepted practice for the past several decades. Although the premise behind these tests seems reasonable, there is an issue of skill and training that must be considered when developing tests for this purpose.

Findings: Can the physical requirements of demanding jobs be learned or met in a reasonable period of time with minimal practice or training? If so, does this mean that there is an inherent bias in the test that will make it difficult to support in a legal challenge? As was demonstrated in the case *Berkman v. the City of New York* (1987), a learned skill can be interpreted as strength and agility. In this case, only one female applicant was able to complete a test requirement, climbing an eight-foot wall. Her testimony indicated that she had learned a special technique to enable her to complete the task. What was originally perceived as strength and coordination was revealed, instead, to be a learned skill.

In another case, 269 individuals in an automobile plant underwent preemployment strength testing (Rollins, 1984). Seven women were unable to pass the strength portion of the test. Under the conditions of this study, the participants who failed were allowed to retake the test after a period of training. All seven of these participants ultimately were able to pass; subsequent, they handled their jobs without difficulties.

This example illustrates a very important concept: Training and practice may offset poor performance in a strength test. This concept is particularly pertinent for women, who historically have performed less well in strength testing than men (Ward, 1978) and have a high probability of being screened out for physically demanding jobs. Caution must be exercised so that preemployment tests do not unduly screen out individuals who legitimately may be able to handle jobs once they have had reasonable practice and training. Building these concepts into the test design may minimize this potential source of error.

Objective Evaluation of Job Functions

The Premise: One of the more recent uses for preemployment testing has been to help guide employers in making objective, job-related decisions for hiring. Movement in this direction has been largely influenced by the Americans with Disability Act, which allows employers to use preemployment tests, provided the exams are job related and consistent with business necessity (EEOC, 1992). Employers can test applicants on their abilities to perform the essential functions of jobs to determine if they can hire these individuals with or without reasonable accommodation. This type of testing is theoretically designed to minimize the subjectivity of hiring decisions. On the surface it appears to be reasonable.

The Findings: Although it is perfectly legitimate for employers to want the best qualified applicants for their jobs, it is not acceptable to automatically assume that a disabled individual cannot handle the work requirements and design a test to screen him or her out. It is possible to mitigate this potential bias by carefully designing tests and building reasonable accommodations into the hiring analysis. These steps promote careful consideration of the disabled applicant and ensure that the test is not just used to keep him or her out of the workplace.

To summarize, preemployment testing should not be used for the purpose of reducing the incidence or cost of workplace injury. Studies have not supported the assumptions underlying this practice. If the test is to be used for public safety or to minimize the subjectivity of the hiring process, it is important to minimize any inherent test bias by considering the following:

- The use of practice before the test
- Opportunities for failed applicants to retake tests after they have had a chance to build strength and flexibility
- Reasonable accommodations for qualified disabled applicants

RELIABILITY AND VALIDITY

Reliability and validity are critical issues when evaluating any testing methodology. In the preemployment testing arena, these concepts are held to an even higher standard because of the legal ramifications of hiring decisions.

To develop a test that does not unfairly screen out qualified applicants, two basic elements in the test design must be present: (1) test outcomes must be consistently repeatable and not subject to influence by the test administrator or other outside factors (test reliability), and (2) a test must measure what it is supposed to with a high degree of scientific certainty (test validity). So, in designing a test for warehouse workers, it is critical to determine that the test actually measures the ability of the worker to adequately perform the job. What if the test were given to an existing workforce, and only 60% of the workforce could pass it with the standards that had been set? Wouldn't this tell us that the test is clearly not measuring the true demands of the job because all of the current employees are actually handling the work requirements? Even if the test appears to be valid on the surface, face validity has historically been insufficient as a defense in a court challenge offered under a discrimination lawsuit (Perry, 1991).

The Equal Employment Opportunity Commission (EEOC) is the governing body for Title VII of the Civil Rights Act of 1964 and the Americans with Disability Act of 1991. As such, it has set forth requirements for test design, including test validation requirements for exams used for employment purposes (EEOC, 1978). The EEOC strictly guides employers and test developers in the determination of test validity, based on the guidelines found in the Principles for the Validation and use of Personnel Selection Procedures (1978). These documents provide guidance in drawing up acceptable validity standards. In order for a test to be fair and able to withstand a legal challenge under Title VII, it should meet one of the validity standards and be shown to be reliable.

Reliability. Reliability, an important element for a test design, is the demonstration of repeatable measures over multiple testings. Demonstrating reliability ensures that test outcomes will not be dependent on the individual administering the test or other outside, uncontrollable factors, and that scores will be consistent with multiple testings. The EEOC requires proof of reliability in a test design.

Validity. The EEOC outlines three types of acceptable validity measures: criteria, content, and construct validity. It is only required that a test meet one of these validity measures. All three validation techniques require documentation that demonstrates the methods and process of the validity study. (See Table 9.1 for a summary of validity types.)

Table 9.1. Validation Measures

Validity type	Explanation	Example
Criterion-related validity	Demonstrates that the selection procedure is predictive or significantly correlated with critical elements of work behavior.	Individuals who are able to adequately perform all test elements on preemployment strength test are shown to have a reduced incidence of injury compared with those who do not perform well on the test.
Construct validity	Demonstrates that identifiable job characteristics are important for successful performance of the job.	Individuals with good eye/hand coordination are shown to be more successful on an assembly line operation.
Content validity	Demonstrates that the content of the selection procedure is representative of important aspects of performance of the job.	A job requires lifting a bag from the floor and carrying it four times per hour. The exact replication of these activities is shown to adequately and precisely measure these demands.

As defined in the *Uniform Guidelines on Employee Selection Procedures* (1978), criterion-related validity demonstrates that the selection procedure is predictive of, or significantly correlated with, critical elements of work behavior. For example, does a particular preemployment strength test accurately predict who will successfully be able to handle the job without injury?

The second type of validity, content validity, is the weakest form of validation. It indicates that the content of a selection procedure is representative of important aspects of performance of the job. A panel of independent, objective experts can issue an opinion of content validity (Lechner, Roth, & Straaton, 1991). So, for example, are the test elements in a preemployment test truly representative, accurate, and precise enough to measure the demands of a particular job?

The third type of validity is construct validity, which demonstrates that identifiable job characteristics are important for successful performance of the job. An example might be testing an individual's decision-making skills for a leadership position.

TESTING METHODOLOGIES

With the onset of the Americans with Disabilities Act, there has been an increased focus on job-specific, functional testing. This section will discuss the methods most frequently used to determine if an individual can handle the physical requirements of a job, most notably strength testing methodologies, because this is an area very commonly handled by physical and occupational therapists. It is important to keep in mind that there are other components of evaluation, such as cardiovascular fitness and aptitude testing, that may also be used.

Physical and occupational therapists typically use three different testing methodologies either individually or in combination in preemployment strength testing: isometric or static strength testing, isokinetic strength testing, and dynamic strength testing. The validity of some of these tests for preemployment purposes has been critically challenged in the scientific literature, yet their usage continues. When designing a strength selection model, the pros and cons of these testing methodologies relative to validity and reliability need to be understood. (These pros and cons are summarized in Table 9.2.)

Isometric Strength Testing

Isometric strength testing, largely patterned after work done by Chaffin (1975) and Chaffin, Herrin, and Keyserling (1978), has been commonly used for preemployment testing. Isometric strength testing is popular because of its reliability, ease of use, and low injury rate (Keyserling, Herrin, & Chaffin, 1980). In this type of test, the individual pushes, pulls, or lifts up on a stationary handle connected to a strain gauge or load cell. The test position is chosen to model a real work activity. Because a strain gauge set up is economical and transportable, it can be convenient to use, especially if tests are done on-site for an employer.

Early research reported promising results regarding the reliability and validity of static strength testing for preemployment purposes (Biering-Sorenson, 1984; Cady et al., 1979; Chaffin et al., 1978; Keyserling et al., 1980). Chaffin and colleagues' (1978) landmark study of 551 employees revealed that for workers whose job strength requirements

Table 9.2. Pros and Cons of Testing Methodologies for Preemployment Testing

Pros	Cons
Isometric strength testing	
• easy to use	• questionable validity for preemployment
• relatively inexpensive	purposes
• low injury rate	• conflicting data on relationship to dynamic
• can be done at work site with strain gauge	strength
• good reliability	• may experience difficulty in demonstrating job-
• standardized, well-publicized testing protocols	relatedness for some work activities
Isokinetic strength testing	
• relatively easy to use	• questionable valididty for preemployment testing
• standardized testing protocol	• not job related
	• no demonstrated relationship to functional/
	dynamic activities
	• relatively expensive equipment required
	• results difficult for lay people to understand
Dynamic strength testing	
• can easily be adapted to be job specific	• limited evidence of validity
• easy to implement (can be done at the work	• little standardization of testing protocols
site)	
• inexpensive	
• some evidence of content validity	
• results can be readily understood by lay people	
• results can be easily used to help make	
decision about reasonable accommodations	

approached or exceeded their isometric strength, their injury frequency and severity rates increased by a 3:1 ratio. There are some questions, however, about the conclusions drawn from some of these early studies that cast doubts on the efficacy of isometric strength testing for preemployment purposes. For example, in a study done by Biering-Sorenson (1984), it was found that the results of isometric strength tests were of no significance in predicting a first-time occurrence of low back pain, but were more predictive of a recurrence of low back pain. However, it is questionable whether the reduced postinjury isometric strength was residual weakness from the first back injury or the cause of the second injury.

Two other more recent studies with large sample sizes further questioned the use of isometric strength testing for preemployment purposes. Batti'e, Bigos, Fisher, Hansson, Jones, and Wortley (1989) evaluated 3,020 individuals at an aircraft plant and conducted a four-year follow-up. They found no correlation between strength and subsequent complaints of back pain and, in fact, found that if the data were not age adjusted, individuals with the strongest strength measurements were more likely to have complaints of back pain. The authors also concluded that isometric strength testing is influenced by many individual factors, including height, weight, and especially gender. Even when they evaluated individuals within the same job categories, they found that employees reporting back injuries had strength comparable to their uninjured co-workers. They concluded that isometric strength testing is ineffective in identifying individuals at risk for industrial back problems. This finding was supported by Troup and colleagues (1987) who found no predictive value for isometric strength testing unless it was paired with knowledge of a previous back injury.

The two studies cited used standard positions for isometric strength testing and were not job specific, factors which could have had a bearing on the results. However, in spite of these shortcomings, the results of these tests, combined with the weaknesses found in some of the early studies and disagreement over the degree of correlation between static and dynamic test results (Campion, 1983), put a high degree of uncertainty on the use of isometric testing for preemployment purposes. Although static strength tests are reliable, easy to use, safe, and convenient, their validity as a predictor of job performance or risk of injury is not supported.

Isokinetic Testing

Isokinetic testing has been a popular testing alternative because of its perceived reliability, validity, and ability to effectively and objectively measure physical impairment. This testing method has made its way to the preemployment testing arena through commercially available testing systems.

There have been numerous articles written on the use of isokinetic testing in making hiring decisions. Perhaps one of the best summaries of this literature was written by Newton and Waddell (1993). In this study, 108 published articles on isokinetics and preemployment testing (through March of 1992) were reviewed. Most notable were findings on reliability and validity. Newton and Waddell found inconsistent support of test reliability and determined that test reliability is very dependent on the position of the joint and the speed tested. They also found a very strong learning effect and described a tendency for underestimation of trunk function when a single testing session was used. In the area of validity, the authors found no direct evidence of a relationship between the results and actual muscle strength or functional capacity in realistic activities. They also found evidence that test results may be affected by secondary factors, such as psychosocial functioning. Contrary to popular perception, Newton and Waddell found inadequate scientific evidence to support the use of isokinetic testing in *any* evaluative format, especially preemployment testing.

Confirming these results, Deuker, Ritchie, Knox, and Rose (1994) looked at prehire isokinetic and dynamic strength in 230 applicants for heavy labor positions in a steel mill and then followed the employees for 5.5 years. They found no predictability between isokinetic strength and dynamic lifting and no relationship between isokinetic strength and work-related low back injuries. They concluded that isokinetic testing is not a valid measure for preemployment testing. Very clearly, research suggests that isokinetic testing should not be used for preemployment testing.

Dynamic Strength Testing

Dynamic strength testing has gained increased popularity because of its easily recognizable relationship to actual work. If an individual is required to lift a bag of flour, testing this method using the actual activity feels more "real" than lifting up on a stationary handle or bending and extending the trunk in a repetitive fashion. However, in a legal situation, this face validity is insufficient.

Although there are abundant claims of the reliability and validity of dynamic strength testing, there are very few published, peer-reviewed studies supporting these assertions. Lechner and colleagues (1991) reviewed ten popular functional capacity testing methodologies that incorporated dynamic strength testing, only to find that all of them lacked the critical components of test reliability and validity. In a preemployment testing situation, where this burden of proof is critical to a successful discrimination defense, this deficiency takes on a new level of significance. A universal standard for administering these tests does not exist. This situation has resulted in almost as many variations of dynamic testing as there are industrial rehabilitation clinics.

There has been one promising study that addresses the issues of reliability and validity in dynamic testing. Lechner, Jackson, Roth, and Straaton (1994) looked at the reliability and validity of a functional capacity evaluation known as the Physical Work Performance Evaluation (PWPE). In this study, 50 working volunteers were tested on the PWPE over a two-year period. Two different administrators per evaluation were used, each establishing his or her own rating on each test item. The evaluators were blinded to the participant's work status. Interadministrator reliability was evaluated as well as the validity between actual and predicted work levels. The study results demonstrated good interadministrator reliability and moderate test validity. The study participants were actually shown to be working above their predicted work level 14%–18% of the time. The authors explained this finding by concluding that their test was designed to predict a maximal level of safe work performance instead of an absolute level of work that is influenced by other unrelated factors. This study raises an important question relative to the possibility of dynamic testing's underpredicting work function. In a preemployment situation, a 14% to 18% rate of underprediction is significant. Further evaluation is needed to determine the prevalence of underprediction and whether its cause is related to test design or other less controllable factors. How prevalent or real is this effect? Is its cause one of test design or of other, less controllable factors? These questions need to be evaluated in further detail for their implications for the selection process.

In summary, dynamic strength testing has received the strongest support for use in preemployment testing. It must be understood, however, that this testing procedure is in its early stages of development and has only rudimentary support. A close eye must be kept on further developments to determine if it will hold up in the long term as a valid testing method.

LEGAL ISSUES

A challenge when using preemployment testing is understanding its relationship to the complex judicial statutes that govern employer hiring practices. Two key legal doctrines govern this domain: Title VII of the Civil Rights Act of 1964 and the Americans with Disabilities Act of 1991. (Table 9.3 summarizes the selection procedure requirements for these statutes.)

Title VII of the Civil Rights Act of 1964

Title VII of the Civil Rights Act of 1964 was developed to eliminate discriminatory hiring preferences and to establish fair employment practices. It prohibits an employer from discriminating against applicants on the basis of race, color, religion, sex, or national origin. The significance of Title VII and its relationship to preemployment testing has primarily been realized with women, as it has been used to severely challenge the legality of preemployment testing for this population.

The court uses a three-part test to determine if disparate impact on a protected

Table 9.3. Legal Statutes Governing Preemployment Testing

Statutes	Who protects	Selection procedure requirement
Title VII Civil Rights Act of 1964	Groups of individuals based on race, color, religion, or sex	Selection procedure must meet one of three criteria • test validation requirements • be shown to be of business necessity • be a bona fide occupational qualification
Americans with Disabilities Act of 1991	Qualified individuals with a disability	Selection procedure must be • consistent with business necessity • job related (if a qualified individual cannot demonstrate the ability to perform an essential job requirement, reasonable accommodations must be considered)

group exists. The first part of the test requires that the individual claiming discrimination show that it occurred. Only a discriminatory effect is required. Proving intent is not required. The EEOC's *Uniform Guidelines on Employee Selection Procedures* (1978) have determined that a selection rate for any race, sex, or ethnic group that is less than four fifths (or 80%) of the rate for the group with the highest rate will generally be regarded as evidence of adverse impact. For example, if the hiring rate for females is 10%, but it is 70% for males, this condition would meet the first challenge. Because of the courts loose standards for defining a discriminatory effect, it is not difficult for plaintiffs to meet this first court challenge.

Once a discriminatory effect has been established, the burden of proof is shifted to the employer. In the second part of the test, the employer must show that legitimate nondiscriminatory criteria were used in the selection procedure. The employer has three lines of defense: job-relatedness, business necessity, or bona fide occupational qualifications.

In the first line of defense, an employer must show that a test is job related and can adequately measure job performance. These criteria generally must be met in strict accordance with the EEOC guidelines, which are very difficult to meet, particularly in the area of test validation. Face validity is insufficient to meet this burden, and only sufficient evidence of criterion, content, or construct validity will suffice. A thorough, well-performed job analysis is critical to any attempt to demonstrate validity. Test developers must establish this requirement even if the employer did not request that the test be validated.

The second line of defense is to show that the test in question is a business necessity. This defense has three elements (Conway, 1987);

1. The business necessity must override the social harm that results from discrimination.
2. The employment practice must fulfill the alleged purpose.
3. There must be no alternative practice that would better fulfill this need.

Even in the event that a test meets all the validation requirements, if it can be shown that an employer was able to successfully hire candidates prior to the initiation of the strength test, the courts would likely find that this practice is not a business necessity (Canton, 1987). If there is a high degree of risk involved, the courts may be more lenient, but this defense is usually utilized in cases in which public safety is involved (Conway, 1987).

The third line of defense for an employer is to show that the hiring procedures are a bona fide occupational qualification (BFOQ). To do so "requires that a reasonable determination that all, or substantially all, women would be unable to perform the job safely and efficiently because strenuous manual labor is required" (Conway, 1987). a BFOQ is a statutory exception to Title VII that is applied very narrowly by the courts. Employers are very limited in their use of this defense (Perry, 1991).

Many court challenges have been found in favor of the plaintiff because of the difficulty employers have in meeting the defense's burden of proof. If, however, an employer can satisfactorily meet this challenge, the burden then shifts back to the plaintiff for the third part of the three-part test. The plaintiff must demonstrate that there is another selection device that is not discriminatory in nature but equally valid and job related. This requirement is extremely difficult to meet.

The EEOC does not prohibit the use of preemployment testing, nor does it require that the testing be valid unless adverse impact is shown to exist (EEOC, 1978). However, if employers wait until after they are challenged, it is unlikely that they will be able to adequately defend their testing practice.

In summary, Title VII governs preemployment testing in cases of adverse impact. The requirements for good test design and validation are very clear. If the test does not meet these requirements, chances are that the testing practice will not withstand a legal challenge.

Americans with Disabilities Act of 1991

The Americans with Disabilities Act (ADA) of 1991 established that it is unlawful to discriminate against individuals with a disability (as defined by the act) solely based on that perceived or obvious disability. In the hiring arena, this act presents a new set of requirements to ensure that employment discrimination based on a disability does not occur. The ADA does not prohibit an employer from developing job qualifications to ensure that the most qualified individuals are selected to perform a job effectively and safely (EEOC, 1992). Any qualification standards or selection criteria that tend to screen-out an individual with a disability must, however, be job related and consistent with business necessity. Even so, if it screens out an individual with a disability on the basis of that disability, the employer must consider whether the individual could meet the standard with reasonable accommodation (EEOC, 1992).

Preemployment tests are not considered to be medical examinations under the ADA and may be performed at either the preoffer or postoffer phase. A preemployment test is defined as a test in which an applicant demonstrates his or her ability to perform actual or simulated job-related tasks (essential or marginal) (EEOC, 1994). For example, if a job requires an individual to frequently lift a heavy bag, this activity can be tested because it is job related. However, looking at heart rate before and after the procedure is a medical test and cannot be included in a preoffer test. Also, if a preemployment test is performed preoffer, it cannot require that a medical screen be given prior to the preemployment test unless it responds only to the question of whether the applicant can safely perform the preemployment test (EEOC, 1992). The ADA does not require that a qualification standard apply only to the essential functions of the job. However, an individual with a disability cannot be screened out because of his or her inability to perform a marginal function; the individual must be judged solely on the ability to perform the essential functions of the job, with or without accommodations (EEOC, 1992).

According to the EEOC *Technical Assistance Manual* (1992), the same business necessity standard as that seen in Title VII of the Civil Rights Act is applied, except that under the ADA this standard is applied to an individual rather than a class of individuals. Because the ADA protects individuals with disabilities (versus groups of disabled people), the *Uniform Guidelines on Employee Selection Procedures* (1978) do not apply under the ADA selection procedure. Therefore, the validation requirements discussed under Title VII are not necessary. Frierson (1992) pointed out that the qualification test must measure a job applicant's or employee's abilities to perform the job, not his or her abilities to take a certain type of test. Also, the format of the test should never disqualify the individual.

According to the EEOC *Technical Assistance Manual* (1992), an employer may require that an individual not be a direct threat to the health and safety of himself or herself or others as long as the standard is applied to all applicants. However, the interpretation of this guideline in a defense situation is often narrow. A high probability of significant risk for substantial harm that is current and not predictive in nature is required. For example, if an individual with a history of low back pain meets the essential requirements of a job, with or without accommodations, he or she cannot be denied access to the job because there is speculative risk of future reinjury. Even if the risk of substantial harm is real, the employer must consider eliminating or minimizing the risk below the level of direct threat through reasonable accommodation.

Case law examining how the court will interpret these standards still does not exist. For this reason, the application of these concepts for developing preemployment tests are speculative in nature, and clinicians will need to closely follow future developments to further clarify the issues. What does seem clear at this point is that preemployment testing can be done at any stage of the hiring process, but it must be job related and consistent with business necessity. Preemployment testing can evaluate essential and marginal functions, but an individual with a disability cannot be screened out because of her or his inability to perform a marginal function. If an applicant protected under the ADA cannot perform an essential requirement of the job, then a reasonable accommodation must be considered.

Legally, there are two key requirements for preemployment strength testing: (1) Make sure your test has been validated, and (2) make sure your test is job specific and is testing the essential job requirements.

DEVELOPING A PREEMPLOYMENT TEST

There are thirteen steps that should be followed to construct a preemployment test that is valid and meets legal guidelines (see Figure 9.1). These steps summarize what is currently known about strength selection testing and are subject to change with new research and developments.

Step 1. Work with the employer to determine the purpose for implementing preemployment testing, and discuss the pros, cons, and likely outcomes, particularly if the goal is to reduce injuries. Employers who have a realistic expectation of outcomes are more likely to be satisfied with the progress in the long term.

Step 2. Perform a thorough job analysis and determine the essential and marginal functions of the job. Carefully document this information, and keep it on file to show the logic used to develop the test.

Step 3. Work with the employer and his or her legal resources to help them determine if the selection process is a business necessity. If it is not, discuss other strategies to evaluate employee potential; such as utilizing the probationary period to evaluate strength capabilities and phasing in job duties to help employees adjust to the demands of the job. Ergonomic principles can also be looked at to help design the job so that the majority of people can meet its demands.

Step 4. If there is a business necessity for a hiring selection process, design a test that is job related and measures the essential functions of the job. Utilize dynamic testing as your testing methodology. The test can be done on- or off-site, and should be done with actual work materials where available. All instructions, test elements, rest periods, and discontinuation criteria should be standardized. If one is using a predeveloped evaluation system, make sure the test is job specific. If it is not, it should not be used.

Step 5. Validate the test design. If an evaluation is purchased, request information on validity and reliability. Remember that there is liability involved in using evaluations that have not established validity and reliability. If a provider is developing its own evaluation, it is important to validate the test.

The simplest but weakest form of validation is content validation. At a bare minimum, at least two independent reviewers should critically review a preemployment test to determine if the test elements precisely and accurately measure the essential elements of the job. A more substantial measure of content validity involves evaluating existing employees in particular jobs to accurately ascertain the abilities necessary to perform those jobs. Once this step has been completed, the tests may be administered to potential applicants. In jobs that are very physically demanding in which there is a possibility of an adverse impact on a women, a higher standard of validity (criterion or predictive validity) is advised. Assistance from professional test developers or researchers may be warranted. This process is expensive and time consuming. The costs associated with this process must be weighed against the anticipated benefits.

Step 6. Work with the employer to determine if the evaluations will be administered preoffer or postoffer. If the test is performed preoffer, it should not contain any medical procedures (such as taking blood pressure measurements) and should not inquire into the past medical history of the applicant. It is appropriate to ask the applicant if there is any known reason why she or he may not be able to complete the test safely. A medical screen is only appropriate if it very narrowly evaluates the applicant's ability to safely engage in a physical strength test.

Step 7. Develop information flow procedures. It is recommended that the employer be given the test results to determine if they meet or do not meet the job requirements. This procedure will put the hiring responsibility on the employer, allowing him or her to decide if reasonable accommodations are necessary.

Step 8. Develop tracking procedures to look at pass/fail frequency; the applicant's demographic information, such as gender and age; and reasonable accommodations considered for failed applicants. Also track any test injury data to make sure that the test design is safe.

Step 9. Perform the evaluations. Act as a resource for employers if reasonable accommodations are being considered.

Step 10. Routinely check with the employer to make sure that essential job functions that would likewise require a change in the evaluation procedure have not changed.

Step 11. Routinely review the aggregate test results to determine if there are any signs of adverse impact (selection rate for females of less than 80%) or a consistent ne-

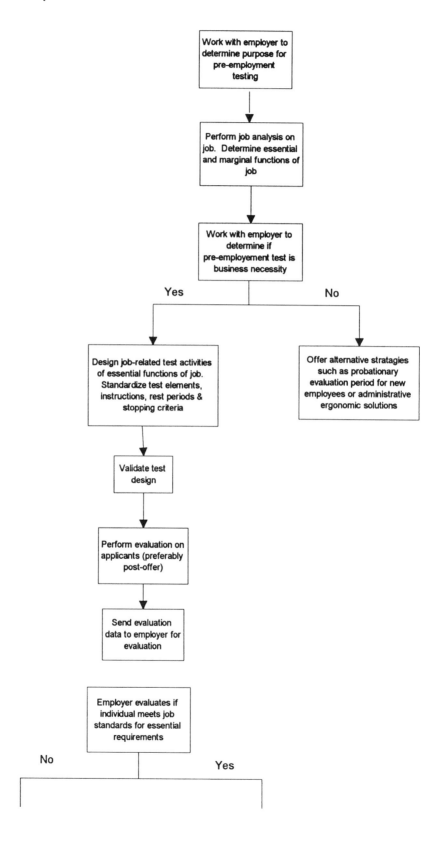

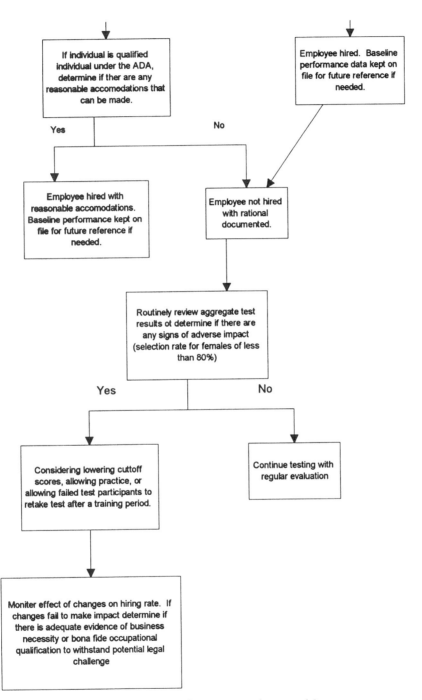

Figure 9.1. Preemployment strength test model.

glect of reasonable accommodations where appropriate. If there are signs of adverse impact, consider lowering the cutoff scores or allowing failed applicants to retake the evaluation after a period of training.

Step 12. Monitor the effect of any changes on the potential of adverse impact for women. If these changes fail to positively influence the results, have the employer and legal counsel revisit the concepts of business necessity and evidence of a bona fide occupational qualification to ensure that there is adequate evidence to support a legal challenge.

Step 13. If there is inadequate support for business necessity or a bona fide occupational qualification, consider ceasing the selection testing for that job.

If these thirteen steps are followed, it is likely that the preemployment test will meet the current challenges. These steps can be difficult and costly, but they are important. It is imperative that providers using preemployment testing focus on establishing the validity and reliability of dynamic testing methods. It is also important to follow legal precedence, especially in new developments with the ADA, in order to determine its impact upon selection testing.

REFERENCES

American Psychological Association, Division of Industrial Organizational Psychology. (1980). *Principles for the validation and use of personnel selection procedures* (2nd ed.). Berkeley, CA: Author.

Andersson, G. (1981). Epidemiological aspects on low back pain in industry. *Spine, 6*, 53–60.

Batti'e, M. C., Bigos, S. J., Fisher, L. D., Hansson, T. H., Jones, M. E., & Wortley, M. D. (1989). Isometric lifting strength as a predictor of industrial back pain reports. *Spine, 14*, 851–856.

Berkman v. City of New York, 1987, F. Suppl. 536.

Biering-Sorenson, F. (1984). Physical measurements as risk indicators for low back trouble over a one year period. *Spine, 9*, 106–119.

Bigos, S. J., Spengler, D. M., Martin, N. A., Zeh, J., Fisher, L., & Nachemson, A. (1986a). Back injuries in industry: A retrospective study III. Employee-related factors. *Spine, 11*, 252–256.

Bigos, S. J., Spengler, D. M., Martin, N. A., Zeh, J., Fisher, L., Nachemson, A., & Wang, M. H. (1986b). Back injuries in industry: A retrospective study II. Injury factors. *Spine, 11*, 246–251.

Cady, L. D., Bischoff, D. F., O'Connell, M. S., Thomas, P. C., & Allan, J. H. (1979). Strength and fitness and subsequent back injuries in firefighters. *Journal of Occupational Medicine, 21*, 269–272.

Campion, M. A. (1983). Personnel selection for physically demanding jobs: Review and recommendations. *Personnel Psychology, 36*, 527–550.

Canton, D. (1987). Adverse impact analysis of public sector employment tests: Can a city devise a valid test? *Cincinnati Law Review, 56*, 683–709.

Chaffin, D. B. (1975). Ergonomics guide for the assessment of human static strength. *American Industrial Hygiene Association Journal, 36*, 505–511.

Chaffin, D. B., Herrin, G. D., & Keyserling, W. M. (1978). Preemployment strength testing: An updated position. *Journal of Occupational Medicine, 20*, 403–408.

Conway, J. M. (1987). Title VII and competitive testing. *Hofstra Law Review, 15*, 299–322.

Deuker, J. A., Ritchie, S. M., Knox, T. J., & Rose, S. J. (1994). Isokinetic trunk testing and employment. *Journal of Occupational Medicine, 36*, 42–48.

EEOC. (1978). *Uniform guidelines on employee selection procedures*. Washington, DC: Author.

EEOC. (1992). *Technical assistance manual of the employment provisions (Title I) of the Americans with Disabilities Act*. Washington, DC: Author.

EEOC. (1994). Enforcement guidance on preemployment inquires under Americans with Disabilities Act. *Equal Opportunities Commission Daily Labor Report, 96*, 1–36.

Frierson, J. G. (1992). *Employers guide to the Americans with Disabilities Act*. Washington, DC: BNA Books.

Keyserling, W. M., Herrin, G. D., & Chaffin, D. B. (1980). Isometric strength testing as a means of controlling medical incidents on strenuous jobs. *Journal of Occupational Medicine, 22*, 332–336.

Lechner, D., Jackson, J. R., Roth, D., & Straaton, K. (1994). Reliability validity of a newly developed test of physical work performance. *Journal of Occupational Medicine, 36,* 997–1004.

Lechner, D., Roth, D., & Straaton, K. (1991). Functional capacity evaluation in work disability. *Work, 1*(3), 37–47.

Newton, M., & Waddel, G. (1993). Trunk strength testing with iso-machines: Part I. Review of a decade of scientific evidence. *Spine, 18,* 801–811.

Perry, L. L. (1991). Preemployment strength testing: Implications in sex discrimination. *Work, 1*(3), 32–36.

Rollins, A. J. (1984). *The use of dynamic strength testing to assist in the selection of individuals for heavy manual materials handling jobs.* Unpublished master's thesis, University of Cincinnati, Cincinnati, Ohio.

Snook, S. H., Campanelli, R. A., & Hart, J. W. (1978). A study of three preventive approaches to low back injury. *Journal of Occupational Medicine, 20,* 478–481.

Troup, J. D. G., Foreman, T. K., Baxter, C. E., & Brown, D. (1987). The perception of back pain and the role of psychophysical test of lifting capacity. *Spine, 12,* 645–657.

Troup, J. D. G., Martin, J. W., & Lloyd, D. C. E. F. (1981). Back pain in industry: A prospective survey. *Spine, 6,* 61–69.

Ward, J. S. (1978). Sex discrimination is essential in industry. *Journal of Occupational Medicine, 20,* 594–596.

10

Surveillance and Survey Techniques

Lawrence P. Hanrahan

SURVEILLANCE

According to the *American Heritage Dictionary* (1991), the word *surveillance* comes from the Latin verb *viglare* (to be watchful), and the French verb *surveiller* (to watch over). As a medical term, surveillance is defined as watching or monitoring (*Dorland's Illustrated Medical Dictionary*, 1988). The notion of surveillance as it relates to the goals of occupational and public health is probably best illustrated by analogy to the concept of *immunological surveillance*:

> A hypothesized monitoring function by which the immune system protects against cancer. According to the theory, tumor cells constantly arise throughout life by malignant transformation of normal cells, but almost all are recognized and destroyed by the immune system. Only a few somehow escape or circumvent immune surveillance to grow and become clinically detectable cancers. (*Dorland's Illustrated Medical Dictionary*, 1988)

Like the immune system, surveillance systems monitor the occurrence of adverse events (disease, injury, or health hazards), direct activities to control and eliminate them, and oversee the efficacy of the control activities. Ideally, it is a continuous, adaptive, and compensatory process, marshaling resources when and where needed to maintain and improve health. In this way, public health surveillance has been defined (Klauke et al., 1988) as "the ongoing and systematic collection, analysis, and interpretation of health data in the process of describing and monitoring a health event. This information is used for planning, implementing, and evaluating public health interventions and programs."

Lawrence P. Hanrahan • Wisconsin Division of Health and Departments of Industrial Engineering and Preventive Medicine, University of Wisconsin–Madison, Madison, Wisconsin 53703.

Sourcebook of Occupational Rehabilitation, edited by Phyllis M. King. Plenum Press, New York, 1998.

EPIDEMIOLOGY

Epidemiology is defined as

> the science concerned with the study of the factors determining and influencing the frequency and distribution of disease, injury, and other health-related events and their causes in a defined human population for the purpose of establishing programs to prevent and control their development and spread. Also, the sum of knowledge gained in such a study. (*Dorland's Illustrated Medical Dictionary*, 1988).

Epidemiology studies the health and disease status of human populations. According to Kleinbaum, Kupper, and Morgenstern (1982), epidemiologic research can be experimental (includes randomization and experimental regulation of the study factor), quasi-experimental (experimental regulation of the study factor without randomization), and observational. Observational epidemiologic research can be either descriptive (e.g., estimate disease rates, ascertain populations at greatest risk, etc.) or analytic (e.g., test hypotheses, postulate new causal factors and mechanisms, or new preventive intervention techniques).

Epidemiology for occupational health entails studying disease and injury occurrences that result from workplace hazards. Analytic epidemiologic studies use investigational techniques such as cross-sectional studies (disease and hazard prevalence, relative risk, hypothesis development), cohort studies (disease incidence in exposed groups compared with disease incidence in unexposed groups, hypothesis testing), and case referent studies (exposure odds in diseased persons compared with the exposure odds in disease free individuals, hypothesis testing). These study types define exposures at work that are postulated causal factors for injury and disease. For example, to date over 30 analytic observational studies have shown increased risks for carpal tunnel syndrome (CTS) resulting from occupational exposures to highly repetitive hand movements, forceful hand movements, and vibration (Bernard, 1997).

RELATIONSHIP BETWEEN SURVEILLANCE AND EPIDEMIOLOGY

Epidemiology as a research function provides the science base for effective surveillance action (Hanrahan & Moll, 1989). Surveillance is a sensing and signaling system; epidemiology helps to decode its meaning. Epidemiology is an integrative and interpretive function, responding to the surveillance information of illness, injury, or hazard. Once an adverse trend or incidence of injury is detected, the surveillance system signals that something should be done. It is at this point that epidemiologic activity may come into play. The phases of this response could include (a) conducting more surveillance (better data collection and descriptive epidemiologic analysis of events); (b) instructing a formal epidemiologic study of events (e.g., cross-sectional, cohort, and case-referent studies to propose and then test hypotheses to ultimately define causes); (c) planning and implementing interventions to modify or eliminate causes (i.e., experimental intervention trial); and (d) assessing the effectiveness of interventions through ongoing, continuous surveillance (i.e., observe shifting or lowering in the frequency of events: disease, injury or exposure to health hazards). Surveillance can also marshal preventive activities by simply distributing surveillance information to effectors of change.

PROCESS OF SURVEILLANCE: METHODS

In the past, surveillance programs have been characterized as either active or passive. Passive systems often depend on reporting laws (e.g., communicable disease reports), but they can also rely on data collected for administrative, billing, and other purposes (e.g., death certificates, hospital discharge billing data, workers' compensation data). Active systems seek information from event reporters by contacting them and using data collection instruments specifically designed for the surveillance activity (Sullivan, Gibbs, & Knowles, 1994).

Passive and active systems each have their own strengths and weaknesses. Compared with active systems, passive systems often possess greater completeness of case ascertainment when administrative databases are used. For example, all of the compensated work-related back injuries can easily be found in a state's workers' compensation database. However, because the data collected are for another purpose (prompt and fair compensation of the injured worker), there is usually little information of surveillance utility beyond basic case demographics. For instance, workers' compensation information systems usually contain the case's industry, occupation, age, and gender information, but often contain little or no data about the exact medical diagnosis and treatment for the injury and the types of rehabilitative therapies used (to indicate which ones were effective), and no detailed information about the workplace hazards that were causal factors for the event. In contrast, passive systems relying on disease-reporting laws often have incomplete case ascertainment because of case detection problems. For example, a clinician must remember to report a case that for any practitioner is a rare occurrence.

Active systems are superior to passive ones to the extent that the exact data needed is asked for and obtained on the report form. However, active programs often require substantially more resources for proper implementation than do passive ones. Potential case reporters must be routinely contacted by the central office. Because of this, an active program is limited because of reporting burdens (e.g., additional paperwork for clinicians and their office staffs, or (the "one-time" set-up and use of a costly data collection instrument) and the need for more system management resources. Because of these issues, active systems are often characterized by incomplete case ascertainment—only selected reporters can be contacted because of time and financial cost. A final consequence is that more often than not data collection is periodic and not continuous.

In summary, passive and active surveillance systems may be conceptually distinguished as push (passive) or pull (active). Passive—push—systems are akin to broadcasting. Data collection has been routinized by reporting laws or administrative functions. Because of this, health information can be readily transmitted (broadcasted) from the local level to those performing the centralized surveillance function. On the other hand, active—pull—systems involve search and polling routines, through which a central office contacts local reporting units.

A third or hybrid type of surveillance is the push-pull system. A push-pull surveillance program relies on a passive administrative database for case ascertainment. Once cases are detected in the passive system, an active surveillance process feeds the cases back to the treating practitioner to obtain the necessary surveillance data. Each of these three techniques plays a part in the discussion of the evolution of the Wisconsin Carpal Tunnel Syndrome surveillance program that follows.

SURVEYS AND DATA COLLECTION INSTRUMENTS

Good survey design is a key component to any successful surveillance program. Although a discussion on the comprehensive design of survey data collection instruments is beyond the scope of this chapter, the reader is referred to the seminal work by Dillman (1978). Dillman described the process of using his "total design method" (TDM) to construct effective mail and telephone surveys so that people will respond (yield a high response rate) and give quality answers to the questions posed. Dillman covered important issues, such as obtaining representative samples and accurate answers to all questions; the principles of question writing, wording, and structure; pretesting; and survey administration in detail.

Finally, Ehrenberg and Sniezek (1989) provided a good overview for a standard questionnaire that can be used for routine occupational health surveillance. Questionnaire modules to consider include case demographics, occupational history, medical/symptom and environmental history, and personal risk factors as well as a condition-specific question module. The appendix contains an example of a short follow-back questionnaire for occupational carpal tunnel syndrome surveillance.

DATA ANALYSIS TECHNIQUES

In their simplest form, surveillance data analyses produce basic, descriptive statistics to characterize time (trends in injury rates), place (industries and occupations with a high rate of cases), and person (age and gender-specific risks) (Cates & Williamson, 1994). Along with simple case frequency measures, one basic statistical measure is the disease or injury rate. It is essentially a ratio—the number of persons injured divided by the number of persons at risk for the injury during a specified time period. Often surveillance data analyses will then examine injury rates that change over time and describe injury-rate differences according to place and person risk factors. When rates are computed, one is able to ascertain who, where, and when increased risks occured. One statistic—the relative risk—compares the disease or injury rates of one group with those of a referent group. It is a simple measure that describes increased or decreased risk for the group of interest. For example, if the annual carpal tunnel syndrome surgery rate was 200 per 100,000 females and 100 per 100,000 males, then the female to male relative risk would be 2 (200/100), indicating that females have twice the annual surgery rate of males.

Because injury and disease do not distribute randomly in the population, a principal goal of surveillance is to determine where these nonrandom, increased risks occur. However, these differences must often be accounted (adjusted) for in the surveillance analyses to insure proper interpretation of the data. To illustrate, suppose that a particular injury is due to a workplace hazard, that the rate also increases with a person's age, and that the injury rate is higher for females. Suppose further that we have tracked the population rate for over 30 years, and we have noted a steady increase in the rate, but we also know that the workforce has aged, and more women are now in the workforce. With only a crude rate (number of events/number of workers at risk), we would not know if the change were due to an increase in the number of workplace hazards, or simply due to the aging of the workforce and an increasing number of women entering the workplace.

Any of several methods may be employed to adjust for factors that obscure surveillance analyses, including stratified analysis, rate standardization, and multivariate regression. In the earlier example, one could adjust for age and gender factors by doing a stratified analysis. Tables of age- and gender- specific rates could be constructed for each of the 30 years, and then year-to-year changes in the rates could be directly examined for each specific age and gender group. Rate standardization is another adjustment method. Using this technique, summary injury rates are calculated by adjusting for the confounding variables (age and gender), allowing one to obtain an undistorted view of the effect of time on the rate. Another more sophisticated analytic method involves the use of multivariate regression techniques (Kleinbaum, Kupper, & Morgenstern, 1982). These techniques can examine an exposure–injury relationship while simultaneously adjusting for many confounders in the analysis. An especially popular procedure is logistic regression. It is often preferred because the logistic function is ideally suited for estimating and predicting risks. Logistic regression software is also readily available for personal computers, and it can also be used to approximate the Poisson regression analysis of rates (SAS Institute, 1989).

Other statistical techniques are available for surveillance analyses but they have yet to be routinely and extensively used in the field. These techniques include all of the statistical procedures employed in the fields of quality improvement and statistical quality control (Box, Hunter, & Hunter, 1978; King, 1995). Statistical quality control techniques include elementary graphical analyses (Pareto and Ishikawa charts), control charts, and automated process control techniques (Shewhart and Cusum techniques, forecasting, and autoregressive integrated moving average—ARIMA—models), capability analyses, and process optimization through designed experiments (King, 1995). Although these techniques are important tools for providing a comprehensive understanding of surveillance data, they have not been widely used because more often than not, surveillance data are of insufficient quantity (and quality) to successfully employ the more advanced of these methods.

OCCUPATIONAL DISEASE AND INJURY SURVEILLANCE

In 1987, the National Academy of Sciences conducted an in-depth study of the problems surrounding occupational injury and disease surveillance (Pollack & Keimig, 1987). The study noted several problems and challenges. For example, surveillance is hampered by latency between exposures and disease outcomes. In addition, many of the conditions caused by occupational exposures may also be caused by other nonoccupational factors. This situation may mislead the clinician making the diagnosis. It also may make it difficult to link workplace exposures to disease. Finally, there is no single information system that fully describes the impact of occupational disease and injury in the United States.

Rutstein, Mullan, Frazier, Halperin, Melius, and Sestito (1983) developed one way of handling the problems of occupational health surveillance. They established the concept of the sentinel health event: "preventable disease, disability, or untimely death which is occupationally related, and whose occurrence may provide the impetus for epidemiologic or industrial hygiene studies, or serve as a warning signal that materials substitution, engineering controls, personal protection, or special medical care may be required" (Rutstein et al., 1983). So although a sentinel health event signals a failure of public health prevention efforts, it also represents an opportunity to prevent further disease occurrences.

In 1987, the Centers for Disease Control's (CDC) National Institute of Occupational Safety and Health (NIOSH) instituted the Sentinel Event Notification Systems for Occupational Risk (SENSOR) program as a means of doing occupational disease and injury surveillance (Baker, Honchar, & Fine, 1989). The SENSOR program is conducted by state health departments; its primary goal is to prevent occupational disease and injury. More generally, SENSOR programs seek to

- identify new (or unrecognized) conditions (i.e., occupational diseases, injuries, and hazards).
- identify "sentinel" conditions that represent failures of occupational health prevention.
- determine the extent and distribution of occupational conditions.
- track trends over time.
- target occupations, industries, and workplaces for preventive consultations.
- disseminate information to assist decision-makers.

The steps for conducting occupational health surveillance include the following:

- Establish a case definition (i.e., event to be monitored).
- Develop a case ascertainment and data management system.
- Establish interventions, such as publications and educational efforts for affected industries, workers, and health practitioners, for the immediate and long-term prevention of the condition.
- Conduct worksite visits for hazard abatement and co-worker screening.
- Make regulatory agency referrals.
- Conduct investigations to develop control technology.
- Conduct data analyses to ascertain trends, patterns, and provide intervention guidance.
- Disseminate surveillance information to contribute to occupational disease and injury prevention.
- Ensure that surveillance protocols protect patient rights and confidentiality.
- Evaluate surveillance and intervention efforts.
- Standardize surveillance protocols.

THE EVOLUTION OF OCCUPATIONAL HEALTH SURVEILLANCE PRACTICE—PROJECT SENSOR/CTS IN WISCONSIN

Wisconsin was one of 10 states initially selected by CDC-NIOSH to participate in the SENSOR program. From 1987 through 1991, a passive surveillance activity was undertaken, analyzing the Wisconsin workers' compensation file for "probable" occupational carpal tunnel syndrome (OCTS) cases. In addition, the sentinel event-sentinel reporter active surveillance technique was used to obtain cases of OCTS (Hanrahan, Higgins, Anderson, Haskins, & Tai, 1991). Starting in 1993, the SENSOR-CTS program employed the passive-active technique. An administrative database—hospital discharge records—was searched for CTS surgery cases. The physicians treating the cases were then actively surveyed to obtain surveillance information (Hanrahan, Higgins, Anderson, & Smith, 1993).

Passive Surveillance

Time trends and risks by industry and occupation were determined from the Wisconsin workers' compensation data (Hanrahan, Higgins, Anderson, Haskins, & Tai, 1991). From case reviews, "probable" OCTS cases—those classified "disease of peripheral nervous system at the wrist"—were selected. A significant, five-fold increase in the OCTS rate was seen from 1983 to 1988 (from 25 to 115 cases per 100,000). For the entire time period, the overall rate for OCTS was estimated at 70 per 100,000 Wisconsin workers, while in high-risk industries, such as poultry and meat processing, the rates were 820 and 740 per 100,000 workers, respectively. As expected, occupations with highly repetitive, manual tasks were at highest risk. Those at risk included dental hygienists, data entry keyers, electronic equipment assemblers, sewing machine operators, assemblers, butchers, and workers employed in hand-cutting occupation (Hanrahan & Moll, 1989).

Although trends and high-risk industries and occupations could be identified, this surveillance activity was limited because of its use of "probable OCTS" cases. That is, this was information obtained from the workers' compensation first report of injury. It was not a diagnostic abstract filled out by a treating physician. In addition, the analyses could be further limited because of other aspects of the workers' compensation system. For example, the data may have also underreported the number of conditions because Wisconsin has a three-lost-work-day waiting period requirement to qualify for workers' compensation, self-employed workers may not be required to carry workers' compensation insurance, and covered workers may wish to forgo collecting compensation because it may be perceived as a threat to job tenure.

Active Surveillance

For active surveillance, approximately 25 clinicians were enrolled as reporting partners. The limitations of this active program were obvious. There were only 796 cases reported in the five-year period from 1987 to 1992, with less than 400 cases meeting the NIOSH SENSOR case definition (Matte, Baker, & Honchar, 1989) of CTS symptoms, objective clinical diagnostic findings, and work-relatedness. Because only a very small number of reporters were involved, this approach was unable to track time trends or estimate the magnitude of the OCTS burden by industry, occupation, age, or gender. In a very limited sense, it could identify individual candidate worksites for preventive consultations however.

Passive-Active Surveillance

Carpal tunnel release surgery was made a reportable outpatient procedure in June 1990, with over 9,000 episodes performed annually in Wisconsin (Hanrahan, Higgins, Anderson, & Smith, 1993). The Office of Health Care Information (OCHI) maintains the inpatient and outpatient discharge data. Data are based on hospital billing information. In conjunction with CDC-NIOSH, the OCTS case definition was modified in 1993 to capitalize on the surgery data newly available to the SENSOR program (see Table 10.1). CTS cases were defined as outpatient and inpatient discharges, with a diagnostic mention of carpal tunnel syndrome and a procedural mention of carpal tunnel release. Because of the tremendous case volume, one year's data were selected for active surveillance follow-

**Table 10.1. Wisconsin SENSOR Carpal Tunnel Syndrome
Surveillance Case Definition (1993–1997)**

Classification	Code	Description
		Diagnosis
ICD9-CM*	354.0	Carpal tunnel syndrome
		Procedure
ICD9-CM	04.43	Carpal tunnel release
CPT-4**	64721	Neuroplasty and/or transposition; median nerve at carpal tunnel
CPT-4	29848	Arthroscopy, wrist, surgical; with release of transverse carpal tunnel ligament

International Classification of Diseases: Clinical Modification (9th revision).
**Physician's Current Procedural Terminology* (4th edition).

up. That is, cases meeting the diagnostic and procedural criteria were selected and descriptively analyzed (passive surveillance). Once cases had been selected, physicians were contacted to obtain additional case information (active surveillance).

The active surveillance component was done by developing a follow-back form with CDC-NIOSH technical assistance (see appendix). Hospital discharge case identifiers were "mail-merged" to the form. The medical record number, hospital, attending physician name and license number, and surgery date were listed on each report form. In addition, all known patient identifiers, such as the first initials of the last and first name, the date of birth, age at surgery, gender, race, and ethnicity, were included. Forms were then mailed to the attending physician's office for completion. The information requested included the patient's full name and address, phone number, usual occupation and job duties, place of employment and kind of business, date and locus of CTS diagnosis and surgery, origins of CTS (work or nonwork cumulative trauma, acute trauma, 17 preexisting conditions [and others]), workers' compensation status, and comments.

For analysis purposes, work-related cases were determined by either a designation of case payment for workers' compensation (from OHCI or the attending physician), or the surgeon's determination that the case was work related. In addition, because all CTS surgery cases for one year were enrolled in the surveillance system, absolute CTS surgery risk could be determined by age, gender, industry, and occupation irrespective of the work-relatedness opinion.

CTS Surgery Surveillance—Analysis of Data

Four quarters of hospital discharge data were followed (July 1993–June 1994). A total of 9,359 surgical episodes were identified for 7,853 patients. Approximately 94% indicated carpal tunnel syndrome as the principal diagnosis, and 95% had carpal tunnel release as the principal procedure. The crude annual surgical rate was 173 per 100,000 persons. For women, the rate was 207 per 100,000, while for men, it was 138 per 100,000. The ratio of these two rates (207/138) produced a relative risk of 1.5. Thus, females had a 50% higher surgical rate when compared with males. (The distribution of CTS surgery rates by age and gender is displayed in Figure 10.1.) Surgery risks increase dramatically in both genders after age 24.

These surgeries were performed by over 400 physicians. When follow-up forms

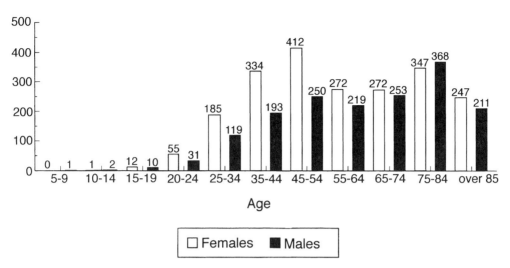

Figure 10.1. All CTS surgery rates / 100,000: Wisconsin (July 1993–June 1994).

were mailed to the patient's attending physician, 5,588 surgical reports were returned (59.7% response rate), representing 4,779 patients (60.9% response rate). In 33% of cases, the surgeon indicated that the CTS was caused or exacerbated by work, with 31% of the patients filing for workers compensation, and 30% were caused by work-related-cumulative trauma. An additional 17% were classified as possibly due to work related cumulative trauma. (Note that percentages should not add up to 100% because multiple categories may have been checked.) Using the aforementioned definitions for work-relatedness, an estimated 44% of cases were found to be job related (see Figure 10.2). Males had a higher percentage of work-related cases, and work-related percentages decreased with age for both males and females.

For 8% of the cases, non-work-related cumulative trauma was indicated as a cause, while 3% were thought to be due to acute trauma. Only 4% of the cases listed an underlying comorbidity as a potential cause of CTS. In approximately 39% of cases, the etiology was unknown.

Figures 10.3 through 10.5 depict work-related percentages for a subset of cases in industries and occupations that were coded as of April, 1996. Figures 10.3 and 10.4 display the percentages of cases listed as work-related by industry and gender groups. Work-relatedness was highest for those patients working in manufacturing (90% females, 81% males), retail trade (61% females, 72% males), and transportation (74% females, 50% males). Males in the construction industry also had a very high percentage of work-relatedness (81%). Males and females who were, machine workers, precision production and craft workers, laborers, and transportation operatives had nearly all CTS cases listed as work-related (see Figure 10.5). In contrast, professionals, executives and farmers had a much lower rate of work-relatedness (see Figure 10.6). Interestingly, male and female sales workers and administrative support workers demonstrated very different OCTS percentages. Males were relatively low (18% sales, 33% administrative support), while females were much higher (75% sales, 67% administrative support) (Figure 10.6).

Using the 44% work-related case rate, and weighting cases to adjust for nonresponse,

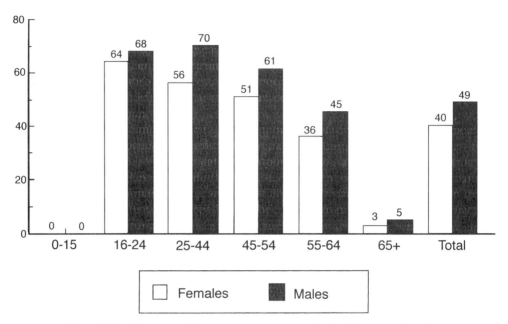

Figure 10.2. Wisconsin CTS surgery: Percentage work related by age and gender.

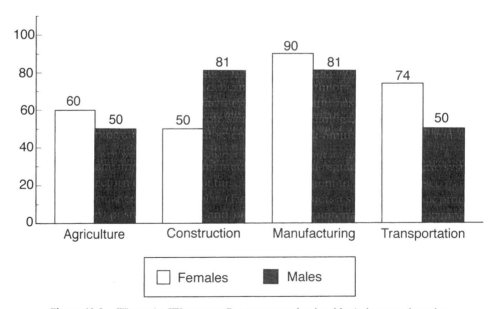

Figure 10.3. Wisconsin CTS surgery: Percentage work related by industry and gender.

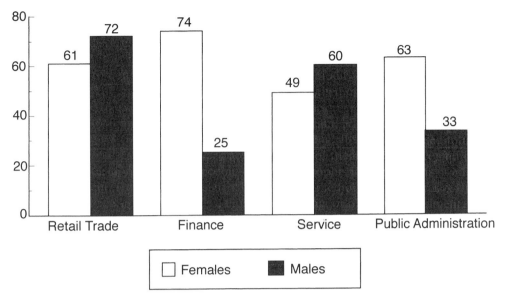

Figure 10.4. Wisconsin CTS surgery: Percentage work related by industry and gender.

resulted in a crude annual surgery incidence of 143 per 100,000 Wisconsin workers for OCTS (116/100,000 for males, 175/100,000 for females). Annual age-specific and gender-specific OCTS surgery rates were calculated for Wisconsin (shown in Figure 10.7). The figure also included the nation's objective for the year 2000 as a reference (60 per 100,000 workers *for all cumulative trauma disorders*, as set by the U.S. Department of Health

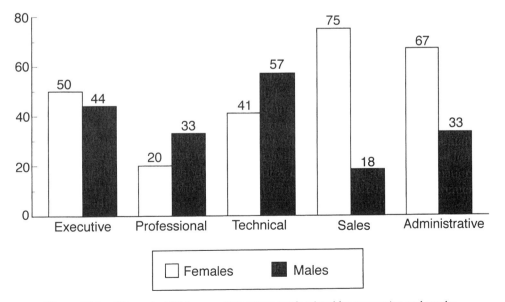

Figure 10.5. Wisconsin CTS Surgery: Percentage work related by occupation and gender.

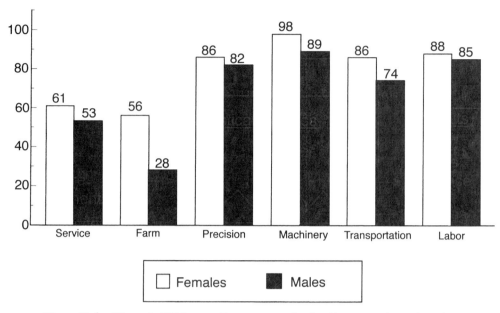

Figure 10.6. Wisconsin CTS Surgery: Percentage work related by occupation and gender.

and Human Services, Public Health Service, 1991). Only Wisconsin workers aged 16–24 are below the national objective: 38 (females) and 22 (males) OCTS cases per 100,000 workers. The rate of OCTS for working women aged 25–44 and 55–64 is over three times greater than the target, while for women 45–54, it is nearly five times greater than the target of 60 per 100,000 for all work-related cumulative trauma disorders. Men experienced somewhat lower risks than women, but here again after age 24, each rate was higher than the year 2000 objective.

These data were used to approximate the magnitude of the OCTS problem in the United States. When these age-specific and gender-specific rates are projected onto the United States working population (see Figure 10.8), it is an estimated that 336,000 patients with occupational CTS will require surgery annually. Case frequencies peak for both genders in the 25–44-year-old age group, and thereafter steadily decline with age. Only a small number of OCTS surgery cases occur among 16–24 year olds and among those aged 65 and older.

Surveillance Information Dissemination

These initial descriptive analyses will be elaborated on with incidence rate studies by the SENSOR program. These SENSOR incidence rate investigations will pinpoint high risk industries and occupations and adjust for age and gender groups. Based on these results, higher risk industries and occupations will be targeted for comprehensive surveillance information dissemination activities and consultative interventions. At risk populations in Wisconsin will be ranked according to relative risk and size. Groups at the top of this ranking will be invited to participate in prevention seminars. They will receive a surveillance information bulletin that will underscore their risk profiles and point out

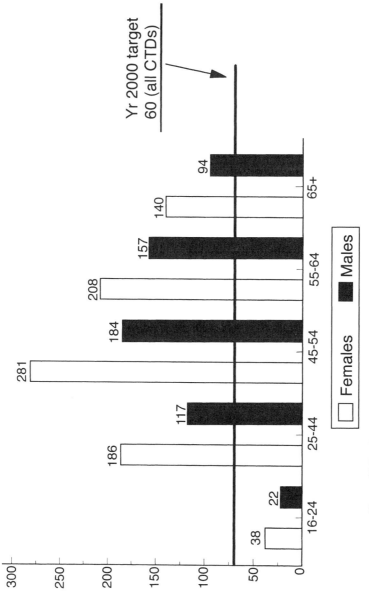

Figure 10.7. Wisconsin annual CTS surgery rates / 100,000: Work related by age and gender.

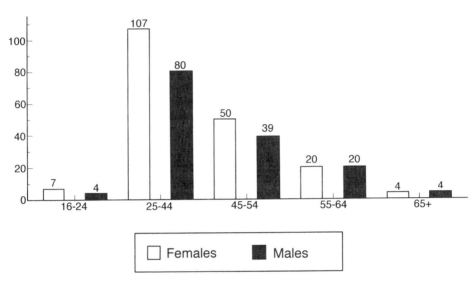

Figure 10.8. CTS surgery: Work related U.S. annual estimates, in thousands.

opportunities for CTS prevention. These analyses will also be used to direct on-site intervention programs that will provide technical assistance for the prevention of OCTS.

THE FUTURE OF SURVEILLANCE

Information Revolution

Surveillance, like epidemiology, is fundamentally an information science. Computers, or more correctly, personal computers, represent the "big bang" for both health science fields. Before computers, epidemiology and surveillance activities were conducted in a "dark void" of intensive manual labor. The number of data elements and questions asked were limited, owing to the tremendous cost of collecting and analyzing the resulting information. Statistical analyses were simplified out of necessity. Indeed, all of the sophisticated analytic tools commonly available today (and all of which are now easily run on ordinary desktop computers) were only uncommonly available on large and expensive-to-run mainframe computers less than 20 years ago. In the past, more advanced statistical analysis tools had to be developed "in-house." Less than 20 years ago, logistic regression programs would run only on large mainframe computers. In contrast, the home computers of today have essentially the computing power of mainframes of less than a generation ago.

The formation of the Internet, or World Wide Web (www), a global network to connect local area networks, mainframes, and personal computers, is the second stage in the evolution of health information systems. It may well play the dominant role in the future collection, analysis, and dissemination of surveillance information. The creation of the World Wide Web has solved two important problems for surveillance: information connectivity and information compatibility. Because of the web, data systems and information products no longer need be isolated on stand-alone computer systems that have custom access methods. Instead, information can be managed so that those who need access to it can obtain it, regardless of where the information and the user reside. The second problem, compatibility, has been solved by the web's use of standards that may be implemented on virtually all operating systems and hardware platforms. Thus, even though individual, corporate, and government data systems may use differing information "currencies," web software systems have developed "currency exchange protocols" that allow disparate information sources to be linked and processed.

Indeed, many word-processing and statistical analysis software programs now include features that allow the user to easily post documents or analyze output via the web. For example, the SAS Institute ("What an (un)tangled Web, We Weave," 1997) has just released web-enabled applications for its statistical analysis product. These application allow users to routinely post static web pages from analysis programs that are routinely run (daily, weekly, etc.). One can also create dynamic web pages from users' interactive queries and requests for analyses of databases.

Another important web development is the push server. Push servers are systems through which users receive information automatically from a network server (Spangler, 1997). Under this arrangement, the needed information finds the user. Thus persons requiring routine access to data in the future will subscribe to the surveillance information channel. Each user will then receive updated information on a periodic basis in one of two ways: the user's client software will poll the server for an update, or the server will always be broadcasting, while the client software will be constantly in a listening mode.

Using these tools and others, health data systems that are web-enabled will participate in the automation of surveillance data collection, analysis, dissemination, and evaluation. In this way, surveillance will be closely integrated into clinical and rehabilitative practice for the improvement of all levels of care and, ultimately, of public health.

In contrast, clinical links to current health information systems are still largely designed for billing purposes and not ongoing process improvement. The Wisconsin SENSOR-CTS experience of the past five years has shown that for may clinicians surveillance activities represent an intrusion into the work of providing the best possible clinical care to their patients. This attitude stems from the fact that even though CTS cases have been identified by passive, electronic administrative databases, clinic staff must, in the "active-pull" phase, review patient charts and abstract information for surveillance forms and then mail the forms to the surveillance center. The world wide web holds the promise of eliminating this and other inefficiencies. A description of how such a system could function follows.

The web-enabled, clinical health information systems of tomorrow will automatically flag cases meeting epidemiologic study and surveillance-reporting criteria. Web-enabled surveillance and epidemiologic study forms will link up with the patient at the time of diagnosis and treatment. Patients, will then "opt-in" to epidemiologic study protocols and surveillance systems, with the help of the clinic staff at the point of health care service delivery. In hospitals, clinics, and practitioner offices, patients will access health data kiosks to provide surveillance information and interview data for epidemiologic studies aimed at determining causal factors. In this way, the burden of case reporting for clinical practitioners will be reduced, and surveillance data collection cycle time will be reduced vastly.

Once the surveillance or epidemiologic data are collected by the clinic's intranet, it will be encrypted and all personal identifiers removed. This processed information then will be securely transmitted to a surveillance center or epidemiologic study web site (e.g., managed care organization, state health department, university research center, CDC). Once at the center, web-enabled analysis tools will process the input and dynamically update the surveillance or web page. The updated surveillance information will then be "pushed" by the server back to surveillance or study data users. Thus, through web technologies that are available today, all aspects of surveillance (collection, analysis, dissemination) and epidemiologic research can be easily automated.

A number of challenges confront the evolution of this system. These challenges include guaranteeing absolutely secure transactions to protect patients' rights and confidentiality, data validation, data sharing among competing managed health care plans, and patient participation.

Perhaps the most important of these is patient education. Education is needed to secure patient participation at a sufficient response level to make the effort worthwhile. The patient will need to fully understand the importance of surveillance and participation in epidemiologic studies. This education should bring about a new patient attitude toward and participation in health care by instilling in the patient the feeling that his or her health care is deficient if he or she has not been asked to provide information that aids in health process improvement.

This cybernation of health care, or process control by computer, holds the promise for a vast improvement in all stages of health care delivery and public health. The key is the technologic revolution of informatics described here, and all that it implies for surveillance and epidemiology. This evolution will serve as the technologic basis for the emerging field of health systems cybernetics.

Health Systems Cybernetics: Surveillance, Epidemiology and Health Care in the Twenty-First Century

Health systems cybernetics represents the fusion and synthesis of a number of fields, including (a) cybernetic control and systems theory; (b) information science (informatics); (c) statistical quality control and process improvement techniques; and (d) public health surveillance and epidemiology. These fields are interrelated. Cybernetics will provide the overriding theory of this emerging field, while informatics will determine how it will be physically executed. Statistical quality control techniques will provide the necessary analytic tools for governing process, while surveillance and epidemiology provide the necessary health sciences context.

Cybernetics (and systems theory) is concerned with the study of control processes in electronic, mechanical, and biological systems, and especially the analysis of information flow in such systems. Advanced cybernetic control theory largely developed out of research conducted during World War II (Smith, 1945) and has since been applied to a broad range of fields, including the physical sciences, biology, psychology, human behavior and physiology, and the social sciences (Smith & Smith, 1966, 1973; von Bertalanffy, 1972).

Feedback is one important control mechanism in self-regulating cybernetic systems. Feedback, or the return of a portion of the output of a system to its input, is used to maintain system performance or to control it. (Figure 10.9 depicts a simple feedback process.) Thermoregulation, postural control, and blood sugar maintenance are all examples of feedback control mechanisms that function in biologic systems. The household thermostat is a mechanical example. It too functions as a closed-loop feedback control system: A temperature target is set; the ambient temperature is analyzed; and the furnace is

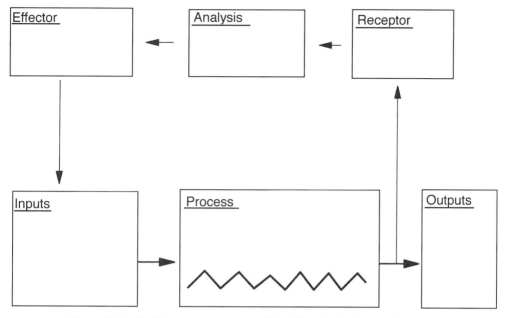

Figure 10.9. Health systems cybernetics: Closed-loop feedback control process.

switched on until the desired warmth is reached. Once the target is reached, the system switches the furnace off. The thermostat monitors the ensuing temperature drops and switches the furnace back on when the lower temperature limit is reached. Through this process, a steady-state ambient temperature is achieved in the home.

Similarly, in health systems cybernetics, surveillance functions as a sensing and analyzing function in a closed-loop feedback control process (se Figure 10.10). Outputs (e.g., injuries, diseases, hazards) are detected and fed into the surveillance analysis center. Once analyzed, this information is transmitted to effectors (epidemiology—ascertain causal factors to control, intervention trials, etc.) to modify the inputs (person, task, environment). The success or failure of this process is then monitored relative to a preset target value (e.g., 60 cases of cumulative trauma disorders per 100,000 workers).

With the total automation of the health data stream, advanced statistical process control techniques (Deming, 1992; Ishakawa, 1985; King, 1995) can be used to understand the root causes of systems variations and control them. Surveillance and epidemiologic investigations then can become much more sophisticated in terms of information development. That is, using design of experiments methods (Box, Hunter, & Hunter, 1978; King, 1995; SAS Institute, 1994), directed sampling, or planned experimental runs may be developed from the observational surveillance case data. Using this scientific, statistical experimentation methodology, complex causal and risk-factor information can be more rapidly obtained. And this, in turn, can bring about a more rapid improvement to population health.

In the health systems cybernetics model, surveillance functions as a closed-loop feedback control tracking system. But instead of achieving a homeostasis or steady state, its goal is the management of system inputs to continually lower disease and injury rates (or conversely, continually improve health). This process of control functions at every

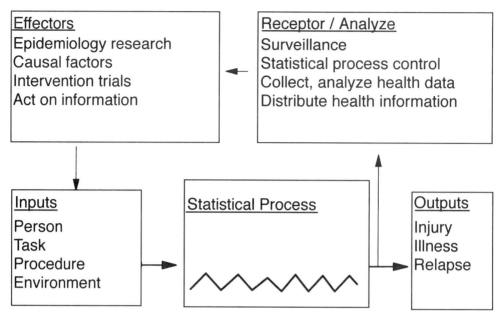

Figure 10.10. Health systems cybernetics: Surveillance, feedback control process.

level of the health care system (see Figure 10.11). Here, all levels of the process are improved. In primary tracking control, job risk factors and hazards are eliminated. In secondary tracking control, the process improves the early diagnosis (detection) and treatment (outcomes research). In tertiary tracking control, the process improves injury case management, rehabilitation, and reintegration into the workforce.

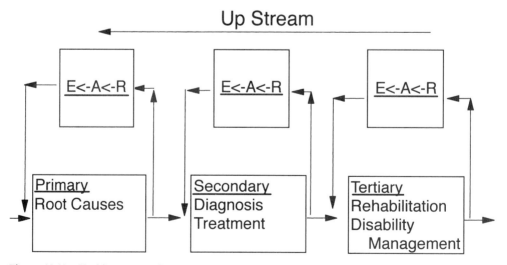

Figure 10.11. Health systems cybernetics: Receptor-analysis-effector feedback control (primary, secondary, and tertiary process improvement).

Surveillance activities have long been the sole province of public health agencies. However, changes in our health care system, including the movement toward health maintenance and managed care organizations, have begun to expand the focus of clinical-based systems. Because they are no longer simply individual treatment based, these systems will increasingly take on a population health perspective. This perspective is a most necessary one if the process of care is to be scientifically improved and result in perhaps the best of all methods for containing costs. Cost containment should lead to the widespread implementation of surveillance activities in the private health care sector. Indeed, one major nongovernmental initiative is the National Committee for Quality Assurance's (NCQA) Health Plan Employer Data and Information Set (HEDIS) system, which provides quality of care targets that examine the health care system from a population perspective. With these targets in place, cybernetic health systems will be needed to track successful compliance with target goals.

The Significance of Surveillance to Occupational Rehabilitation

Surveillance is important to the field of occupational rehabilitation in the following ways: First, surveillance allows us to understand the sources of patient injury (i.e., the occupational hazards that injure workers and the personal characteristics that place individuals at increased risk for injury). Through surveillance we can also determine the factors that need to be modified in the workplace, so that once a worker is returned to the job, she or he is not reinjured because of reexposure to a health hazard. Second, surveillance and epidemiologic analysis is also important to the occupational rehabilitation process itself. For example, surveillance activities can be implemented as part of the clinical rehabilitative process. When these functions are linked the epidemiologic analysis of patient outcomes, they can perform a vital function in improving the success rate of care and reintegration into the workplace. That is, through surveillance one can determine which rehabilitative treatments and placements work best, and through epidemiology why certain practices may have a less than desirable positive outcome rate. In this way, surveillance and epidemiologic analyses can serve as techniques to improve the process of occupational rehabilitative practice.

WISCONSIN DIVISION OF HEALTH - CARPAL TUNNEL SYNDROME SURVEILLANCE CASE REPORT
INSTRUCTIONS TO PROVIDERS

The Wisconsin Department of Health and Family Services (DHFS) requests surveillance reporting of all cases of carpal tunnel syndrome. All data will be held in strict confidence [Wisconsin SS Chapter 250.04(3)(b)(3)]. Because aggregate information is the goal of the project, patient names and any other identifiers will not be utilized in any manner for the analysis. All results will be published only as statistical summaries. These data will be available, upon request, to your facility for your use. According to Wisconsin Statutes, Chapter 146.82(2)5, DHFS may have access to a patient's medical records without the patient's prior consent. The agency (DHFS) must submit a written request, which this correspondence serves as, and be performing public health research or an investigation as an authorized function [Chapter 140.05 (1 and 14) Wisconsin SS].

The following case of surgical treatment for carpal tunnel syndrome has been reported to the Wisconsin Division of Health. Please complete our surveillance on this case by filling in the blanks. If you have any questions, please contact Jeanette Tierney (608) 266-7298 or Larry Hanrahan at (608) 267-7173. Please place reports in the postage paid envelope provided. We appreciate your cooperation. Note: Some of the fields will be filled out for you. If any are incorrect, please cross out the information and fill in with corrections. Please complete the patient's name; only their initials are currently known.

MEDICAL RECORD #: 000000001

HOSPITAL: General Surgery Hospital, Inc.

ATTENDING PHYSICIAN: Jay Smith, MD   LICENSE #:0000000   SURGERY DATE: 9/1/96

Check here if CTS was caused or exacerbated by work: ____Yes. ____No.

PATIENT INFORMATION:

DATE OF BIRTH: 5/10/66   AGE: 30   GENDER: Male   RACE: White   ETHNICITY: _____

LAST NAME: A_____   FIRST NAME: B_____   MI: _____

ADDRESS: _____

CITY: _____   STATE: _____ ZIPCODE: 55555

PHONE: (____)_____

USUAL OCCUPATION: _____

USUAL JOB DUTIES: _____

EMPLOYER NAME: _____

EMPLOYER ADDRESS: _____

EMPLOYER CITY: _____   STATE: _____ ZIPCODE: _____

EMPLOYER PHONE: (____)_____   TYPE OF BUSINESS: _____

CLINICAL DIAGNOSIS: Please circle each diagnosis you made and indicate the date:

CTS Right Wrist: Yes   No   Date: _____

CTS Left Wrist: Yes   No   Date: _____

SURGICAL TREATMENT on **9/1/96** was for:

Right hand CTS release surgery   Yes   No

Left hand CTS release surgery   Yes   No

(OVER, PLEASE)

FOR OFFICE USE ONLY: DATE: YEAR AND QUARTER: HDSNUM:00000001
                       9/15/97   3/96

ORIGINS OF CARPAL TUNNEL SYNDROME: This particular case of CTS was related to the following risk factors **(indicate all that apply by circling Yes, No or Possible).**

CTS as a consequence of work related cumulative trauma.	Yes	No	Possible
CTS as a consequence of non-work related cumulative trauma.	Yes	No	Possible
CTS as a consequence of acute trauma (eg., fall; crushing injury).	Yes	No	Possible
CTS as a result of aggravation of a pre-existing condition (eg. diabetes).	Yes	No	Possible

If yes or possible to pre-existing conditions, please check all that apply below:

___ 1. Diabetes
___ 2. Oral contraceptive use
___ 3. Post menopausal estrogen use
___ 4. Natural menopause
___ 5. Obesity
___ 6. Presently pregnant
___ 7. Gout
___ 8. Rheumatoid arthritis
___ 9. Arthritis

___ 10. Congenital defects: _____
___ 11. Osteo arthritis
___ 12. Ganglions
___ 13. Myxedema
___ 14. Acromegaly
___ 15. Cervical radiculopathy
___ 16. Thoracic outlet syndrome
___ 17. Pronator teres syndrome
___ 18. Other (specify): _____

CTS etiology is unknown.   Yes   No

PAYOR:

Was a Workers Compensation case filed (please circle)?   Yes   No   Don't Know

ADDITIONAL COMMENTS:

_____
_____
_____
_____
_____
_____
_____
_____

Form Completed by: _____ Date: _____

Daytime Telephone: (_____) _____

Wisconsin Department of Health and Family Services
Division of Health
SENSOR-CTS Project

REFERENCES

Baker, E. L., Honchar, P. A., & Fine, L. J. (1989, December). Surveillance in occupational illness and injury: Concepts and content. *American Journal of Public Health*, 79(Suppl. 12), 9–11.

Bernard, B. P. (Ed.). (1997). *Musculoskeletal disorders and workplace factors: A critical review of epidemiologic evidence for work-related musculoskeletal disorders of the neck, upper extremity, and low back* (DHHS Publication No. 97-141). Washington, DC.

Cates, W., & Williamson, D. (1994). Descriptive epidemiology: Analyzing and interpreting surveillance data. In

S. M. Teutsch & R. E. Churchill (Eds.), *Principles and practice of public health surveillance* (pp. 96-135). New York: Oxford University Press.

Dillman, D. A. (1978). *Mail and telephone surveys: The total design method.* New York: Wiley.

Dorland's Illustrated Medical Dictionary (27th ed.) (1988). Philadelphia, PA: W. B. Saunders.

Deming, W. E. (1992). *Out of the crisis.* Boston, MA: Cambridge Press.

Ehrenberg, R. L., & Sniezek, J. E. (1989, December). Development of a standard questionnaire for occupational health research. *American Journal of Public Health, 79*(Suppl. 12), 15-17.

Hanrahan, L. P., & Moll, M. B. (1989, December). Injury surveillance. *American Journal of Public Health, 79*(Suppl. 12), 38-45.

Hanrahan, L. P., Higgins, D. N., Anderson, H. A., & Haskins, L. K. (1991, February). Project SENSOR: Wisconsin surveillance of occupational carpal tunnel syndrome. *Wisconsin Medical Journal, 90*(20), 39-41.

Hanrahan, L. P., Higgins, D., Anderson, H., & Smith, M. J. (1993, December). Wisconsin carpal tunnel syndrome surveillance: The incidence of surgically treated cases. *Wisconsin Medical Journal* (12), 685-689.

International classification of diseases: Clinical modification (9th revision), 1994 hospital edition, Vols. 1, 2, 3 (1993). Los Angeles: Practice Management Information Corporation.

Ishikawa, K. (1985). *What is total quality control? The Japanese way.* (D. J. Lu, Trans.) Englewood Cliffs, NJ: Prentice-Hall.

King, D. W. (1995). *Statistical quality control using the SAS system.* Cary, NC: SAS Institute.

Klauke, D. N., Buehler, J. W., Thaker, S.B. (1988). Guidelines for evaluating surveillance systems. *Morbidity and Mortality Weekly Reports, 37*(Suppl. 5), 1-18.

Kleinbaum, D. G., Kupper, L. L., & Morgenstern, H. (1982). *Epidemiologic research: Principles and quantitative methods.* Belmont, CA: Lifetime Learning Publications.

Matte, T. D., Baker, E. L., & Honchar, P. A. (1989, December). The selection and definition of targeted work-related conditions for surveillance under SENSOR. *American Journal of Public Health, 79*(Suppl. 12), 21-25.

National Committee for Quality Assurance (NCQA). (1996). *1996 health plan employer data and information set* (Version 3.0) (HEDIS 3.0). Washington, DC: Author.

Palmer, D. H., & Hanrahan, L. P. (1995). Social and economic costs of carpal tunnel surgery. *American Academy of Orthopaedic Surgeons: Instructional Course Lectures, 44,* 167-72.

Physician's current procedural terminology (4th edition) (1993). Chicago: American Medical Association.

Pollack, E. S., & Keimig, D. G. (Eds.). (1987). *Counting injuries and illnesses in the workplace: Proposals for a better system.* Washington, DC: National Academy Press.

Rutstein, D. D., Mullan, R. J., Frazier, T. M., Halperin, W.E., Melius, J. M., & Sestito, J. P. (1983). Sentinel health events (occupational): A basis for physician recognition and public health surveillance. *American Journal of Public Health, 73,* 1054-1062.

SAS Institute. (1989). *SAS/STAT users guide, version 6, volume 2, fourth edition.* Cary, NC: Author.

SAS Institute. (1994). *SAS/QC software: ADX menu system for design of experiments* Version 6, 1st ed. Cary, NC: Author.

Smith, K. U. (1945). *Behavioral systems analysis of aircraft gun systems: Special report.* Washington, DC: US Air Force Air Materials Command.

Smith, K. U., & Smith, M. F. (1966). *Cybernetic principles of learning and educational design.* New York: Holt, Rinehart & Winston.

Smith, K. U., & Smith, M. F. (1973). *Psychology: An introduction to behavior science.* Boston, MA: Little, Brown.

Spangler, T. (1997, June 10). Push servers: The intranet channel. *PC Magazine, 16*(10), 156-180.

Sullivan, K. M., Gibbs, N. P., & Knowles, C. M. (1994). Management of surveillance system and quality control of data. In S. M. Teutsch, & R. E. Churchill (Eds.). *Principles and practice of public health surveillance* (pp. 86-95). New York: Oxford University Press.

U.S. Department of Health and Human Services, Public Health Service. (1991). *Healthy people 2000: National health promotion and disease prevention objectives.* Washington, DC: Author.

von Bertalanffy, L. (1972). *General system theory: Foundations, development, applications.* New York: George Braziller.

What an (un)tangled web we weave. (1997, Quarter 1). *SAS Communications,* 16-21.

III

ASSESSMENT OF WORK-RELATED DISORDERS

11

Functional Capacity Evaluation

Deborah E. Lechner

An automobile mechanic experiences sharp radiating pain down his leg while working over the engine of a small British sports car. He has just finished a course of acute care physical therapy, and his physician is wondering if he is ready to return to work. A licensed practical nurse applies for a job at a nursing home. Her prospective employer offers her the job but wonders if she has the physical abilities to meet the job demands. A steel worker with postpolio syndrome and ankylosing spondylitis finds that with each passing month he is having increasing difficulty completing his physical work responsibilities. He is wondering if it is finally time to apply for disability. An injured construction worker has just entered a five-week course of work conditioning and work simulation. His therapist needs to set work-related goals for the program. All of these individuals could benefit from an objective, reliable, and valid functional capacity evaluation (FCE).

An FCE is designed to determine an individual's ability to perform safely the physical demands of work (Lechner, Roth, & Straaton, 1991). It is an essential evaluation tool for determining readiness to return to work after injury, performing preemployment/postoffer screening, making disability determinations, performing goal-setting treatment planning for industrial rehabilitation, monitoring progress throughout industrial rehabilitation, and determining case closure. The importance of an FCE for effective decision making in an occupational health practice cannot be overemphasized.

Prior to the use of FCEs, return-to-work decisions were based on diagnosis and/or impairment measures. Often physicians merely asked clients if they felt they were ready to resume working. Sometimes decisions were based on observations of client movement or pain behaviors during a brief office visit. Clients were not asked to demonstrate performance of work-related tasks. Instead physicians often used intuitive clinical judgment to make return-to-work decisions. The quality of these intuitive decisions varied greatly from clinician to clinician. The FCE evolved in response to a need for more

Deborah E. Lechner • Division of Physical Therapy, School of Health Related Professions, University of Alabama at Birmingham, Birmingham, Alabama 35294.

Sourcebook of Occupational Rehabilitation, edited by Phyllis M. King. Plenum Press, New York, 1998.

objective, consistent, and accurate observation-based testing. Well-designed FCEs offer distinct advantages to the intuitive and diagnosis-based processes.

FEATURES OF A WELL-DESIGNED FCE

Well-designed FCEs are not unlike other well-designed clinical measures. They should be comprehensive and standardized, yet flexible enough to meet "real-world" clinical demands. They should be safe, objective, feasible, reliable, and valid. Optimally, an FCE's procedures are based on scientific evidence in the literature or research conducted by the test developer.

Comprehensiveness

Clinical measures should cover all the domains of the variable being examined. In an FCE, this means that all 20 physical demands of work as described by the Department of Labor in the *Dictionary of Occupational Titles* (*DOT*) (U.S. Department of Labor, 1991) should be examined (see Table 11.1). An addendum to the *DOT*, the *Revised Classification of Jobs* (Field & Field, 1992), expands the *DOT* classification by describing and defining the intensity and frequency of the demands of work. Materials handling tasks are rated as sedentary, light, medium, heavy, and very heavy (see Table 11.2). Position and mobility demands are rated according to the percentage of the workday that each must be performed: constantly, frequently, occasionally, and never (Table 11.2). Because the categories used to describe the intensity and/or frequency of each of the demands are broad (i.e., a material-handling demand that falls into the medium category can range from 21 lb to 50 lb), there is a need to define more specifically the job demands and client abilities within each category in order to adequately match the worker to the job and prevent injury. Optimally, each client's job demands should be assessed directly rather than by relying on a *DOT* description. Individual jobs are often very different from their *DOT* listing. If a direct observation is not possible or feasible, then a formal written job description based on a previous job-site assessment can be used. Unfortunately, many job descriptions do not provide comprehensive descriptions of the physical demands of the jobs and must be supplemented by verbal descriptions from the client and employer. If neither a direct observation nor a formal written job description is available, a verbal description from the client combined with verification from the employer can be used for comparison. The source of the job description should always be documented in the summary report. If a job-site visit has not been made, the match between the client's abilities and job demands should be described as only an estimate. The examiner can suggest in the report that an on-site evaluation would permit a more precise comparison.

Some therapists include a musculoskeletal evaluation of the client's range of motion, muscle strength, posture, passive intervertebral mobility, sensation, reflexes, and other special tests as part of the FCE process. Their rationale for performing impairment evaluations is that the results can be correlated to function. Some therapists look for consistency between these impairment measures and function as evidence that the client is making a full effort during an FCE. In this author's view, a full musculoskeletal evaluation (including detailed range of motion measures, comprehensive manual muscle testing, joint mobility testing, postural assessment, gait analysis, and sensory testing) for the purpose of correlating impairment date to function is unnecessary. There is considerable evidence in the literature to prove that measures of impairment are not directly

**Table 11.1. Physical Demands of Work Defined
by the *Dictionary of Occupational Titles***

1. *Strength demands*
   Lifting: raising or lowering an object from one level to another
   Carrying: transporting an object, usually holding it in the hands or arms
   Pushing: exerting force on an object so that is moves away from the force
   Pulling: exerting force on an object so that it moves toward the force
   Standing: remaining on one's feet in an upright position without moving about
   Walking: moving about on foot
   Sitting: remaining in a seated position
2. *Climbing*: ascending or descending ladders, stairs, scaffolding, ramps, poles, etc.
3. *Balancing*: maintaining body equilibrium to prevent falling
4. *Stooping*: bending the body downward and forward by bending legs and spine at the waist
5. *Kneeling*: bending the legs at the knees to come to rest on knee or knees
6. *Crouching*: bending body downward and forward by bending legs and spine
7. *Crawling*: moving about on hands and knees or hands and feet
8. *Reaching*: extending arms and hands in any direction
9. *Handing*: seizing, holding, grasping, turning, or working with hands
10. *Fingering*: picking, pinching, or otherwise working primarily with the fingers
11. *Feeling*: perceiving attributes such as size, shape, temperature
12. *Talking**: expressing or exchanging ideas by means of the spoken word
13. *Hearing**: perceiving the nature of sounds by the ear
14. *Tasting/smelling**: distinguishing flavors or odors using the tongue and/or nose
15. *Near acuity**: clarity of vision at 20 inches or less
16. *Far acuity**: clarity of vision at 20 feet or more
17. *Depth perception**: abiity to judge distances and spatial relations
18. *Accommodation**: adjustment of lens of eyes to bring an object into sharp focus
19. *Color vision**: ability to identify and distinguish colors
20. *Field of vision**: observing and area that can be seen up and down and right and left when eyes
    are fixed on a given point

Source: J. E. Field & T. F. Field (1992). *Classification of Jobs* (pp. 3–4). Athens, GA: Elliott & Fitzpatrick. Copyright 1992 by Elliott & Fitzpatrick. Adapted with permission of T. F. Field.
*Demands assessed indirectly or informally during FCE. If problems are apparent, then patients are referred to the appropriate specialist for further evaluation.

related to function (Alexander, Maida, & Walker, 1975; Althouse, 1980; Dueker, Ritchie, Knox, & Rose, 1994; Jette, 1984; Newton & Waddell, 1993).

Consider the example of a client with ankylosing spondylitis whose illness has rendered his entire spine motionless. If one attempts to measure his spine range of motion, one finds that he has 0° of movement, yet he works 60 to 70 hours per week at a heavy level job. He has learned to compensate for his loss of spine motion and is highly motivated to work. At the other end of the spectrum is the client with a hypermobile spine whose range of motion measures are within normal limits, but who guards during functional activity to minimize the pain that results from functional movement. Another client may be fearful and guarded during the spine range of motion measures but more confident performing functional activities. The spine range of motion does not correlate to function in any of these individuals. The client in the first example is clearly not exaggerating his condition. The other two clients, however, are at risk of being perceived as not cooperating fully on either the musculoskeletal exam or the FCE, based on the consistency between the two exams. This assumption may or may not be correct and can label the client erroneously in the eyes of the employer, the physician, the case manager, and the attorney.

Table 11.2. Definitions of Work Intensity and Frequency

STRENGTH DEMANDS

Sedentary: Exerting up to 10 lb of force occasionally and/or a negligible amount of force frequently to lift, carry, push, pull, or otherwise move objects, including the human body. Involves sitting most of the time, but may involve walking or standing for brief periods of time.

Light: Exerting up to 20 lb of force occasionally and/or up to 10 lb of force frequently and/or a negligible amount of force constantly. Even when weight lifted is negligible, a job is rated light when (1) it involves walking or standing to a significant degree; (2) it requires sitting most of the time but involves pushing and/or pulling of arm or leg controls; (3) it involves working at a production rate that requires constant pushing or pulling of materials.

Medium: Exerting 20 to 50 lb of force occasionally and/or 10 to 25 lb of force frequently and/or up to 10 lb of force constantly. Physical demand requirements are greater than that required for Light work.

Heavy: Exerting 50 to 100 lb of force occasionally and/or 25 to 50 lb of force frequently and/or 10 to 20 lb of force constantly. Physiccal demands are greater than required for Light work.

Very heavy: Exerting greater than 100 lb of force occasionally and/or greater than 50 lb of force frequently and/or greater than 20 lb of force constantly. Physical demand requirements are greater than that required for Light work.

FREQUENCY DEMANDS

Never: Activity or condition does not exist.
Occasionally: Activity of condition exists up to ⅓ of the time.
Frequently: Activity or condition exists from ⅓ to ⅔ of the time.
Constantly: Activity or condition exists ⅔ or more of the time.

SOURCE: J. E. Field & T. F. Field (1992). *Classification of Jobs* (pp. 3–4). Athens, GA: Elliott & Fitzpatrick. Copyright 1992 by Elliott & Fitzpatrick. Adapted with permission of T. F. Field.

Rather than spend valuable evaluation time on measures that do not provide further information regarding function, musculoskeletal, neuromuscular, and cardiovascular screening procedures should be performed primarily on those clients who have "red flags" in their intake interviews. For example, a client who suffers episodes of sharp, burning pain that radiates down the leg as the result of certain movements over a discrete nerve root distribution should be screened for radiculopathy, using a straight leg raise test, slump test, reflexes, and myotomes. If the tests are positive for radicular symptoms, the examiner can proceed with the FCE, but she or he would be advised to discontinue tasks that reproduce the radicular symptoms. If the client reports symptoms of dizziness or blurred vision with neck extension or overhead work, the examiner should screen for vertebral artery insufficiency. If this test is positive, any tasks within the FCE that illicit symptoms of dizziness or blurred vision should be discontinued immediately.

Standardization

The procedures for test administration and scoring should be documented in a "user-friendly" procedure manual. The exact nature of the procedure manual will vary according to the nature of the evaluation. However, some basic elements should be included. The manual should begin with a general introduction to the testing approach and philosophy. In FCE testing, the examiner's attitude toward and interaction with the client can enhance or jeopardize the evaluation. A carefully articulated philosophy can set the tone for this interaction and promote trust between the examiner and client. Development of trust is perhaps the most crucial element for enhancing client cooperation and optimally occurs early in the contact between examiner and client.

Each task of the evaluation should be carefully defined and described according to the equipment needed and the exact procedures to be followed. Standardized verbal instructions are essential for minimizing examiner bias. The manual should also include precise instructions for scoring the client's performance. If the system is based on visual observation and classification of performance by the clinician, operational definitions are imperative. If the scoring system is to be repeatable and accurate, algorithms or formulas for projecting performance from a brief period of observation to an eight-hour day are essential. Without such algorithms, reliability and validity studies performed with one group of therapists cannot be generalized to other therapists.

Objectivity

Too often, objectivity is mistakenly associated exclusively with interval or ratio scales. To be objective, measures do not have to be expressed in terms of inches, foot-pounds of force, joules, degrees, and so on. A measure is objective when it is as free as possible from observer bias (Rothstein & Echternach, 1993). Observation of movement as the means of evaluating client performance also can be objective if the procedures and parameters of observation and the scoring system have been operationally defined. Reliability and validity research establishes the objectivity, consistency, and accuracy of the scoring system. We can never remove clinical judgment from the FCE process, nor would we want to do so. However, we can standardize and objectify the process so that each client receives a consistent, accurate, and unbiased evaluation.

Feasibility/Practicality

For responsible clinicians facing the challenge of providing high-quality service at a minimum cost to the client and to society at large, cost-effectiveness is paramount. The clinician's goal should be to perform no more testing than is necessary to provide accurate results. The clinician does not need to use expensive equipment unless peer-reviewed research demonstrates that using such equipment significantly improves the accuracy of the evaluation. To date, literature has supported the fact that reliable and valid FCEs can be performed using therapist observation and scoring in a one-day, three- to four-hour format (Lechner, Jackson, Roth, & Straaton, 1994). Can the same result be achieved in a shorter time? Would the reliability and validity be enhanced with videography, electromyography, electrogoniometry, or force plate analysis? Currently, there is no peer-reviewed research that addresses these issues.

Most therapists are interested in minimizing the time required for report writing. Most end users of FCEs (case managers, physicians, attorneys, employers, and vocational evaluators) are looking for reports that are understandable and concise, yet contain the necessary information. The primary elements of the report provide information regarding the client's safe level of work, specific limitations within that level, tolerance for an eight-hour day, and level of cooperation in testing, as well as a comparison of the client's abilities with the job demands (if there is a job to which the client can return). Most referral sources also expect a brief summary and recommendations section. Some FCE reports begin with a synopsis of the client's medical history. Others omit this section because this information is usually well known to all parties by the time an FCE is ordered.

There is some controversy surrounding the disciplines of the individuals who are considered qualified to perform FCE. Occupational and physical therapists were the first to perform FCEs. Given their formal educational preparation in the areas of anatomy, physiology, pathology, kinesiology, and pathokinesiology, this author believes that physical and occupational therapists are best prepared academically to perform FCEs. Individuals from other disciplines, such as exercise physiologists, kinesiologists, athletic trainers, and physicians, sometimes acquire the requisite skills and knowledge in movement analysis and pathology through clinical practice and postgraduate specialization. In such cases, these individuals can become competent in performing FCEs. Perhaps this controversy is best addressed by establishing the competencies necessary to safely, reliably, and accurately perform an FCE. Training courses could then require clinicians to demonstrate those competencies, using written and practical tests.

Space requirements for an FCE vary according to the tasks tested and the equipment used. In general, a private area for evaluation is optimal but not required. Dynamic lifting and position tolerance tests, performed using visual analysis, generally require at least a 10-foot-square area to allow for adequate visualization of the entire body. In some cases, it will be important to view the client from a specific perspective. Therefore, having an uncluttered evaluation area is helpful. For carrying, pushing, pulling, walking, and crawling, a 25–30-foot walkway that allows one to step back 8–10 feet from the client in either the sagittal or frontal planes is optimal. Shorter, or more narrow walkways make visual observations difficult and may adversely affect reliability and validity. Access to stairs and adequate ceiling height for ladder climbing are important when assessing potential space for an FCE.

Reliability

Reliability refers to the consistency of a measure. Two types of reliability are important to an FCE: interrater reliability and intrarater or test-retest reliability. Because individual FCE tasks are often selected for job-specific testing, reliability must be established for each individual task and for the test as a whole.

Interrater reliability refers to the ability to achieve similar scores on the evaluation when it is administered by different evaluators (Portney & Watkins, 1993). Given the staffing patterns in many busy clinics, interrater reliability is extremely important. If one therapist administers the evaluation prior to an industrial rehabilitation program, and another therapist administers the evaluation at the conclusion of the program, significant differences in the scores due to the differences in the therapists' test administration and scoring should not occur. Interrater reliability is best established by having more than one therapist simultaneously and independently evaluate the client as he or she performs the tasks of the FCE. Therapists' scores can then be compared using correlation coefficients.

Intrarater or test-retest reliability refers to the consistency of an evaluation performed by the same examiner at different points in time (Portney & Watkins, 1993). If the same examiner administers an FCE to the same client more than once, will the same results be achieved? The answer is affected by several factors: the stability of the client's condition, the time interval between examinations, the memory of the client and the examiner regarding performance on the first test, and the treatment received by the client between examinations. To date, no studies of intrarater or test-retest reliability have been published in the peer-reviewed literature.

To examine intrarater reliability in an FCE, one may want to choose clients who have achieved maximal improvement and are no longer undergoing treatment. Clients may need to be instructed to avoid changing their activity levels and/or provide activity logs for the time intervals between tests. Having clients blinded as to the amount of weight lifted may minimize their learning effect. Allowing several weeks between examinations may be necessary to minimize examiner memory of the initial test scores. However, allowing more than one month to elapse between the two evaluations may permit the client to change significantly in the interim, even if she or he has reached maximum improvement and is no longer being treated.

Validity

Validity refers to the accuracy of the evaluation (Portney & Watkins, 1993) and is much more difficult to address than reliability. In an FCE, the validity question becomes: Can we accurately predict the level of work that an individual can perform safely? There are a variety of ways to demonstrate validity. Some are considered more scientifically rigorous than others.

Content validity refers to the extent to which a test covers all the domains of the variable in question (Portney & Watkins, 1993). In an FCE, content validity refers to the extent to which the evaluation measures all the physical demands of work. The scope of physical demands has been outlined by the *Dictionary of Occupational Titles (DOT)*. The *DOT* defines 20 physical demands of work (Table 11.1). If the examiner wants to perform a comprehensive assessment, then the FCE should include at least one sample of each of these physical demands. Content validity is judged against the *DOT* standards. If the examiner wants to perform an FCE that is specific to a particular job, then the FCE should be tailored to the job demands, and content validity is judged against those job demands. Content validity is typically judged by an independent and objective panel of experts and, as such, is not empirically based. Thus, it is the weakest form of validity and should be supplemented whenever possible by scientific study.

Criterion-related validity refers to the comparison of a newly developed instrument with one that is considered to be the "gold standard" (Portney & Watkins, 1993). In order to be considered gold standard, an instrument must have demonstrated reliability and validity. One possible gold standard in FCE is the work that the worker is actually performing on the job. However, there are problems with using actual work status as a gold standard. Individuals often work at levels above and below their safe maximums.

Consider the example of a young healthy person who performs a sedentary clerical job but on weekends is involved in mountain climbing and weight lifting. The results of an FCE would likely indicate that this individual can perform at least medium or heavy work. The individual's actual work status, however, is sedentary. In this case, the FCE is not inaccurate. Instead, the worker is simply not working in a job that demands his or her full physical potential. At the other extreme are workers who work above their safe level. The classic example is the older worker whose abilities have declined over the years. His work exceeds his safe limits, but he finds ways to compensate, often through assistance from his co-workers. Both examples illustrate the problems inherent in using current work status to validate an FCE. In lieu of a previously validated test, however, this may be the only gold standard available in some instances.

Two types of criterion-related validity include concurrent validity and predictive validity (Portney & Watkins, 1993). *Concurrent validity* refers to a test's ability to determine current abilities. To establish concurrent validity in an FCE, one can compare the

FCE results with the client's current work status. *Predictive validity* refers to a test's ability to determine future abilities (Portney & Watkins, 1993). To establish predictive validity in an FCE, one can determine physical ability to perform work, and then follow workers for a period of time to determine how long they are able to sustain that level of work without injury.

In the absence of an adequate gold standard by which to compare a newly developed instrument, investigators are faced with demonstrating construct validity. *Construct validity* refers to a test's ability to measure an abstract clinical theory (Portney & Watkins, 1993). In construct validity, one must build or develop evidence in support of validity, using one of several methods. In the *known-groups* method, the newly developed test is used to discriminate between groups of individuals that are known to have a particular characteristic (Portney & Watkins, 1993). If an FCE can accurately discriminate between workers who are performing at the sedentary, light, medium, heavy, and very heavy categories (according to *DOT* definitions), then the evaluation could be considered to have construct validity. Or if the FCE can discriminate between those who are working and those who are not, it could be considered to have construct validity.

In the *multitrait-multimethod matrix* method of establishing construct validity, a test is validated by comparing it with other measures that are measuring the same and different constructs (Portney & Watkins, 1993). There are two types of construct validity that must be established in the multitrait-multimethod matrix. *Convergent validity* involves comparing two measures that are expected to correlate positively with each other. *Discriminate validity* compares two measures that are expected to correlate poorly or negatively. To establish convergent validity in an FCE, one might compare FCE results to the results of a self-report measure of work-related function or observation-based measures of activities of daily living. To establish discriminant validity, one might compare the results of an FCE to measures of range of motion, muscle strength, or cognitive ability.

Unfortunately, some therapists confuse validity with the concept of sincerity of effort (see discussion on sincerity of effort later). Their reports state that "this FCE is invalid" or "this FCE is conditionally valid" due to a lack of client cooperation or symptom magnification. Validity is *not* a measure of the client's sincerity of effort. Test validity is established through research and does not change with client cooperation. If the client self-limits on many tasks of the test, then it becomes a test of what the person is willing to do. The result is still what the person will do back at the workplace and, as such, is a valid representation of current abilities. Defining validity as a lack of sincerity of effort is an incorrect interpretation of validity.

THE IMPORTANCE OF RELIABILITY AND VALIDITY

Reliability and validity are not merely academic exercises intended to satisfy intellectual curiosity. They are critical to credibility in the area of physical abilities testing and make a significant difference in real-world practice. Without reliability, the referral source could send the client to a different therapist and get an entirely different result. Without validity, the client, therapist, referral source, and employer could not know if test results are accurate. Medical care practitioners have an ethical obligation to provide reliable and valid assessments. If test results are to be upheld in litigation, they must demonstrate evidence of reliability and validity.

PEER-REVIEWED STUDIES OF RELIABILITY AND VALIDITY IN FCES

The first study addressing validity of a functional capacity evaluation was published by Smith, Cunningham, and Weinberg (1986). Using a prison population, these investigators examined the predictive validity of an FCE. They administered the Smith FCE, a medical history, and a "Client Activity Interview" to 125 prisoners. Using the results from these evaluations, return-to-work predictions were made. A return-to-work questionnaire was then sent to each of the prisoners after release. Forty-two percent of the questionnaires were returned. Of those who returned the questionnaires, 87% of the predictions were correct. The investigators concluded that their FCE had predictive validity.

Several factors threaten the external validity of this study. First, prisoners as subjects are a very unique and unusual group. Can we generalize the results of this study to injured workers? Second, the investigators used several instruments to make their predictions. Therefore, the exact contribution of the FCE to the prediction is unclear. Third, the low rate of return on the questionnaire suggests that the response group may be the more educated and/or motivated group and, as such, was biased toward successful return to work. Despite these shortcomings, this study is an important first attempt to address the validity of an FCE.

The second study addressing validity in an FCE was reported by Dusik, Menard, Cooke, Fairburn, and Beach (1993). They attempted to establish concurrent validity of the ERGOS work simulator by comparing this instrument to a two-week FCE process. They administered the ERGOS, the RTPE (exercise-oriented physical evaluation), and the SHOPS (project-formatted industrial tasks) to 86 subjects. They also administered Valpar Work Sample Tests to a subset of 17 subjects. The number of women in the sample ($n = 8$) was too small for statistical analysis. The study's conclusions, therefore, were drawn from the remaining 78 male subjects. Comparison of the manual materials handling tasks of the ERGOS to the RTPE revealed positive Pearson r correlation coefficients that ranged from .45 to .71, all of which were found to be statistically significant at the $p < .001$ level of probability.

For the remaining physical demands (stooping, kneeling, crouching, reaching above and below shoulder height, and handling), the investigators used kappa coefficients to determine the agreement between ERGOS and the other two assessment methods. The kappa coefficient is a measure of agreement between examiners with the percentage due to chance removed (Fleiss, 1981). (Kappa coefficients are determined on the basis of the suggested reference values listed in Table 11.3) (Landis & Koch, 1977). Dusik et al. (1993) reported kappa coefficients between the non-materials-handling tasks of the ERGOS and the RTPE, VALPAR, and SHOPS in the slight to fair range with only two of the ERGOS tasks being significantly correlated to the other methods ($p < .01$). They found crouching and handling measured by the ERGOS significantly correlated to crouching and handling on the VALPAR and SHOPS. The investigators found that the ERGOS rated subjects as "restricted" more frequently than did the two other assessment approaches (Dusik et al., 1993). The kappa coefficient values for agreement between the ERGOS and the other assessment methods on an overall level of work ranged from .41 to .66 and were found to be significant (p values ranged from $p < .0001$ to $p < .00035$). The investigators concluded that the strength and overall level of work determined by the ERGOS was comparable to the two-week FCE process.

**Table 11.3. Suggested
Reference Values
for Kappa Coefficients**

Less than .00 = poor agreement
.01 to .20 = slight agreement
.21 to .40 = fair agreement
.41 to .60 = moderate agreement
.61 to .80 = substantial agreement
.81 to 1.0 = almost perfect agreement

A major design flaw in this study, however, severely limits the conclusions that can be drawn regarding concurrent validity of the ERGOS. The two-week process, including the RTPE and the SHOPS evaluations, had no previously established reliability and validity. The investigators, therefore, compared the ERGOS to an evaluation process that had not been properly established as a gold standard.

The third validation study was published by Lechner, Jackson, Roth, and Straaton (1994). It examined the interrater reliability and construct validity of a newly developed FCE, the Physical Work Performance Evaluation (PWPE), in 50 clients with musculo-skeletal dysfunction.

To determine reliability of the PWPE, two therapists simultaneously observed and scored clients as they performed the tasks of the test. At the conclusion, each therapist determined client abilities for each task, each section of the test, and for the test as a whole. The two independent scores were compared using a kappa coefficient to deter-mine reliability (Brennan & Prediger, 1981). The investigators found tasks in the dynamic strength section of the test (manual materials handling tasks) to be the most reliable, with all tasks falling in the "substantial" (.61–.80) to "almost perfect" (.81–1.0) categories. Two tasks in the position tolerance section fell into the moderate agreement category; the remaining five tasks fell into the substantial category. In the mobility section, one task, repetitive squatting, fell into the fair range; two tasks fell into the moderate range; and the remaining four tasks fell into the substantial range. The reliability for determining an overall level of work was .83, falling in the almost perfect category. The reliability for determining subject cooperation was nearly perfect for eleven tasks, substantial for seven tasks, and moderate for one task. Thus, this investigation concluded that the results demonstrated high interrater reliability for the PWPE.

To determine the validity of the PWPE, clients completed job-demand question-naires. The examiners were blinded to the results of these questionnaires and to the work status of the clients. The predicted level of work intensity and frequency for each task, each section of the test, and the overall level was then compared with actual work status using a Spearman rho correlation coefficient. Lechner and her colleagues (1994) found moderate positive correlations between PWPE predictions and actual work that ranged from .41 to .55. They also found that only 14% to 18% of the clients were working above the predicted level of work intensity. Given the previously mentioned problems associated with using current work status as a gold standard, the investigators concluded that these results provided evidence in support of construct validity.

A limitation of this study is that the subjects' work status was not in transition nor pending determination. The subjects were either working at least 20 hours per week or not working due to musculoskeletal dysfunction. Their return-to-work or disability decisions had been previously made. In contrast, many workers who undergo an FCE have return-to-work decisions pending. In addition, the mean duration of their problems was eight years, indicating the study subjects represented a chronic population whose condition was very stable. By comparison, some clients who undergo an FCE are less chronic and in the subacute stage of their disease.

In a second study, Lechner, Sheffield, and Page (1998) examined predictive validity in a group of clients who were off work due to a musculoskeletal injury and were covered by workers' compensation insurance. The PWPE was administered to 30 consecutive clients on admission to a five-week work-hardening program. A job-site analysis was performed to determine the physical demands of the job. Any deficits between clients' abilities and job demands were identified as treatment goals. At the conclusion of the program, the clients were retested using the PWPE on the deficit items. The match between client abilities and job demands was used to make return-to-work recommendations. Clients were cleared to return to their full duties at work if their abilities matched all job demands. A recommendation of return-to-work with modified duty was made if the client's abilities were found to be lacking for four or fewer tasks *and* job modification was feasible. A recommendation of no return to work was made if more than four of the client's abilities fell short of job demands, and job modification duty was not feasible.

Kappa coefficients for agreement between recommendations and actual return to work were .74 at discharge, .69 at three months postdischarge, and .70 at six months postdischarge. These results fell into the substantial agreement category for kappa coefficient values. When Lechner, Sheffield, and Page (1998) examined the reasons why clients did not follow their recommendations, they discovered that lack of modified duty was the most frequently cited reason. The study concluded that the results provided strong evidence supporting the predictive validity of the PWPE when used in the context of an industrial rehabilitation program. The primary limitation of this study was that it did not address predictive validity of the FCE outside the industrial rehabilitation process. (Table 11.4 provides a summary of the peer-reviewed research for comparison of methods and results of the reliability and validity research in FCE.)

ASSESSING CLIENT SINCERITY OF EFFORT

One of the most difficult and controversial issues in administering FCEs involves determining the client's sincerity of effort during the evaluation. Because the possibility of secondary financial gain through the workers' compensation system is ever present, some clients are perceived to be exaggerating or fabricating their symptoms to improve the likelihood that they will receive financial remuneration. As a result, many methods of attempting to identify these clients through FCE testing have been developed (see Table 11.5). A thorough discussion of each of these methods and the literature surrounding these approaches is beyond the scope of this chapter and is the subject of a recent critical review (Lechner, Bradbury, & Bradley, 1998). However, a brief review of the issues surrounding the assessment of sincerity of effort is warranted.

Despite the widespread use of methods for detecting sincerity of effort, some of them were not originally developed for that purpose. Waddell's test of nonorganic signs is a classic example (Waddell, McCulloch, Kummel, & Venner, 1980). Waddell developed eight clinical signs or tests that should not produce pain when administered to low back

Table 11.4. Peer-Reviewed Studies Addressing the Reliability and Validity of FCEs

Author/date	Number of subjects	Study design	Reliability results	Validity results
Smith et al. (1986)	125	Used FCE, intake interview, and activity questionnaire to predict RTW* in a prison population. Followed up with RTW questionnaire. Compared predicted to acutal return to work.	None reported.	Found 87% correct predictions.
Dusik et al. (1993)	78	Administered ERGOS Work Simulator to male subjects admitted to work rehab program. Compared results to a 2-hr physical exam (RTPE) and a 2-week job tasks simulation evaluation (SHOPS). Compared results to determine concurrent validity.	None reported.	Pearson *r* coefficient between ERGOS and RTPE for manual materials tasks ranged from .45 to .71 K coefficients between ERGOS and SHOPS fell in "fair" range for stooping, kneeling, crouching, reaching, & handling. K coefficients between ERGOS and RTPE and SHOPS fell in the moderate to substantial range for determining an overall level of work.

	N	Procedure	Results	
Lechner et al. (1994)	50	Administer the PWPE to client with musculoskeletal dysfuction with 2 examiners scoring simultaneously.	K coefficient for agreement on physical abilities of each task ranged from moderate to almost perfect.	Spearman rho correlation coefficients between predicted and actual work ranged from .41 to .55.
		Compared results from the 2 examiners to evaluate reliability.	K coefficient for client cooperation ranged from substantial to almost perfect.	14%–18% working above predicted levels.
		Compared PWPE results to actual work status to determine validity.	K coefficient for overall level of work = .83.	82%–86% correction predictions.
Lechner et al. (1998) (manuscript in preparation)	30	Administered PWPE to clients as they were admitted to a 5-week work-hardening program. Job-site analysis provided information regarding job demands. Retested on deficient tasks at end of program.	85% agreement between investigators and test developer (DL) on 21 major tasks of the test and complete agreement on overall level of work during training prior to initiation of study.	K coefficients between recommended and actual return to work ranged were
		Recommended RTW full duty, RTW modified duty, or no RTW based solely on comparison between client abilities and job demands.		.74 at discharge .69 at three months .70 at six months
		Compared recommendadtions to actual RTW.		Most who did not follow recommendations cited "lack of modified duty" as reason.

*RTW = return to work.

Table 11.5. Widely Used Methods of Determining Sincerity of Effort

Waddell's nonorganic signs (NOS)
Coefficient of variation (CV)
Bell-shaped curve
Rapid exchange grip (REG)
Correlation between musculoskeletal evaluation and FCE
Documentation of pain behavior
Documentation of symptom magnification
Heart rate to pain intensity ratio
Somatic Amplification Rating Scale (SARS)
Pain scores (0–10, with higher pain scores presumed to indicate poor sincerity of effort)
Consistency of performance when functional tasks are repeated

clients. If the client experiences pain and scores positively on three out of the eight signs, he or she is considered to score positively on Waddell's signs. Waddell developed these signs "to help identify clients who require more detailed psychological assessment" (Waddell et al., 1980, p. 117). This explicitly stated purpose does *not* suggest that scoring positively on Waddell's signs means that the client is not giving a full effort on an evaluation (Scalzitti, 1997). Yet, unfortunately, the nonorganic signs have been equated with poor sincerity of effort and outright malingering in clinical practice and in discussions of clinical assessment in the peer-reviewed literature (Lehman, Russell, & Spratt, 1983; Spratt, Lehman, Weinstein, & Sayre, 1990).

Many of the tests used to detect sincerity of effort are not being performed or scored using methods that were established in their published validation studies. Usually the methods are too complex and cumbersome to apply in the clinical setting. Use of the bell-shaped curve is an example. The bell-shaped curve involves testing isometric grip strength at five different handle positions (Stokes, 1983). The expectation is that a graphic plot of the force at the five different positions will produce a bell-shaped curve. As originally developed by the investigators, a complex computerized curve analysis procedure was used to analyze the curve (Robinson, Geisser, Hanson, & O'Connor, 1993; Simonsen, 1995). Most clinicians use visual inspection of the curve, which has been shown to be less reliable and valid (Robinson et al., 1993).

The standardization, reliability, and validity of some of the methods used to determine sincerity of effort are questionable. For example, Waddell's nonorganic signs were described in a manner that has resulted in wide variability in test administration. This lack of standardization may contribute to findings that suggest that some of the signs are unreliable. Korbon, DeGood, Schroeder, Schwartz, and Shutty (1987) found that axial loading, trunk rotation, and overreaction had poor reliability. Other studies that demonstrated good reliability of Waddell's nonorganic signs required considerable training of the examiners by Dr. Waddell prior to data collection (Waddell, Main, Morris, Venner, Rae, Sharmy, & Galloway, 1982; Waddell et al., 1980) or two examiners observing simultaneously rather than two test administrators (Spratt, Lehman, Weinstein, & Sayre, 1990). Given the extent of variability in the administration of Waddell's nonorganic signs, inter-rater reliability may need to be examined with each examiner administering the test.

Measuring the coefficient of variation (CV) typically involves having the client perform three repetitions of a maximum isometric contraction. The CV is calculated by dividing the standard deviation by the mean of the three measures. The underlying assumption is that submaximal efforts will produce greater variability or a higher CV. Poor reliability and a high incidence of false negatives, however, have been reported for this approach to isometric testing (Lin, Robinson, Carlos, & O'Conner, 1996; Robinson et al., 1993). Robinson and colleagues (1993) reported interclass correlation coefficients for maximal and submaximal efforts of isometric grip strength as being from .036 to 0.25, indicating very poor reliability for the CV. They also found a higher percent of false negatives with this approach. Using the ERGOS Work Simulator, Simonsen (1995) examined CVs for eight isometric strength tasks. The results of the study revealed a poor correlation between the CVs of the different tests and concluded that there was no evidence to suggest that CV can be used independently to determine sincerity of effort.

These are but a few examples of a growing body of evidence in the peer-reviewed literature that strongly suggest that we do not have a validated method for determining sincerity of effort in clients who are undergoing an FCE. During FCE performance, the therapists can document whether a client is performing to a maximum effort by comparing a visual observations of signs of effort with the client's willingness to perform. If the client stops himself or herself prior to reaching a maximum effort, however, the therapist cannot determine the reason(s) underlying this self-limiting behavior. The client may be terminating the task because of pain, fear of reinjury, anxiety, depression, poor understanding of instructions, or a conscious or unconscious attempt to manipulate the results of the test. Based on the available peer-reviewed literature, an FCE *cannot* be used to determine which of these factors is underlying the self-limiting behavior, regardless of the methods used.

SAFETY IN FCE

The primary focus of safety in FCE testing is on preventing further injury during the testing process. Injury can occur as a result of placing excessive demands on the client's musculoskeletal, cardiovascular, or neurological systems. Safety is enhanced by stopping the client on tasks at the point at which the activity begins to appear unsafe. The determination of a safe maximal level involves clinical decision making and a therapist's professional judgment. Clear operational definitions and specific decision-making criteria help to standardize the decision-making process and protect the client from overexertion.

Teaching proper lifting techniques prior to testing will also minimize the risk of reinjury during testing. The examiner cannot expect clients to permanently change their lifting techniques or apply newly learned techniques in the work setting after one instruction section. At least, however, clients will be more likely to use better body mechanics for the test, and thus they will be less likely to reinjure themselves during the evaluation. If the client requires instruction in a lifting technique prior to evaluation, the need for further body mechanics instruction should be documented in the summary report so that this issue can be addressed prior to return to work.

Controversy exists surrounding the safety of isometric lift testing. Some examiners insist that isometric lifting is safe. Others report that exertional injuries have occurred secondary to isometric lifting. One possible explanation for the reported injuries is that with isometric lifting the client can build up a significant amount of force with little accompanying observable biomechanical evidence of effort. This lack of visual feedback limits the examiner's ability to stop the client before he or she exceeds a safe maximum.

If the client relates symptoms of intermittent, sharp shooting pain associated with the burning, numbness, or tingling that follows a nerve root distribution, examiners are advised to perform a brief neurological screen prior to the FCE testing. The screen can include neural tension, reflex, and myotome testing. If any of the three tests are positive, it provides supporting evidence that the client may be experiencing irritation or compression of a nerve root from disc material, scar tissue, or osteophyte formation. Any FCE tasks that increase symptoms related to nerve root irritation/compression should be stopped as soon as the radicular symptoms are evident.

If the client relates symptoms of dizziness or blurred vision, particularly with activities that involve neck extension, the clinician should check the patency of the vertebral artery. This testing involves slowly inducing neck extension, side bending, and rotation while observing the clients' eyes for asymmetry in pupil restrictions, nystagmus, or reproduction of the symptoms of dizziness, nausea, or blurred vision (Magee, 1992, pp. 53–54). If the test is positive, the examiner will want to discontinue immediately any FCE tasks that bring on these symptoms.

Clinical experience has heightened this author's awareness of the extent of undiagnosed hypertension in the work-injured population. Therefore, as a safety precaution, blood pressure should be monitored prior to initiating an FCE. The cutoff used by this author is 150–160/100. If the blood pressure significantly exceeds this cutoff, the client should be advised that the FCE cannot be performed due to hypertension, and he or she should be advised to seek medical attention for this problem. Contacting the referring physician to describe the problem and suggesting that an FCE could be performed as soon as the blood pressure is brought under control will help to insure that this problem is addressed. Following up with written documentation is recommended. If the referring physician insists on proceeding with an FCE despite marked hypertension, politely but firmly refusing to do so is in the best interest of the client.

If the client's blood pressure only slightly exceeds the cutoff point, the therapist may try to encourage the client to relax by discussing the testing protocol. Sometimes explanation and reassurance regarding testing procedures will be enough to lower the client's stress level and thus decrease blood pressure. Sometimes initiating physical activity will lower blood pressure. The examiner might evaluate the client's natural lifting style, give feedback regarding lifting technique, and then recheck the blood pressure. If the blood pressure stays the same or decreases with physical activity, the examiner might proceed, checking blood pressure at intervals throughout the evaluation. If blood pressure increases with activity, the examiner should terminate the FCE and contact the physician as described earlier.

Monitoring the client's heart rate with a device that has an upper-limit alarm will help to prevent clients from performing tasks that exceed their cardiovascular capabilities. When clients are taking heart rate suppressing drugs, such as beta or calcium channel blockers, however, heart rate can no longer be used as an indicator of overexertion. Instead, the clinician must rely on the client's perceived exertion level, or on clinical signs of overexertion, including respiratory rate and color, to determine safe exertion levels.

ROLE OF NORMATIVE DATABASES IN FCE

Since the passage of the Americans with Disabilities Act (ADA) in 1992, return-to-work decisions and preemployment/post-offer testing must be made by comparing the client's abilities with the job's demands. Regardless of whether the individual's abilities are in the 5th or 95th percentile of a normative database, if abilities meet the job demands, then the client can return to work or the job applicant can be hired. Therefore, in this author's opinion, normative databases are of relatively little value in FCEs. The one exception is the manual dexterity tests. Results must first be translated into a percentile score and then into an aptitude score for comparison with the Department of Labor's classifications of the dexterity demands of jobs.

JOB-SPECIFIC VERSUS COMPREHENSIVE FCE

Much controversy surrounds the issue of choosing to do a job-specific or generic (comprehensive) FCE. There are advantages and disadvantages to each approach. With the job-specific approach, test time may be reduced, and the test may seem to have more content validity, especially in the eyes of the client and the employer. The apparent content validity may enhance the client's cooperation during testing. The job-specific evaluation, however, needs to be performed using a standardized protocol. Optimally, it should be supported by research demonstrating reliability and validity. To address these issues, the job-specific FCE could be composed of a subset of tasks selected from a larger group that have been individually validated.

One shortcoming of job-specific evaluations becomes evident if the client is not able to return to his or her former job. If only a job-specific FCE has been done, the results will not provide the comprehensive assessment of physical abilities that is optimal for exploring alternative work placement. Often, additional testing is needed. The comprehensive FCE may take longer to perform, but it will provide the information needed should the client not be able to return to his or her former job.

REPORT CONTENT

The major points of interest for the referral source, client, insurer, and employer are the client's safe limits for performing physical work. Most referral sources want to know the answers to the following three questions: What are the client's abilities? Do these abilities meet the job demands? Did the client give maximum effort during the evaluation? If the client's abilities do not meet the job demands, then the referral source will likely want some recommendations of interventions to consider. Therefore, a section regarding recommendations is usually included. Recommendations should be made after consideration has been given to the client's previous treatment. One sure way to alienate referral sources is to recommend treatments that have previously failed.

THE MARKET VERSUS ETHICS

The "market"—those who request FCEs—is applying increasing pressure for clinicians to perform evaluations in less and less time. Peer-reviewed literature suggests that a reliable and valid assessment can be performed in 3 to 4 hours (Lechner et al., 1994). There is no evidence, however, that reliable and valid testing can be done in less time. Also, there is pressure from some referral sources, insurers, and case managers to identify those individuals who exaggerate or falsify injury claims. In at least one state (Oregon

Work Injury Management Association meeting, June 1996), examiners are being pressured to project "real abilities" for those clients who self-limit. To date, we do not have validated methods allowing us to make these types of projections. On all of these issues (length of testing, documenting sincerity of effort, and projecting "real" from self-limiting performance), we need to be aware of the literature and argue our case convincingly to referral sources. In many cases, precedence is set to meet a market demand, regardless of the research evidence. Once a precedence is set, it is difficult to change.

CLINICAL IMPLICATIONS

Regardless of whether the clinician chooses a commercially available FCE system or develops a "homegrown" version, the criteria for sound clinical measurement discussed earlier should be applied. Standardization, reliability, and validity are essential for demonstrating that an FCE is fair and objective. These principles provide guidance for the clinician who is making procedural and equipment decisions. When choosing a commercially available FCE, consider the practical issues and ask to see peer-reviewed literature that supports reliability and validity.

Because of the variety of approaches and testing philosophies used in FCE, there is much confusion among end users/consumers surrounding the interpretation of these evaluations. The professionals who administer FCEs must be able to justify whatever methodology they choose to referral sources, insurers, employers, attorneys, and patients. The goal should be to provide objective testing that is biased neither toward nor against the client.

REFERENCES

Alexander, R. W., Maida, A. S., & Walker, R. J. (1975). The validity of preemployment medical evaluations. *Journal of Occupational Medicine, 17,* 687-692.

Althouse, H. L. (1980). Revealing a true profile of musculoskeletal abilities. *Occupational Health and Safety, 1,* 25-30.

Brennan, R. L., & Prediger, D. J. (1981). Coefficient kappa: Some uses, misuses, and alternatives. *Educational and Psychological Measurement, 41,* 687-699.

Dueker, J. A., Ritchie, S. M., Knox, T. J., & Rose, S. J. (1994). Isokinetic trunk testing and employment. *Journal of Occupational Medicine, 36,* 42-48.

Dusik, L. A., Menard, M. R., Cooke, C., Fairburn, S. M., & Beach, G. N. (1993). Concurrent validity of the ERGOS work simulator versus conventional functional capacity evaluation techniques in a workers' compensation population. *Journal of Occupational Medicine, 35,* 759-767.

Field, J. E., & Field, T. F. (1992). Classification of jobs. Athens, GA: Elliot & Fitzpatrick.

Fleiss, J. L. (1981). *Statistical methods for rates and proportions.* New York: Wiley.

Jette, A. M. (1984). Concepts of health and methodological issues in functional status assessment. In C. V. Granger & G. E. Gresham (Eds.), *Functional assessment in rehabilitation* (pp. 46-64). Baltimore, MD: Williams & Wilkins.

Korbon, G. A., DeGood, D. E., Schroeder, M. E., Schwartz, E. P., & Shutty, M. S. (1987). The development of a somatic amplification rating scale for low back pain. *Spine, 44,* 611-621.

Landis, J. R., & Koch, G. C. (1977). The measurement of observer agreement for categorical data. *Biometrics, 33,* 159-174.

Lechner, D. E., Roth, D. L., & Straaton, K. V. (1991). Functional capacity evaluation in work disability. *Work, 1,* 37-47.

Lechner, D. E., Bradbury, S., & Bradley, L. A. (1998). Detecting sincerity of effort: A summary of methods and approaches. *Physical Therapy, 78,* 867-888.

Lechner, D. E., Jackson, J. R., Roth, D. L., & Straaton, K. V. (1994). Reliability and validity of a newly developed test of physical work performance. *Journal of Occupational Medicine, 36,* 997-1004.

Lechner, D. E., Sheffield, G., & Page, J. J. (1998). Predictive validity of the physical work performance evaluation. Manuscript in preparation.

Lehman, T. R., Russell, D. W., & Spratt, K. F. (1983). The impact of patients with nonorganic physical findings on a controlled trial of transcutaneous electrical stimulation and electroacupuncture. *Spine, 8,* 625-634.

Lin, P. C., Robinson, M. E., Carlos, J., & O'Connor, P. (1996). Detection of submaximal effort in isometric and isokinetic knee extension tests. *Journal of Orthopedic and Sports Physical Therapy, 24,* 19-24.

Magee, D. J. (1992). *Orthopedic physical assessment* (pp. 55-56). Philadelphia, PA: W. B. Saunders.

Newton, M., & Waddell, G. (1993). Trunk strength testing with iso-machines: Part 1. Review of a decade of scientific evidence. *Spine, 18,* 801-811.

Portney, L. G., & Watkins, M. P. (1993). *Foundations of clinical research: Applications to practice* (pp. 60-77). Norwalk, CT: Appleton & Lange.

Robinson, M. E., Geisser, M. E., Hanson, C. S., & O'Conner, P. D. (1993). Detecting submaximal efforts in grip strength testing with the coefficient of variation. *Journal of Occupational Rehabilitation, 3,* 45-50.

Rothstein, J. M., & Echternach, J. L. (1993). *Primer on measurement: An introductory guide to measurement issues* (pp. 78-80). Alexandria, VA: American Physical Therapy Association.

Scalzitti, D. A. (1997). Screening for psychological factors in patients with low back problems: Waddell's nonorganic signs. *Physical Therapy, 77,* 306-312.

Simonsen, J. C. (1995). Coefficient of variation as a measure of subject effort. *Archives of Physical Medicine and Rehabilitation, 76,* 516-520.

Smith, S. L., Cunningham, S., & Weinberg, R. (1986). The predictive validity of the functional capacities evaluation. *American Journal of Occupational Therapy, 40,* 564-567.

Spratt, K. F., Lehman, T. R., Weinstein, J. N., & Sayre, H. A. (1990). A new approach to the low back physical examination: Behavioral assessment of mechanical signs. *Spine, 15,* 96-102.

Stokes, H. M. (1983). The seriously uninjured hand: Weakness of grip. *Journal of Occupational Medicine, 25,* 683-684.

U.S. Department of Labor, Employment and Training Administration. (1991). *Dictionary of Occupational Titles* (4th ed. rev., Vols. 1-2). Washington, DC: U.S. Government Printing Office.

Waddell, G., Main, C. J., Morris, E. W., Venner, R. M., Rae, P. S. Sharmy, S. H., & Galloway, H. (1982). Normality and reliability in the clinical assessment of backache. *British Medical Journal Clinical Research, 284,* 1519-1523.

Waddell, G., McCulloch, J. A., Kummel, E., & Venner, R. M. (1980). Nonorganic physical signs in low back pain. *Spine, 5,* 117-125.

12

Work Analysis

Paula C. Bohr

Work analysis is a critical component of primary, secondary, and tertiary intervention for work-related injuries and illnesses. When work analysis includes the assessment of a person's suitability for work, the match between the worker and the work is maximized. A good match of the worker, work environment, the work demands decreases the risk of injury or illness. If there is a mismatch, the worker may be placed in a hazardous job situation with a high likelihood of injury or illness.

Work analysis has long been that a fundamental part of ergonomics through which the human factors in job performance are clearly defined. Many terms have been used to describe analysis of work. Some of these terms include *job analysis*, *hazard analysis*, *worksite analysis*, *task analysis* and *ergonomic assessment*. Regardless of the term used, work analysis is a formal, systematic way to characterize the parameters of work as they relate to a worker's performance. This chapter will provide an overview of work analysis, including the components of analysis, data collection methods and tools, determination of job demands, and identification of musculoskeletal risks. The approaches and techniques described here are intended to provide a foundation for analysis that can be applied to reducing the likelihood of injury, interrupting or minimizing the progression of an illness, or reducing the resultant disability of an injured worker.

APPROACHES TO WORK ANALYSIS

Work analysis can be viewed from either a systems perspective or from a person-centered perspective. Both approaches have applications in the fields of ergonomics and occupational rehabilitation if the full spectrum of intervention is to be addressed. Each approach has a distinctly different focus and different roots.

The systems approach focuses on the design of work in relation to the capabilities

Paula C. Bohr • Program in Occupational Therapy, Washington University School of Medicine, St. Louis, Missouri, 63108.

Sourcebook of Occupational Rehabilitation, edited by Phyllis M. King. Plenum Press, New York, 1998.

and limitations of people. It has traditionally been within the purview of the human factors engineer. Human factors engineering is concerned with the "application of data and principles of human factors and ergonomics to the design of equipment, subsystems and systems" (Christensen, 1987, p. 8). This approach views the system as being dependent on either modal data for humans or on machine requirements. It tends to be a logical approach that relies on mathematical calculations. The primary application of this approach is to the design of human-machine systems to protect the worker and minimize potential incompatibilities among the components of the system.

The person-centered approach focuses on the person within the context of the work environment and the job demands. It has most often been the avenue for interventions by specialists in the field of rehabilitation ergonomics. According to Matheson, Isernhagen, and Hart (1996), rehabilitation ergonomists "utilize knowledge of functional limitations, work demands, and individual characteristics to optimize the safe work capacity of injured workers and to reduce the incidence and severity of the injury or illness of healthy workers" (p. 223). Branton (1987) supported this approach by defining ergonomics as "the systematic study of the reality of limitations to interaction between humans and their work environment and with each other at work." Because this approach views the individual person within the system, its application usually revolves around early detection and treatment of work injury or illness, accommodation for the worker to slow the progression of an injury or illness, and reduction of the resultant disability. This approach generally includes analysis of risk factors and safe, healthful work practices, as well as an assessment of the severity of injury.

Both approaches are important to the fields of ergonomics and occupational rehabilitation. The approach selected will depend, in part, on the objectives of the work analysis being conducted. If the objective of the analysis is primary prevention, the systems approach affords the opportunity to design or alter work systems to maximize the match between the worker and the system. The person-centered approach is most applicable when the objective is the early identification of the signs and symptoms of a problem or returning the injured worker to the job.

DEFINING WORK ANALYSIS

Terminology related to work analysis is often confusing, especially when terms are used interchangeably as if they were equivalent. In many cases, the terms are not synonymous. Although the analysis process is more important than the term used to describe it, it is important to clarify the terms currently in use.

A *job description* defines the functions of the job. It is intended to provide insight into the purpose of the job and how it relates to other jobs or to the entire operation of the facility. Most job descriptions list the tasks to be performed, both essential and nonessential, and some information about the job's physical demands. The nonessential tasks can be accomplished in other ways, but the essential tasks make up a significant part of the work and cannot be altered without substantially changing the job (Equal Opportunities Employment Commission, 1992). With passage of the Americans with Disabilities Act (ADA) in 1990, it was mandated that job descriptions must include identification of the essential job functions that must be performed as a part of the job. Job demands typically include weights handled, educational level required, body postures necessary for completing the tasks, and duration of tasks.

Job analysis is a term that was coined by the U.S. Department of Labor soon after the passage of the Wagner-Peyser Act in the 1930s (U.S. Department of Labor, 1991). This method was developed to establish a concise, consistent basis for the identification of qualification requirements to be used for the recruitment, selection, placement, and promotion of personnel. The approach uses subjective and objective information to define a uniform occupational language of worker functions that serves as the basis for systematic comparison of job tasks. Job analysis generally defines the activities of a given occupational category or job position and specifically delineates the demands of the job. The demands of the job may include requirements for physical performance, mobility, sensory-perceptual processing, and cognitive abilities. When used in the context of a systems approach, the set of activities that defines the job are viewed as a subset of the total activities that contributes to the organization of a system. The information is utilized in job design or redesign and the development of training techniques that permit workers to function within the system. From a person-centered perspective, the information from a job analysis is used to determine essential job requirements before a new worker is placed, or an injured worker is returned to the job. The job analysis information can also be used to aid in the placement of the injured worker in an alternative work position and train the injured worker to minimize the risk of further impairment.

A *task analysis* is a formal methodology that details the interactions between the worker and the equipment of a system without designating the worker who performs the identified tasks. According to Drury (1987), task analysis involves the "analysis, resynthesis, interpretation, evaluation, and transformation of the task requirement in light of knowledge and theory about human characteristics" (p. 375). Because task analyses are generally used to integrate the human element into a human-machine system, the focus of a task analysis is to define the performance requirements of the worker. The result of a task analysis is a detailed list of the demands of the job that includes such information as the frequency of performance and the strength required for performance.

It is common for the terms task analysis and job analysis to be mistakenly interchanged. Job analysis employs a variation of task analysis, although its definitions of tasks and level of detail differs from those of a task analysis. For example, both task analysis and job analysis include descriptions. A task analysis includes a detailed description of the human task requirements of the system, while the job analysis focuses on a general description of the set of activities that are necessary to complete the work.

Ergonomic assessment is a more generic term used by many practitioners to describe a wide range of work analyses that define work demands and identify risks. Ergonomic assessment implies a process of evaluation without specifying the tools to be used to collect and analyze data. This type of assessment can include biomechanical analyses, physiological assessments, and/or identification of psychological demands. Because the term is broad in perspective, it allows the flexibility to select the assessments tools appropriate to the situation. This term has application to the systems and person-centered approaches.

THE WORK ANALYSIS PROCESS

Components of Analysis

Work analysis is a dynamic process that considers the worker, work environment, and work demands. If the analysis is to be comprehensive, it must contain assessment of all three areas because all are critical to the work being accomplished. Depending on the reasons for completing the analysis, more emphasis may be placed on one area, but all three must be considered because they are closely interrelated. For example, the primary reason for completing an analysis may be to determine the physical demands of the job. However, if those demands are to be used as a basis for determining whether a worker is capable of doing the job, consideration must also be given to the working environment in which the tasks must be completed and to the physical capacities of the individual worker.

Scope and Application of Analysis

Before beginning a work analysis process, it is important to define the objectives and scope of the analysis. If the focus of analysis is the worker, the objectives generally will relate to the suitability of the individual for a particular job or the need for accommodation to allow the worker to complete the job. When the emphasis is on work environment, the focus of objectives is more on the safety requirements of the equipment and tools needed to perform the job and the environmental conditions (temperature, humidity, chemical exposure, noise, radiation, etc.) that can impact worker and system performance. A focus on work demands typically relates to objectives involving the identification of forces, angles, repetitions, stress levels, and so on that are inherent to the jobs being performed as well as the production demands and work routines.

Equally important is the determination of the depth of analysis needed. Depth relates to the amount of detail required but not necessarily to the comprehensive nature of the analyses. For example, an analysis may be considered comprehensive to the extent that it addresses the three components (worker, work environment, work demands), but it may not include the level of detail adequate for the engineering redesign of an entire work system that is having an adverse impact on the workers. Historically, analyses from a systems perspective that emphasize worksite design are very detailed because they must include exact system requirements and engineering specifications. Analyses from a person-centered perspective require varying levels of detail but can be equally as detailed. The more detailed the analyses, the more time and effort that it will require.

The scope and depth of the analysis reflect how the results of the analysis will be applied. The employer might use the results of an analysis for a variety of purposes including the following:

1. To define a hiring process that includes providing information on job demands to perspective employees and objectively and systematically evaluating worker capacities to ensure appropriate placement of the individual worker
2. To identify potentially risky jobs that might lead to costly injury or illness
3. To ancitipate the impact of applying new technology in an existing work system
4. To determine when changes in production requirements are needed
5. To design and implement new systems or work procedures

The employee is more likely to apply the results of an analysis to the following:

1. To increase his or her understanding of the job and its demands prior to beginning work
2. To minimize the risks of injury or illness by learning alternative work practices
3. To facilitate a return to work after injury or illness.

The rehabilitation professional applies the analysis results in establishing realistic treatment goals that are specific to the injured worker's job demands and work environment and recommending job modifications or accommodations that address the mismatch between the job and environment demands and the abilities of that worker. The engineer applies the analysis information to the design or redesign of jobs, tools, and equipment in order to decrease costly worker problems.

Defining an Analysis Plan

Once the objectives of the analysis process have been identified, the next step is to define a plan for completing the analysis. Ideally, the plan will include a listing of the specific methods and measurement equipment to be used for documenting worker characteristics and abilities, work environment, and work demands. Including all three components ensures that the analysis reflects the interrelationships of these components and accurately represents the work process. If the job or worksite is unfamiliar, detailing the methods necessary to assess the three components may be difficult. Preparation of the analysis plan may require the evaluator to research the industry or the job tasks to gain an understanding of the characteristics of that industry or the job being evaluated and technologies being used. Whether or not the work process is familiar, it is helpful to identify (a) the steps in the process being evaluated; (b) the materials, tools, equipment, and environment required for the work to be accomplished; and (c) the worker(s) performing the job.

To avoid any misunderstanding, the analysis plan should identify the activities to be completed and the individual(s) responsible for completing them. It should also include a time line for completing the analysis, an estimated cost of the analysis, and the type of information that will be reported on completion of the analysis.

Obtaining Facility and Management Support

Gaining the support of the facility and its management can greatly aid in the collection of data. Support must be garnered from all levels of management prior to the on-site visit. Upper-level management may approve and support the analysis process, but without the support of such individuals as the supervisors in the work area being assessed, the safety personnel, and the operations manager or the personnel director, the analysis process can be stymied.

It is advisable to arrange a time to meet with management representatives, including the department heads, supervisors, and anyone else involved in the process, prior to the on-site visit. If possible, the meeting should be face-to-face. Telephone conferencing is an option, but it doesn't facilitate recognition of key personnel at the time of the data collection.

The primary purpose for meeting is to gain management support throughout the process, clarifying responsibilities and authorities to minimize the opportunities for misunderstandings to occur. Meeting also provides a chance to relate information about the process and evaluation methods that will be used and obtain information about workers' characteristics, injury statistics, personnel policies and procedures, and specific jobs. The meeting is an opportunity to determine the methods by which workers will be informed about process, secure permission to photograph and/or videotape job tasks, determine areas of highest priority to analyze, and confirm the plan and schedule for completing the analysis. It may also be an opportunity to request an orientation tour to familiarize oneself with the overall picture of operations, the general work flow for individual areas, and the resource people who may be helpful during the process.

Once the meeting has concluded, the plan for completing the analysis process should be submitted to the facility in writing for verification and approval. Obtaining written approval may prevent misunderstandings later in the analysis process.

Selection of Data Collection Methods

Traditionally, work analysis has been associated with data collection methods defined primarily by engineers (systems approach) or by rehabilitation specialists (person-centered approach). Regardless of the approach used, the methods of data collection that are appropriate to the objective of the work analysis must be selected based on a clear understanding of how and by whom the analysis results are to be used. Specific methods will be discussed later in this chapter, but at this point it is important to establish criteria for the selection of methods. First, it must be determined whether the methods to be used will be quantitative or qualitative in nature. According to Isernhagen (1995, p. 70), quantitative analysis involves "measurement of such parameters as weights, distances, forces, repetitions, speed, productivity, and timing (M[ethod]T[ime]M[easurement])," while qualitative analysis goes beyond the quantitative methods by "imparting logic, order, evaluation, or recommendations to the data analyzed" (p. 71). Quantitative methods are formal measurement processes that rely on technical skill in using the tools available to record measurements and analyzing those measurements mathematically and scientifically. Qualitative methods rely on the synthesis of technical data, descriptive information, research results, and professional judgment to describe parameters that cannot be easily quantified, such as job processes and work flow, work stress, or motivation. Both quantitative and qualitative methods are important to a comprehensive work analysis.

Second, selection of methods is evaluator-dependent. Many analysis methods require a level of familiarity and skill to complete. If the evaluator is unfamiliar or unskilled with the technique or tools being used, there is the possibility that data will be incorrectly recorded, or interpretations of the results may be inappropriate to the particular work situation. When the method is critical to the analysis, the evaluator should seek assistance from professionals who have expertise with the needed tool or method.

Third, the data collection methods must be efficient ways of obtaining the desired level of detail. The methods selected should enable the facts to be obtained quickly, accurately, and comprehensively. For example, it may be possible to gather the necessary level of detailed information from well-written questions on worker surveys rather than from individual worker interviews, which are very time-consuming.

Data Collection

Documentation Review

Surveillance. Surveillance is a mechanism that provides accurate data when developing and implementing interventions. It is a process of collecting, organizing, and disseminating the data that work facilities must maintain in accordance with federal, state, and local regulatory mandates. Surveillance occurs through monitoring hazards in the work environment and the health of workers (Baker, Melius, & Millar, 1988).

Hazard surveillance has been an integral part of compliance with the Occupational Safety and Health Administration (OSHA) mandates (OHSA, 1970). Hazard surveillance includes review of OSHA records and direct hazard surveys. Evaluation of hazards involves "judging the magnitude of the chemical, physical, biological, or ergonomic stresses" (Olishifski & Plog, 1988, p. 21) and deciding how the stresses compare with hygienic guides, threshold limit values, OSHA permissible exposure levels, and/or reports in the literature.

In contrast to hazard surveillance, health surveillance identifies the occurrence of work-related conditions through review of existing health records. Health effect outcomes often rely on data from systems that were created for purposes unrelated to the identification and prevention of musculoskeletal injuries. Data bases typically accessed include workers' compensation records, accident-on-duty logs, medical records, and insurance claims records. These records may provide clues to the incidence and severity of work injuries, which may then lead to the identification of high-risk work areas and populations. The incidence rate is computed based on the number of new cases in a population per specified unit of exposure time (based on full-time employees working 40 hours per week, 50 weeks per year for an exposure time of 2,000 hours per year and an OSHA defined standard unit of exposure time of 200,000 hours) (Putz-Anderson, 1988). The calculated incidence rate may serve as evidence of an existing problem or the early indicator of an emerging problem. Rodgers (1992) suggested that the incidence rate be considered along with the total number of people exposed when determining the jobs that should be evaluated.

Severity.   Severity describes the seriousness of an injury or illness in terms of cost to the employer. There is no standard way to calculate cost to the employer. Common methods include determining cost based on (a) the number of work days lost during a calendar year per million hours worked, (b) the number of work days lost per employee (or per 100 employees) per year, and (c) the cost of workers' compensation per employee (or per 100 employees) per year. In some cases it may be advisable to determine severity based on the type of injury or illness. Regardless of the method used, identification of severity indicates the seriousness of the work-related problem and is useful in establishing the priorities for interventions.

Other records that may provide insight into the problems identified are the records for production. These records often suggest relationships between injury or illness and changing production demands or the implementation of new technology on worker performance. Additionally, these records identify the expectations for worker and system performance. If, for example, the incidence of carpal tunnel syndrome increases when the production rate increases, consideration should be given to any changes in work performance that occur when the demands for production exceed the capacities of the workers.

Although the discussion of data here reflects the identification of problem work areas, these same measures can also serve as outcome measures to determine the effectiveness of interventions over time or the need for further intervention.

Human Resources Data.   Reviewing human resources policies and practices often provides insight into the recruitment, selection, retention, advancement, and termination of workers. Information about the following may be helpful in understanding the nature of the problems that have prompted the worksite analysis:

1. Hiring requirements for workers, including hiring of minority and disadvantaged workers
2. Identification of entry level jobs
3. Sources for the recruitment of workers
4. Practices for training new employees and maintaining the skill level of current employees
5. Job restructuring
6. Changes in workforce demographics and distribution throughout the facility
7. Opportunities for career lattices, promotion, and retirement

When these records are paired with surveillance data, it may be possible to determine whether the occurrence of high worker turnover, decreased worker motivation, or worker stress is related to the demands of the work or to existing policies. For example, surveillance data may suggest an increase in musculoskeletal complaints and/or an increase in lost work days, but when it is paired with personnel data, it may be possible to determine whether the increases reflect boredom or dissatisfaction with an entry-level job rather than its excessive physical demands.

Job descriptions with the associated essential job demands are usually maintained by the human resource personnel. Prior to visiting the work facility, reviewing documented job descriptions is helpful in understanding the mechanics of the job or the abilities the worker must possess to perform the job. They can also provide some guidance to the evaluator in determining the types of analyses that may be required.

Questionnaires

Questionnaires are easily administered, voluntarily completed instruments that are "intended to elicit the evaluations, judgments, comparisons, attitudes, beliefs and opinions of personnel" (Moroney & Cameron, 1995). Questions must be unambiguous and unbiased. Allowing the respondent's identity to remain confidential or anonymous facilitates completion of a questionnaire. In the work setting, confidentiality is a critical issue. If workers are fearful of losing their jobs or of being penalized in some way for answering questions honestly, they will often refuse to participate or provide responses that are not honestly reflective of their opinions. This activity is especially likely to occur when questions relate to worker satisfaction or the psychosocial work environment.

Discomfort questionnaires are commonly used as a part of work analysis to detect symptoms of musculoskeletal stress that may lead to worker injury. Discomfort can be measured on either numeric or visual analogue scales. Often a numeric rating scale is used because it is less cumbersome, though it may not be as sensitive as a visual analogue scale. Ideally, the questionnaire is composed of three questions related to discomfort: (1) How often did you experience aches, pain, or discomfort? (Never, occasionally, several times per week, every day); (2) If you experienced aches, pain, or discomfort, how uncomfortable was it? (Slightly uncomfortable, moderately uncomfortable, very uncomfortable); and (3) If you experience aches, pain, or discomfort, did it interfere with your ability to work? (Not at all, slightly interfered, substantially interfered). For all three questions, the respondent is asked to rate discomfort for individual body parts during a specified period of time (usually in the last week or in the last month). Additional questions related to mental and physical fatigue may also be included.

Interviews

Interviewing is a subjective method for obtaining information about workers and jobs. If they are to be effective data collection tools, the interviewer must have an understanding of the job and the workers performing the jobs. Interviews provide an opportunity to verify job data regarding routine and infrequent job tasks, to gain an understanding of work flow patterns and sequences, and to obtain worker perspectives of physical and mental work stresses.

An interview of a worker should only be conducted with the permission of the worker's supervisor. Even when the supervisor grants permission, the worker may be reluctant to share information with the interviewer, especially if there is fear of salary or time repercussions. For this reason, it is critical that the interviewer clearly articulate the purpose of the interview. In most cases, the interviewer provides a structure that will help the worker think and talk according to the sequence in which duties performed, or in a functional manner if his or her duties are not performed in a regular order. Having a working knowledge of the trade or industry terms that the worker may use will facilitate the recording of interview information. That information should include only the facts about the job. The emphasis should be on the work performed and worker traits involved in completing job tasks. Notes on interviews should be complete, legible, and contain data that will be necessary for the work analysis. Organizing the data in a logical manner, either according to job tasks or categories of information, is helpful. All information recorded should be verified by the worker and the worker's supervisor.

Observations

Observations of work provide valuable information about the techniques used to perform job tasks as well as an understanding of work flow and pace and environment in which the work is performed. From these observations it is possible to document task descriptions, provide a general layout of the work area, describe equipment and identify processes involved, body postures, body movements, and task outcomes. Additionally, general observations can be made regarding special conditions, such as slippery surfaces or radical environmental conditions.

Observing work for the purposes of identifying potential risk factors that can lead to musculoskeletal injury is a typical component of a work analysis. General risk factors have been identified for cumulative trauma disorders, back and lower extremity disorders, and manual materials handling. Identification of risk factors serves as a basis for either a quick fix of the problem or indicates the need for a more thorough job analysis. Checklists, such as the Risk Factor Checklists prepared as a part of the proposed OSHA Ergonomics Standard (OSHA, 1991), may be useful tools. Risk factors for upper extremity injuries include repetition, hand forces, awkward postures, contact stress, vibration, environmental conditions, and loss of control over work pace. Risk factors for lower extremity injuries include awkward postures, contact stress, vibration, push-pull forces, and loss of control over work pace. Manual materials handling risk factors are frequency of the lift, the lifting zone, and the weight of the object. Knowing these risk factors aids the evaluator in targeting specific jobs or tasks that must be analyzed further.

Observations require some method of note taking. The traditional means of note taking are pencil and paper and audio recording. The observer who uses these traditional methods must develop an efficient technique for recording information. Handwritten notes must be complete, organized, and legible if they are to be useful at a later time. In some cases, it may be advisable to use a checklist format, which can be completed quickly. The one disadvantage of a checklist is that there is often insufficient room to write additional notes at the level of detail required for later analysis. Audio recordings are efficient means of entering the needed information on-site, but they require additional time for someone to transcribe the dictation.

Another method for gathering information about the work area is videotaping. The advantage of using a video camera is that it records information that can be analyzed later in a more controlled environment at the evaluator's own pace. The biggest disadvantage is that a video camera sometimes misses what the observer sees on-site because the camera is only able to translate the three-dimensional event into a two-dimensional image. It is not possible to capture all of the information about the task with just one camera. For example, when shooting from the side using one video camera to record the actions of someone moving a box from a conveyor belt onto a palate, it may not be possible to document the amount of spinal rotation occurring during the lift. To some extent this problem can be addressed by shooting the action from several different positions (front, side, overhead, back) and shooting the full body and tight shots of hands, arms, knees, or feet. Normally, the evaluator uses only one video camera, which means that subsequent shots must be taken over several repetitions of the same task. If the worker performs the tasks in the exact manner each time, there is usually not a problem. However, if the worker's technique changes from time to time, some of the information needed for a thorough analysis may be lost. The more complex the job, the more video-taping will be required. It is important to shoot only as much footage as will be needed for later analysis. The more footage shot, the more that will have to be examined later.

Many evaluators use still cameras to record postures and working conditions. Instant cameras (such as a Polaroid) are sometimes preferred because they allow the evaluator to know almost immediately if the desired information has been captured. Thirty-five milli-meter cameras may provide good documentation of work, but the evaluator does not know until sometime after leaving the worksite whether or not the appropriate informa-tion has been recorded.

The skills of the evaluator and the level of detail required will determine the method for recording observations. Pencil-and-paper and audio methods allow the evaluator to record detailed observations about environment exposures (temperature, noise, radia-tion, humidity, chemical contact, etc.) that cannot be captured accurately by two-dimensional visual methods. Visual methods capture more environmental information but may not capture the three-dimensional detail of the activity. Most evaluators use more than one method of recording their observations during an on-site visit. In some work settings, however, the evaluator is restricted to recording information on paper or audiotape because the facility or the individual worker does not grant permission to make a video record. Although videotaping as a part of work analysis is becoming more widely accepted by work facilities, the evaluator should not assume that recording information by any visual means will be possible. Permission to record should be ob-tained prior to the on-site visit.

Formal Measurement

Formal measurements focus on the physical demands of the job tasks, including weights of objects handled (carried, pushed, pulled), dimensions of objects handled, dimensions of work areas, forces (push, pull, grip, pinch), vibration, and general and specific body postures and movements. In addition, it may be necessary to quantify the environmental conditions, such as temperature, lighting, and noise, that might impact performance of job tasks.

Weights of Objects.   Object weights are easily measured with either an analog or digital scale. If the worker handles objects of a consistent weight, it is usually only necessary to determine the weight of one sample of the object. Weighing the object several times ensures accurate and consistent results. On the other hand, if the worker is handling objects that vary in their weights, the range of object weights must be measured. If the weight of the heaviest object is equal to or below an accepted standard, the worker would be at minimal risk for injury. It is inappropriate to average the weight for comparison to accepted standards. If an average were calculated to be equal or slightly below the accepted standard, it would mean that part of the time the worker is handling objects that are heavier than acceptable, and she or he would be at an increased risk for injury.

Databases of acceptable weights to be handled have been constructed based on epidemiological, biomechanical, psychophysical, and physiological design approaches (Mital, Nicholson, & Ayoub, 1993). These databases reflect what the literature has determined to be acceptable weights for the design of manual materials handling jobs. The epidemiological design approach suggests that limiting the maximum load that can be handled to 60 lb (27.24 kg) significantly decreases back problems. The biomechanical design criterion, based on lumbar spinal compression, also indicate the maximum accepted load for males to be 60 lb (27.24 kg); for females, the accepted load is approximately 44.1 lb (20 kg). It should be noted, however, that the biomechanical criterion applies primarily to infrequent lifts. The physiological design criterion, based on energy expenditure rates of 4 kcal/min for males and 3 kcal/min for females over an eight-hour workday, applies to "repetitive lifting where the load is within the physical strength of the worker" (Mital et al., 1993, p. 38), and endurance is the primary consideration. The psychophysical criterion relies on the worker's self-selection of acceptable loads, which are typically lower than those determined for the physiological and biomechanical approaches. Based on the various approaches, Mital et al. (1993) have compiled a series of tables that contain criteria for two-handed symmetrical lifting based on the frequency of the lift and the size of the object. Multipliers are included for calculation of asymmetrical lifting, load asymmetry, coupling, load placement clearance, and heat stress using the table values. Mital et al. (1993) also published tables for acceptable maximum frequencies (cycles/min) for one-handed horizontal lifting based on the research required for the lift and the weight of the load.

Another approach to determining acceptable weight limits for manual materials handling is to use the NIOSH Lifting Equation, which aims to reduce low back pain and injuries attributed to manual lifting. The first equation for calculating a recommended weight limit for specified two-handed, symmetrical lifting was published in 1981 (U.S. Department of Health and Human Services, 1981). More recently, the equation has been revised to reflect new findings and provide methods for the evaluation of asymmetrical lifting tasks and lifts of objects involving less than optimal coupling between the object and the worker's hands (Waters, Putz-Anderson, & Garg, 1994). The current equation is based on a load constant of 51 lb (23 kg), which is considered to be the acceptable maximum load under ideal lifting conditions, and a series of multipliers that account for the horizontal and vertical components of the lift, as well as the distance the object is moved, the trunk rotation required for lift completion, the frequency of the lift, and the coupling. Although the revised equation has not been fully validated, it is considered to be consistent with the literature (Waters, Putz-Anderson, Garg, & Fine, 1993).

Dimensions.   Recording the dimensions of objects and the work area is a routine part of work analysis. The types of measurements taken vary tremendously according to the tasks involved in performance of the job and the characteristics of the workforce. Dimensions may relate to the work area itself—height, depth, and width of the work surface—or the confined space in which a task must be performed. They may also relate to the worker performing the task, including the horizontal distance during manual materials handling, the reach to perform operations, or the distance walked to perform a task.

Recorded dimensional data are usually compared to data from anthropometric tables for purposes of determining whether the work area dimensions are able to accommodate a percentage of the workers who are likely to perform the job. In this design context, determinations may include acceptable ranges of adjustability, ideal work heights, clearances, optimal tool handle size, ideal reach envelopes, or visual task parameters (Eastman Kodak Human Factors Section, 1983; National Aeronautics and Space Administration, 1978). The data are used primarily to minimize the physical stresses on the worker during performance of the job tasks.

In evaluating existing work areas, dimensional data are collected for purposes of redesigning the area to accommodate the limitations of an individual worker or decrease the injury or reinjury of workers performing risky job tasks. When accommodating the individual worker, it is necessary to record existing work area dimensions and the worker's dimensions. Measuring both allows the worker and the work to be optimally matched.

Forces.   Forces are a function of the weight and friction that impact the body in various ways. During manual materials handling, forces depend on whether the objects (tools, boxes, containers, handcarts, etc.) are pushed, pulled, lifted, or carried. During manipulation activities, forces relate primarily to the use of tools or handling objects that require grasping or pinching. Forces in the hand are generally increased when gloves are used or by other factors, such as work flow, production rate, and use of manual tools.

The types of forces measured include static holding and dynamic muscle contractions. Static strength studies have identified forces that should not be exceeded for different muscle groups or tasks (Rodgers, 1985, 1987). Dynamic forces are of concern for ergonomic analysis because the limits are generally lower than are those for static holding. General static and dynamic forces for all areas of the body may be the focus of a risk assessment for musculoskeletal disorders. More specific ergonomic analysis may be needed to determine the impact of specific forces on individual body parts.

Forces can be measured by weighing objects with a weight scale or by using force-gauge dynamometers. Force-gauge dynamometers include handheld dynamometers for measuring grip-and-pinch strength, such as the Jamar dynamometer and B&L pinch gauges, and push-pull forces, such as Chatillon strength dynamometers. The type of dynamometer used will depend on the forces to be measured. As with any instrument, each dynamometer should be calibrated often to ensure the accuracy of measurements.

Current designs of grip-and-pinch dynamometers do not allow accurate, direct measurement of forces during activity. When force transducers are placed on hand surfaces for direct measurement, the results are less than desirable because the addition of the "equipment" often changes the way the worker performs the task. Some practitioners have found it more acceptable to estimate grip-and-pinch forces by having the worker reproduce the forces on Jamar dynamometers and B&L pinch gauges immediately after completing the forceful exertion during the work task. Current research is focusing on the reliability of this procedure to predict the hand forces required during activity.

Measurement of push-pull forces requires a handheld dynamometer that acts like a scale to measure pushing and pulling forces in pounds or kilos. According to Burke (1992), "the trickiest part of this operation is trying to attach the force gauge in a way that closely simulates the normal hand and body part coupling with the object" (p. 97). Use of the dynamometer requires practice to ensure that the instrument is in line with the angle of force, and that it is truly measuring the push or pull force being generated to move the object.

Several measurements of push-pull forces should be taken. One accepted technique is to take three measurements and average them. Data recorded for push-pull forces should include the initial force (maximum force that sets an object in motion), the sustained force (maximum force that keeps the object in motions), and the maximum isometric force exerted. Force measurements should be taken on the various surface types where the activity occurs. If the activity involves the use of a cart, measurements should be taken both with the wheels parallel to the direction of push or pull and perpendicular to the direction of push or pull. The recommended levels of initial, sustained, and maximum isometric force are based on psychophysical design data that are adjusted so that physiological design criteria are not violated (Mital et al., 1993). Biomechanical design criteria are not used because they are not sufficiently limiting when pushing and pulling activities occur on a frequent basis. Most available data is based on two-handed push or pull, but there is some limited data available for one-handed push or pull.

Computerized force prediction programs are currently being developed to estimate the forces exerted during tasks. These programs may be valuable for estimating forces exerted by different body parts. It should be noted, however, that these programs rely on mathematical principles and limited knowledge about how the human body generates and responds to forces under controlled conditions. These types of programs may be useful in the future, but currently they are less practical and harder to use than the manual means described earlier.

Vibration. Vibration is classified as whole body vibration and segmental vibration. Whole body vibration is transmitted to the entire body through a support, such as a seat or the floor. Semi-trailer drivers often experience whole body vibration that is transmitted to the entire body through the vehicle's seat. Segmental hand-arm vibration is usually associated with the use of vibrating hand tools.

Measurement of hand-arm vibrations is a difficult task because it is a vector quantity, and measurements must be obtained by using the standardized system developed by the International Standards Organization (ISO 5349). Under ideal conditions three accelerometers that use biodynamic and biocentric coordinate systems are used to record vibrations. The results are compared with threshold limit values for exposure of the hand to vibration developed by the American Conference of Governmental Industrial Hygienists (ACGIH) and based on epidemiological studies. It is not practical to use this method during an on-site visit to a facility.

In a more practical sense, the existence of vibration should be noted even if it cannot be easily quantified. Worker's subjective complaints of intermittent tingling and/or numbness in the fingers or intermittent blanching and cyanosis of one or more fingertips are good indications that there is a problem with vibration that should be addressed by more a comprehensive, specialized evaluation.

Body Postures and Movements. Body postures are documented in terms of the position of joints or deviations from neutral position. Movements are described in terms of range of motion and direction of motion. Measurement devices, such as goniometers, allow quantification of postures and movements. If the postures are static, direct measurement may be possible. For static postures, the length of time the posture is maintained and the specific joint angles should be recorded. Dynamic postures or movements are more difficult to measure because postures change quickly. The range of movement can be determined by documenting the initial and terminal positions for the particular motion. If it is not possible to measure movement directly on the worker, the worker should be videotaped to capture the motions for later analysis. When videotaping is used, the recorder should be positioned to capture the planes of motion (i.e., directly to the side to capture motions of flexion and extension, from the front or back to capture abduction and adduction motions, and overhead to capture rotations). Often, motions do not occur in pure anatomical planes, thus videotaping may not be ideal for some work situations. However, when used, the videotape can be reviewed, and frames frozen to measure postures and the angles of the various joints.

The repetitive nature of movement patterns should be also quantified. The number of repetitions usually reflect production quotas, machine pacing, and work incentives. Measurement of repetitiveness is based on time-and-motion study. The simplest way to measure repetitiveness is to simply count the number of cycles of the motion that occur during a specified length of time (typically a work shift). The shorter the cycle, the more repetitive the job will be because the worker will repeat the cycle more often during the work shift. For hand and wrist motions, a cycle time of less than 30 seconds, which would mean that the job has at least 1,000 cycles per work shift, is considered highly repetitive (Armstrong, 1984). The time over which the cycle is performed (duration) should also be defined. Konz (1995) suggested that short duration be defined as less than 1 hour per day, moderate as 1 to 2 hours, and long as more than 2 hours.

In some cases, simply counting the number of cycles of motion may not be sufficient if the cycle time is greater than 30 seconds. In these cases, fundamental cycles are defined as the set of repeated motions or elements within a cycle. The cycles may be significantly less for the entire work shift, but the fundamental cycles are repeated at a level consistent with the 1000 cycles per work shift identified by Armstrong (1984).

Another way to measure repetitiveness is to count the number of movement or posture changes per shift. This method places the emphasis on the actual movements not the speed at which the worker is performing. Examples of recorded information include the number of times the worker must squat to perform tasks, the number of times the worker must lean forward from the waist, the number of reaches that must be performed, and the number of times the worker must move from sitting to standing.

Environmental Conditions. Industrial hygienists traditionally have evaluated environmental conditions such as temperature, radiation, chemical exposure, illumination/glare, ventilation, and noise. Evaluation of some of these areas (temperature, illumination/glare, noise) must be considered to be part of an ergonomic analysis because these factors often have an impact on the performance of job tasks.

The evaluation of temperatures in the work area should include the ambient air temperature as well as the temperature radiated from work surfaces and equipment used. The ambient air temperature of the work area can have a significant impact on energy expenditure levels, and it can pose a direct hazard to body tissues. Temperatures radiating from work surfaces and equipment may also pose a direct hazard to body tissues. When ambient air is cold, protective clothing must be worn. Thus the manner in which tasks are completed may be altered because motions are restricted by clothing. In cold temperatures, the exposed hands may become desensitized and cause the worker to grip objects harder than necessary. Gloves worn to protect the hands may require that additional force be used to close the hand or may reduce the coefficient of friction between the gloved hand and the objects that must be manipulated. In hot environments, the worker's perspiration will increase, and more force may be applied to tools as a result of slippage from sweaty hands. If heat is extreme, the need for work-rest schedules should be evaluated as a part of the work analysis.

Illumination/glare can be evaluated in terms of quantity and quality. The degree of accuracy required for job tasks will determine the quantity of lighting necessary in a particular work area. Brightness is needed to optimize viewing conditions for high-accuracy tasks. The quality of the light (glare, color, diffusion, direction, uniformity, and brightness) affects the worker's ability to see easily, accurately, and quickly. Specific, detailed procedures for measuring illumination/glare levels can be found in industrial hygiene literature along with the recommended lighting levels developed by the Illuminating Engineering Society of North America. If documentation of illumination or glare is a necessary part of a work analysis, they can be measured using a light meter.

Noise is unwanted sound. In noisy work environments, it is not unusual to hear workers yelling to be heard above the noise. When hearing protection is required because hazardous levels of noise are present in the work environment, it has an affect on communication. Compliance with the OSHA Noise Standard, 29 CFR 1910.95(a) and (b) (Occupational Safety and Health Administration, 1971), which defines permissible noise exposures in the work environment, is the employer's responsibility. Measurement of noise is determined by using a wide assortment of equipment, including sound survey meters, sound level meters, and octave-band analyzers. The sound level meter is the most basic instrument used to measure sound pressure variations in the air. As with other instruments, the sound level meter should be calibrated for accuracy of measurements.

ENSURING QUALITY AND ACCURACY OF ASSESSMENTS

Quality and accuracy of data are absolute necessities for drawing conclusions about the work environment, worker, and job tasks. Recommendations for change must be based on well-documented data gathered on-site and precise analysis of the data. If there is any reason to suspect inaccuracies, measurements should be rechecked. Likewise, calculations should be checked and double-checked. A slight error in calculation may mean that a hazard is incorrectly identified or is overlooked.

Once calculations are completed it is imperative that the data be compared with appropriate data sources for recommended limits. Sources for data are numerous. Most strength-related data sources are separated for males and females. Metabolic guidelines are different for males and females. Anthropometric data is available for military as well as nonmilitary populations. The data sources used should be comparable to the work population or work environment being analyzed.

REPORT PREPARATION

The report should be typed and carefully edited for spelling and grammar errors. Spelling and grammar errors often influence whether the report is viewed as credible. Inappropriate use of trade terminology may also lead to questions of credibility. When photographs and diagrams are included, they should be clearly labeled and referenced in the report. Appendices that contain reference information or data should also be clearly referenced in the report. Each section of the report should be written so that it is understandable and does not require the reader to flip back and forth between pages or sections of the report.

Preparation of the report of analysis depends on how and by whom the information will be used. Generally, long reports are only read by those who have specific need of the details in the report. It is advisable to provide a summary of the report that can be quickly read in addition to the detailed report. The summary should contain the highlights of the report, including an overview of the data collected, a listing of problems identified, and the recommendations for addressing the problems. Recommendations should be specific. It is often a good idea to offer options or staged solutions for addressing the problems. These actions are especially important when the recommended solutions require large capital expenditures or a great deal of time to implement.

REFERENCES

Armstrong, T. (1984). *An ergonomic guide to carpal tunnel syndrome*. Akron, OH: American Industrial Hygiene Association.

Baker, E. L., Melius, J. M., & Millar, J. D. (1988). Surveillance of occupational illnesses and injury in the United States: Current perspectives and future directions. *Journal of Public Health, 9*(2), 198–221.

Branton, P. (1987). In praise of ergonomics: A personal perspective. *International Reviews of Ergonomics, 1*, 1–20.

Burke, M. (1992). *Applied ergonomics handbook*. Boca Raton, FL: Lewis Publishers.

Christensen, J. M. (1987). The human factors profession. In G. Salvendy (Ed.), *Handbook of human factors* (pp. 3–16). New York: Wiley.

Drury, C. G. (1987). Task analysis. In G. Salvendy (Ed.), *Handbook of human factors* (pp. 370–401). New York: Wiley.

Eastman Kodak Human Factors Section. (1983). *Ergonomic design for people at work* (Vol. 1). New York: Van Nostrand Reinhold.

Equal Employment Opportunities Commission. (EEOC). (1992). *A manual on the employment provisions (Title I) of the Americans with Disabilities Act*. Washington, DC: Author.

Isernhagen, S. J. (1995). Job analysis. In S. J. Isernhagen (Ed.), *The comprehensive guide to work injury management* (pp. 70–85). Gaithersburg, MD: Aspen Publishers.

Matheson, L. N., Isernhagen, S. J., & Hart, D. L. (1996). Rehabilitation ergonomics: A client-centered ecological approach. *Work, 8*(2), 223–225.

Mital, A., Nicholson, A. S., & Ayoub, M. M. (1993). *A guide to manual materials handling*. London: Taylor & Francis.

Moroney, W. F., & Cameron, J. A. (1995, October). *Questionnaire design and use: A primer for practitioners*. Workshop presented at the 39th meeting of the Human Factors and Ergonomics Society, San Diego, CA.

National Aeronautics and Space Administration. (NASA). (1978). *Anthropology research project/Webb Associates: Anthropometric sourcebook* (Vols. 1–3). Houston, TX: NASA Scientific and Technical Information Office.

Occupational Safety and Health Administration. (1970). *OSHA Act of 1970, Section 6: Occupational safety and Health Standard* [WWW document]. URL:http://www.osha-slc.gov/OshAct_data/100006.html.

Occupational Safety and Health Administration. (1971). *Occupational noise exposure standard* [WWW document]. URL: http://www.osha-slc.gov/OshStd_data/1910.0095.html.

Occupational Safety and Health Administration. (1991). *Draft ergonomic protection standard* [WWW document]. URL http://www.ergoweb.com/Pub/info/oshaopts.html.

Olishifski, J. B., & Plog, B. A. (1988). Overview of industrial hygiene. In B. A. Plog (Ed.), *Fundamentals of industrial hygiene* (3rd ed., pp. 3–28). Washington, DC: National Safety Council.

Putz-Anderson, V. (1988). *Cumulative trauma disorders: A manual for musculoskeletal diseases of the upper limb*. New York: Taylor & Francis.

Rodgers, S. H. (1985). *Working with backache*. Fairport, NY: Perinton Press.

Rodgers, S. H. (1987). Recovery time needs for repetitive work. *Seminars in Occupational Medicine, 2*(1), 19.

Rodgers, S. H. (1992). A functional job analysis technique. *Occupational Medicine: State of the Art Reviews, 7*(4), 679–711.

U.S. Department of Health and Human Services. (1981). *Work practices guide for manual lifting* (NIOSH Technical Report No. 81-122). Cincinnati, OH: National Institute for Occupational Safety and Health.

U.S. Department of Labor. (1991). *Dictionary of occupational titles* (4th ed.). Washington, DC: U.S. Government Printing Office.

Waters, T. R., Putz-Anderson, V., & Garg, A. (1994). *Applications manual for the revised NIOSH lifting equation* (DHHS/NIOSH) Publication No. 94-110). Cincinnati, OH: National Institute for Occupational Safety and Health.

Waters, T. R., Putz-Anderson, V., Garg, A., & Fine, L. J. (1993). Revised NIOSH equation for the design and evaluation of manual lifting tasks. *Ergonomics, 36*(7), 749–776.

13

Disability Evaluation

Gunnar B. J. Andersson

All physicians with interest in musculoskeletal disorders will encounter some aspects of impairment and disability evaluation. Many are unprepared for this obligation. Sometimes, it is even an unpleasant experience because of the social, occupational, and legal ramifications that are part of the compensation programs making requests to determine impairment. Workers' Compensation and Social Security Disability Insurance offices most commonly request these evaluations, but private disability insurance companies and personal injury litigation cases often require information of this nature.

To standardize the process and the reporting of impairment and aid those making the final disability decisions, the American Medical Association (AMA) first published *Guides to the Evaluation of Permanent Impairment* in 1958. It is now in its fourth edition. Although not the only evaluation system in current use, it is by far the most commonly used in the United States. The *Guides* should be read in its entirety; it is not suitable for summarization.

The purpose of this chapter is to review definitions used in the disability evaluation arena, discuss alternative systems used to determine impairment, outline the physician's responsibilities in the process, and introduce the principles used to determine impairment of the upper extremity, lower extremity, and spine as indicated in the fourth edition of the *Guides*.

HISTORY

The concept of compensation has a long social and legal history of Western civilization. Workers' compensation laws date back to Roman times; by Roman law, a worker could claim compensation for an accidental injury from an employer and a fellow employee.

Gunnar B. J. Andersson • Department of Orthopedic Surgery, Rush-Presbyterian-St. Luke's Medical Center, 1653 West Congress Parkway, Chicago, Illinois 60612.

Sourcebook of Occupational Rehabilitation, edited by Phyllis M. King. Plenum Press, New York, 1998.

Although some compensation laws existed during the Middle Ages, it was not until the industrial revolution that compensation for negligent accidental injury became a significant issue. Thus, the first successful personal injury case in an English High Court dates back to 1836. Proof of negligence was necessary, and litigation was invalid if there was contributory negligence, or if the accident was caused by "ordinary risk." By the following year, however, the fellow-servant doctrine, stating that an employer was not responsible for negligence on the part of another employee or "fellow-servant," was accepted in English courts. Another step toward modern compensation laws was England's "Fatal Accident Act," which required compensation to the family of a person killed by accident. At about the same time, German law made railway companies responsible for any accidents on the Berlin–Potsdam Railroad.

Parallel development in Germany and England during the 1880s resulted in more comprehensive insurance laws. Bismarck introduced a comprehensive social insurance system in Germany, which included workers' compensation; compulsory insurance was introduced in England through the Employer's Liability Act (1880). Up until this time, fault had to be proved by the injured worker. This requirement was abolished in England by the Workman's Compensation Act (1887), which by 1911, covered all workers, not only those injured in accidents, but also those with industrial diseases and sickness as well.

In Europe, industrial liability was part of a comprehensive social security and welfare system, whereas acceptance of employer responsibility in the United States developed as a separate, no fault system. In 1908, the Federal Employees Compensation Act was passed; in 1911, Wisconsin enacted the first state workers' compensation law; in 1914, the California Industrial Accident Act was passed. Employers were sold on insurance coverage by the promise of immunity from liability suits on behalf of the employees. By 1949, workers' compensation systems existed in all states. In 1954, the Social Security Disability Act was passed, creating a second major disability compensation system.

DEFINITIONS

The term *impairment* denotes a physical or mental limitation of function that is the result of a disease or injury. Impairment is a quantifiable anatomic or functional loss, which can be permanent or temporary. Permanent means that the impairment is unlikely to change substantially over the next year with or without treatment. Impairment is determined by a physician.

Disability, on the other hand, is a reduced capacity to meet personal, social, or occupational demands. In the workplace, disability is the loss of capacity to be gainfully employed as a result of an impairment. *Disability*, therefore, is a broad term and includes not only the physical or mental impairment, but also motivation, education level, work experience, psychological factors, age, socioeconomic factors, and financial status. Disability reflects the interaction between the impairment and external job requirements. The determination of disability is ultimately an administrative one, often made by an agency and based on information other than a physician's measure of impairment. It is important to realize that an impaired individual does not have to be disabled. A determination that a person is "disabled," depends on occupational requirements.

A *handicap* is a disadvantage resulting from impairments and disabilities, described in terms of the interaction between the impaired person and his or her environment relative to peers and social norms. It focuses on social roles, including physical independence mobility, occupation, social integration, and economic independence. A handicap can be overcome by accommodation to the impairment. The Americans with Disabilities Act (ADA) mandates reasonable accommodation to the needs of permanently handicapped workers.

A peculiarity of some impairment evaluation systems is the "whole man" concept. Using this principle, a certain percentage is assigned to different impairments as they relate to different parts of the body. For example, in the AMA's *Guide to the Evaluation of Permanent Impairment* (Doege, 1993) amputation of a ring finger at the proximal interphalangeal joint represents an 80% impairment of the finger, 8% of the hand, 7% of the upper extremity, and 4% of the whole person. A person assessed to have complete loss of lower extremity function, that is, a 100% impairment, has a 40% impairment of the "whole man."

IMPAIRMENT EVALUATION SYSTEMS

For the musculoskeletal system, function is difficult to quantify. Different parts of the body interact differently depending on requirements, and adaptation frequently occurs. To address these difficulties, three different impairment evaluation methods, which are sometimes used separately and are sometimes combined, have evolved (Andersson, 1991, 1996).

Anatomic Systems

The anatomic approach to disability evaluation (based on examination) started with the recording of amputation, ankylosis, and fixed deformity. Later, it came to include weakness, loss of sensation, and measurement of range of motion (ROM). Although amputation, ankylosis, and deformity can be accurately, reproducibly, and objectively determined, weakness, loss of sensation, and ROM are more difficult to measure. These conditions are subjective in the sense that they all rely on the participation of the person being evaluated. Furthermore, it can be argued that weakness and ROM are indicators of function and are, in fact, functional rather than anatomic measures. The reason why these additional measures were included was that amputation, ankylosis, and deformity cover only a small part of impairment disorders. A pure anatomic system, therefore, would be useless for the majority of evaluations. The AMA's *Guides to the Evaluation of Permanent Impairment* initially used a modified anatomic approach, which included the measurement of ROM. In the most recent edition, diagnostic features have been included for the lower extremities and the spine. This change is an example of how impairment systems develop, not by holding to one methodological principle, but by combining different evaluation principles.

Diagnostic Systems

A diagnostic system is based on agreed-upon diagnostic groups (pathologies) to which impairment percentages are assigned. The advantages of the system are simplicity and reproducibility if criteria for the groups are clear, objective, and enforced. Deciding on criteria appears simple on the surface, but consider the difficulty in diagnosing certain spinal conditions, such as a herniated disc or low back strain. In at least 25% of the cases where anatomic evidence of herniated discs is present, those presenting this evidence have never experienced back pain or sciatica and have no disability or impairment. For clinical (as distinct from anatomic or radiologic) diagnosis, a herniated disc seen on an MRI, for example, is not sufficient evidence to make a diagnosis. There also must be appropriate symptoms and signs. Furthermore, a narrow spinal canal accentuates the clinical syndrome of disc herniation, but it can also correctly be diagnosed as spinal stenosis. Low back sprain, the most common back diagnosis, is a diagnosis by exclusion, which many physician's question. Any patient who complains of back pain can be fitted into this category if no other is applicable. The difficulty in developing diagnostic criteria is not the main weakness of a diagnosis-based system, however. Rather, it is the fact that the actual disability, as it relates to a diagnosis, is variable, which is the problem (McBride, 1963). For those reasons, a diagnosis-based system often needs to be combined with other measurements. An expanded diagnosis-based system is currently used by the Social Security Administration (1979; U.S. Bureau of Disability Insurance, 1970) and for Workers' Compensation Disability Evaluation in Minnesota (MMA, 1984). The Social Security Administration combines diagnosis with history, physical examination, and laboratory tests (when applicable), while the MMA system combines diagnosis with history, physical examination, pain complaints, and X-ray evaluation. (The fourth edition of the AMA *Guides* includes aspects of a diagnosis-based system.)

Functional Systems

There is currently no pure functional system in use, although conceptually a functional system would be the best method to evaluate impairment and disability. The difficulty lies in measuring function. Several functional indicators can be measured, but their relationship to overall function remains uncertain. These functional indicators include range of motion — the most frequently used functional estimate, and the easiest to obtain — strength, endurance, and coordination. The California Industrial Accident System includes functional parameters. Estimates are made by patients, however, without objective verification (Clark et al., 1988). The Social Security Administration (SSA) determines abilities to perform basic work activities and residual functional capacities for work, but SSA depends on medical reports for its review and rarely ever directly measures physical capacities. Requiring a sophisticated, objective measurement of various functions is impractical and costly, and the methods used are not so technically advanced that levels of function can be precisely determined.

THE PHYSICIAN'S RESPONSIBILITIES

The physician has at least four responsibilities in the disability evaluation process. The first is to establish the relationship between the injury event and the resulting impairment. This process is important in workers' compensation and personal injury cases, but it is not central to Social Security disability. A causal relationship can be direct, or it can be the result of aggravating an existing condition. The physician's responsibility is to record the events as they occurred. At a minimum the physician's record must contain a description of the alleged accident, including information about where and when it occurred. The problem of establishing causality for many musculoskeletal disorders is well established. *Aggravation* refers to the worsening of a preexisting medical condition. Aggravation may involve occupational and nonoccupational disorders and can be temporary or permanent.

The second responsibility is to determine when the healing period, the time beyond which no reasonable progress toward resolution will be made, will end. This end time is referred to as the point of maximum medical improvement or MMI. It is important that the physician and patient understand that this definition does not imply that normal function has been restored. Unfortunately, with many soft tissue injuries, the healing period is poorly defined. The physician should avoid prolonging the healing period "to be on the safe side," which can lead to deconditioning and chronic pain.

The physician's third responsibility is to determine if at the time of maximum medical improvement, any impairment exists, and if so, to rate this impairment. Regardless of the system that is used, the contribution of a preexisting condition (apportionment) must be assessed at this time. An impairment rating can be legally challenged by a injured worker, employer, or insurance carrier, who can request an independent medical examination (IME). The physician providing the IME examines the patient (claimant) to provide a second opinion on causation, treatment plan, ability to work, permanence of disability, and rate of impairment. Treatment is not assumed. In some states, impairment can only be rated by certified evaluators.

The fourth responsibility relates to work capacity. Often, the physician will be asked to estimate work capacity and outline restrictions, whether they are temporary or permanent. The quality of this information will vary greatly, because the physician's ability to determine work capacity is limited. A simple statement such as "light duty" is not adequate because it is open to a variety of interpretations. More specific restrictions often require a functional capacity evaluation.

THE AMA *GUIDES*

The musculoskeletal system is covered in a single chapter in the *AMA Guides to the Evaluation of Permanent Impairment* (4th ed., 1993). The chapter is divided into three parts: the hand and upper extremity, the lower extremity, and the spine. In general, the use of the *Guides* requires obtaining the patient's complete medical history and performing a physical examination. The history, physical, and other diagnostic information are then analyzed and compared with the criteria specified for the body part in question in the *Guides*.

For the upper extremity, ROM measurements are rounded to the nearest 10° and converted to percentages, using tables. Amputation of all or some part of the arm is added, as is sensory loss in the digits, when present. Separate sections deal with impairment due to peripheral nerve disorders, vascular disorders, and other disorders of the upper extremity. To evaluate the last of these, which include bone and joint disorders, arthroplasty, musculotendinous disorders, and loss of strength, ROM measurements are combined with crepitation, deformity, stability, and strength. The combined values chart, designed to combine impairments of the upper extremity contributed by the hand, wrist, elbow, and shoulder regions, is an important feature. This method is used for the lower extremity as well.

Lower extremity impairment can be evaluated by ROM, and diagnostic and functional criteria, but in general only one of these methods is used. Physical examination items used to assess impairment include limb length discrepancy, gait derangement, muscle atrophy and weakness, range-of-motion measurements, ankylosis, and amputations. In the case of arthritis, joint space, determined radiographically, is also used. With certain diagnostic groups, if the physician determines that a diagnosis provides the best estimate of the patient's impairment, estimates can be based on this diagnosis. Skin loss, peripheral nerve injuries, causalgia, reflex sympathetic dystrophy, and vascular disorders are separately evaluated. Combined value charts are used (as they are with the upper extremity) when several impairments of the same lower extremity or impairments of both extremities are present. The final impairment estimate cannot exceed 100% of the lower extremity (amputation) or 40% of the person.

For the spine, two alternatives for impairment evaluation exist. When using the "injury model," the patient is assigned to one of eight categories on the basis of clinical findings. The "range of motion model" is only used if the patient's condition cannot be assigned to one of the eight diagnostic categories, or if more clinical data are needed to categorize the spine impairment. The ROM model includes a diagnosis-based component that is combined with the range-of-motion-based estimates and a component based on any spinal nerve deficit. In most cases, the injury model also referred to as the "diagnosis-related estimates (DRE) model" will be used.

An evaluation of impairment using the *Guides* is only valid when the impairment is permanent, that is, well stabilized, unlikely to change substantially within a year, or amenable for further medical or surgical therapy.

DISCUSSION

The ideal impairment and disability evaluation system would include the features listed in Table 13.1. The most important of these is validity because any system should, of course, actually measure impairment/disability. The rating should also be consistent when the same impairment is evaluated by the same evaluator (intraindividual reliability). Furthermore, when the impaired person is evaluated by several evaluators, the rating should be the same (interindividual reliability). Wide variations in impairment ratings made by different physicians have been reported, particularly for spinal conditions (Brand & Lehmann, 1983; Clark et al., 1988; Greenwood, 1985; Lehmann & Brand, 1992).

Practicality is an important consideration in impairment evaluation because of the size of population evaluated. Over 4 million Americans receive support from Social Security Disability Insurance (SSDI) and Supplemental Security Income (SSI) programs (about 1.5 million claims are made each year), and each year there are more than 2 million examinations for workers' compensation disability claims related to the musculo-

Table 13.1. Characteristics of an Ideal Impairment and Disability Evaluation System

1. Valid (actually measure impairment disability)
2. Reproducible (interindividual reliability)
3. Practical (office setting)
4. Discriminating (among levels of impairment)
5. Quantifiable (for administrative and computer purposes)
6. Acceptable to all (workers' compensation systems, Social Security, goverment, private insurance, etc.)
7. Based on current understanding of pathophysiology

skeletal system. Given these numbers, it is important that the evaluation be done in a physician's office.

Ability to define different levels of disability—to discriminate—is another important feature. Discrimination presents difficulties when using a pure diagnostic system because the same disease can cause different levels of impairment, and the same impairment different levels of disability. Quantification is another important feature. It is necessary for administrative purposes makes possible the computerization of impairment evaluations. It is advantageous to all if authorities requesting impairment evaluations use the same systems. It would then be possible to perfect a system and better train impairment evaluators. Finally, impairment ratings should reflect pathology whenever possible. Basing an impairment rating on subjective complaints alone, without disease verification, raises issues of fairness.

CONCLUSION

The perfect impairment rating system does not now exist. Anatomic systems alone cannot measure impairment in large groups of people when such measurements are required. Diagnostic systems suffer from a lack of agreement on diagnostic criteria and an inability to discriminate between levels of impairment among individuals with the same diagnosis. Function-based systems are not realistic at the present time because the technology is not available to realize them. Combining different features of different systems currently is the only realistic solution. Developing methods that quantify pain, determine function, and relate impairment to disability are challenges that merit further attention.

REFERENCES

Andersson, G. B. J. (1991). Impairment evaluation, issues, and the disability system. In T. G. Mayer, V. Mooney, & R. J. Gatchel (Eds.), *Contemporary conservative care for painful spinal disorders* (pp. 531–535). Lea & Febriger.

Andersson, G. B. J. (1996). Generic rating systems for musculoskeletal impairment. In S.Demeter, G. B. J. Andersson, & G. Smith (Eds.), *Disability evaluation* (pp. 90–92). St. Louis, MO: Mosby.

Brand. R. A.. & Lehmann. T. R. (1983). Low back impairment rating practices of orthopedic surgeons. *Spine, 8*, 75–78.

Clark, W. L., Haldeman, S., Johnson, P., Morris, J., Schulenberger, C., Trauner, D., & White, A. (1988). Back impairment and disability determination: Another attempt at objective, reliable rating. *Spine, 13*, 332–341.

Doege, F. C. (Ed.). (1993). *Guides to the Evaluation of Permanent Impairment* (45th ed.). Chicago: American Medical Association.

Greenwood, J. G. (1985). Low-back impairment-rating practices of orthopedic surgeons and neurosurgeons in West Virginia. *Spine, 10*, 773–776.

Lehmann, T. R., & Brand, R. A. (1982). Disability in the patient with low back pain. *Orthopedic Clinics of North America, 13*, 559.

McBride, E. (1963). *Disability evaluation.* Philadelphia, PA: J. B. Lippincott.

Minnesota Medical Association. (1984). *Workers' compensation permanent partial disability schedule.* Minneapolis, MN: Author.

Social Security Administration. (1979). *Disability evaluation under social security* (pp. 1–22). Washington, DC: U.S. Government Printing Office.

U.S. Bureau of Disability Insurance. (1970). Disability evaluation under social security. A handbook for physicians. Washington, DC: U.S. Government Printing Office.

IV

REHABILITATION OF WORK-RELATED DISORDERS

14

Work Hardening and Work Conditioning

Phyllis M. King

Since their inception in the late 1970s, work-hardening and work-conditioning programs have undergone metamorphoses. They have become less distinct and now offer more diverse services. This is primarily due to the ever-changing environment of health care, and the need to adapt to new consumer needs. Insurance demands, reimbursement issues, health care service trends, the adoption of disability management practices, and employee–employer relations are just a few variables influencing the practices of work-hardening and work-conditioning programs.

As programs have evolved to meet the needs of consumers, so has confusion over terminology, guidelines, and standards of practice. Terms such as *work hardening, work conditioning, functional restoration, work retraining, return to work,* and *work rehabilitation* have been used to describe programs that rehabilitate the injured worker. These differences in terminology make it difficult to distinguish among programs that may be very similar in structure, content, and goals. In this chapter, the term *occupational rehabilitation program* will refer to work hardening, work conditioning, or both.

This chapter will review the origins and evolution of occupational rehabilitation programs. Common practices, including program development, program operation, and program evaluation, will be discussed. A chapter-ending case study will illustrate the concepts presented.

ORIGINS OF OCCUPATIONAL REHABILITATION PROGRAMS

The concept of occupational rehabilitation originated in the late 1970s and grew out of a recognized need for better management of compensable work injuries. Prior to

Phyllis M. King • Occupational Therapy Program, University of Wisconsin–Milwaukee, Milwaukee, Wisconsin 53201.

Sourcebook of Occupational Rehabilitation, edited by Phyllis M. King. Plenum Press, New York, 1998.

this time, typical work injuries appeared to be the result of acute trauma due to an accident or environmental hazard. Most such injuries were successfully treated with medical interventions (Niemeyer, Jacobs, Reynolds-Lynch, Bettencourt, & Lang, 1994). However, an interesting phenomenon occurred over the past two decades. The incidence of repetitive strain or cumulative trauma injuries affecting joints, tendons, muscles, and nerves began to rapidly exceed acute trauma injuries. Low back pain and upper extremity cumulative trauma disorders were of particular concern. This increase in injuries gave rise to the diagnostic category of chronic pain and other musculoskeletal disorders. At the same time, researchers were finding that a significant percentage of those individuals with cumulative trauma disorders who were treated with a purely biomedical approach were not returning to work but were remaining disabled for years after injury (Niemeyer et al., 1994).

Work Hardening

Work hardening, a concept first described by Leonard Matheson (Matheson, Ogden, Violette, & Schultz, 1994), was an approach created to fill the gap between medical intervention and return to work. It was described as interdisciplinary, based on "evidence that suggested disability following an occupational musculoskeletal injury/illness was the consequence of a complex interaction of medical condition, physical capabilities, ergonomic demands, and a variety of psychosocial issues" (Feuerstein, 1991, p. 9).

Because different disciplines were involved, including occupational therapists, physical therapists, vocational evaluators, psychologists, and others, programs initially lacked consistency in definition and practice. In 1989, the Commission on Accreditation of Rehabilitation Facilities (CARF) officially defined work hardening as "a highly structured, goal-oriented, individualized treatment program designed to maximize the individual's ability to return to work" (Commission on Accreditation of Rehabilitation Facilities, 1988, p.69). Their guidelines recommended work-hardening programs be interdisciplinary in nature and be capable of addressing the functional, physical, behavioral, and vocational needs of the person served. CARF suggested the use of real or simulated work activities in conjunction with conditioning activities to improve biomechanical, neuromuscular, cardiovascular/metabolic, behavioral, attitudinal, and vocational functioning. (Figure 14.1 illustrates the use of a simulated shoveling activity, for example.)

In order to be accredited by CARF, programs must conform to CARF standards for administration and organization. Many practitioners found these standards to be burdensome and not necessarily related to quality of care. For this reason, many programs chose not to seek accreditation.

In 1991, a subcommittee of the American Physical Therapy Association (APTA) responded to the impact CARF standards were having on work-hardening programs and developed alternative guidelines for clinics that did not want to assume the costs of the administrative standards set forth by CARF. These guidelines identified two types of services: work hardening and work conditioning (Helm-Williams, 1993).

Work Conditioning

The APTA guidelines define work conditioning as a program with an emphasis on physical conditioning, which addresses issues of strength, endurance, flexibility, motor control, and cardiopulmonary function (Helm-Williams, 1993). Exercise equipment (such

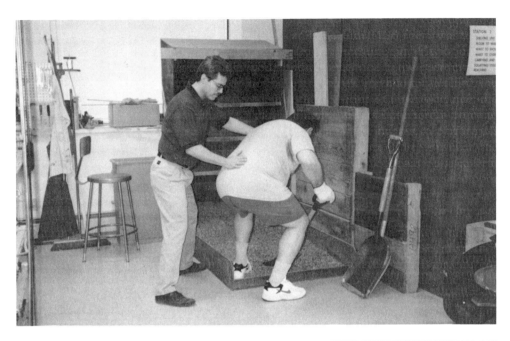

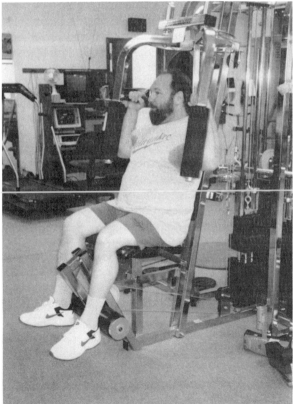

Figures 14.1, 14.2. Simulated work activities are used in conjunction with conditioning activities in work-hardening programs. (Photographs provided courtesy of Dean Hanus.)

**Table 14.1. Similarities and Differences
Between Work-Hardening and Work-Conditioning Programs**

SIMILARITIES

- Both are work-oriented with specific work goals.
- Both are initiated with an appropriate evaluation and concluded with a return-to-work-oriented discharge evaluation.
- Both have limited duration.
- Both interface with other "players" on the team (physicians, employers, insurance representatives, rehabilitation consultants.)

DIFFERENCES

Work conditioning	Work hardening
1. Uses exercise, aerobic conditioning, education, and limited work tasks	1. Uses work simulation as the primary modality
2. One or two disciplines	2. Multidisciplinary
3. Weak vocational component	3. Strong vocational component
4. Usually a half-day program	4. Half- to full-day programs
5. Moderate space allocation	5. Large amount of space allocated
6. More successful with early referrals or uncomplicated psychological or vocational cases	6. Best for the spectrum of work-injured clients

as that shown in Figure 14.2) is commonly used. The objective of work conditioning is to restore the client's physical capacity and function to allow a return to work. (Table 14.1 depicts the major similarities and differences between work hardening and work conditioning.)

EVOLUTIONS IN PRACTICE

The traditional medical model of practice has given way to new approaches that bridge the gap between medical management and return-to-work requirements and processes, enlarging the sphere of involvement for occupational rehabilitation professionals. Other trends, such as managed care and the development of ergonomics and disability management programs by employers, have greatly influenced occupational rehabilitation practices.

Managed Care

In the 1990s, workers' compensation reform came into the national spotlight. Poor rehabilitation outcomes were believed to be the result of conflicting agendas and messages from health care providers, organized labor, legal counsels, employers, claimants, and compensation or insurance agencies. In an effort to increase the need for accountability for the quality, effectiveness, and cost of care, and ensure that resources were directed to cost-effective treatments, workers' compensation began to follow the precedent of managed care set by other health care delivery systems in the United States (Niemeyer, Foto, & Holmes-Enix, 1994). *Managed care* is defined as "an integrated financing and delivery system for health care benefits characterized by: selection standards for providers, contractual payer-provider relationships, and formal processes for monitoring the efficiency and effectiveness of provider networks" (Simental, 1993, p. 26). The major goal of this approach is to influence patient care decision making through individual case assessments to determine the appropriateness of care prior to service delivery.

This managed care scenario presents risks for occupational rehabilitation programs. If programs cannot demonstrate cost-effective services, they might be excluded from provider networks; and if programs do not provide information to guide managed care providers, they can lose control over what becomes incorporated into standards of care.

The pressures of managed care have forced occupational rehabilitation programs to form partnerships with insurance companies and employers. As a result, greater importance is often given to outcomes studies than to the rehabilitation process. Programs have developed an internal system of utilization management, paralleling systems used by insurance agencies.

Ergonomics

As ergonomics became increasingly more accepted by the industrial and occupational medicine communities as a concept for preventing and reducing work-related injuries, occupational rehabilitation programs expanded their practices to include these services. Ergonomics is considered in the assessment of functional capacity and disability, work-injury rehabilitation, return-to-work activities, proactive injury prevention, and wellness efforts. Ergonomic interventions include, but are not limited to, training of workers in body mechanics, posture, and lifting techniques; basic methods of injury prevention and education; the introduction of exercise programs; task and workstation redesign; and general environmental changes in the workplace (Smith, 1989).

Ergonomics practices provide a window of opportunity for occupational rehabilitation programs to provide services at the workplace. Requests by employers and insurance companies for ergonomics services vary. Some employers desire the development of comprehensive ergonomics programs, which requires a collaborative and cooperative effort among the medical, safety, engineering, production, and workers' compensation departments, as well as between top management and labor. Smaller or less invested companies are more interested in educational seminars and/or periodic worksite analyses, often prompted by incidence of work-related injuries and encouragement from insurance carriers. These requests give rise to consultation contracts between employers, insurance companies, and occupational rehabilitation programs. Regardless of the requests, ergonomics has become an avenue by which occupational rehabilitation programs form closer working relationships with industries in order to effectively join medical and productivity considerations.

Early Return-to-Work Programs

Generally, empirical evidence and widely held convictions among medical and rehabilitation professionals support the belief that early intervention is the key to rehabilitation outcome (Shrey, 1995). Because this belief was substantiated time and time again (Gardner, 1987; Pati, 1985; Rundle, 1983; Scheer, 1990; Weiler, 1986), early intervention strategies were developed by occupational rehabilitation programs. Developing such programs necessitates close collaboration among a number of key personnel within industry. Disability management practices advocate interventions that demonstrate effective control of employer costs and protection of the employability of workers. Among the interventions that fall within the domain of occupational rehabilitation programs are the following:

> Functional job analyses
> Functional capacity evaluations
> Physical reconditioning
> Worker retraining
> Return-to-work transitioning
> Ergonomic program development and job modifications
> Modified duty assignments
> Work-injury prevention education
> Work station modifications
> On-site rehabilitation services

The "partnership movement" between occupational rehabilitation programs, industry, insurance providers, and other vested parties has significantly changed the structure, practices, and approaches of traditional work-hardening and work-conditioning programs. An example of this is reflected in the latest issue of CARF standards (1995), which replaces the term work-hardening programs with occupational rehabilitation programs. This document describes three types of occupational rehabilitation programs:

1. Acute Occupational Rehabilitation Programs
2. Work-specific Occupational Rehabilitation Programs—Category One
3. Work-specific Occupational Rehabilitation Programs—Category Two.

OCCUPATIONAL REHABILITATION PROGRAM DEVELOPMENT

Market Analysis

Before establishing an occupational rehabilitation program, it is wise to complete a careful market analysis to determine the demand for such services. Demographics and statistics pertaining to competition, community unemployment rates, industrial growth rates, and local industry mix can provide important information on the future demand for occupational rehabilitation services.

Selection of Location

Selecting an appropriate site is a critical decision. Referral sources prefer nearby locations, and clients' travel distances affect their compliance with attendance requirements once they are in the programs. Facilities should be easily accessible from major highways, and within a 30-minute drive of those they intend to serve (Key, 1996).

Not long ago, it was believed there were two basic choices for locations of occupational rehabilitation programs: either within an established hospital or rehabilitation facility or a freestanding rehabilitation center. As programs proliferated and diversified, occupational rehabilitation programs moved to industrial parks, strip shopping malls, and office complexes. Today, employer-based programs, often referred to as on-site programs, are being promoted as an alternative that not only provides a more realistic environment, but also has the additional benefit of placing the employee back at work and in close communication with the employer. (Chapter 15 provides specific information related to on-site program practices.)

Space

Space requirements vary depending on the length of the program and the amount and size of equipment specified. The client base often determines the equipment mix.

The average size space for a work-conditioning or work-hardening center is 2,500 square feet (Hazard, Matheson, Lehmann, & Frymoyer, 1991). Work-hardening programs accommodate exercise equipment, a work-simulation area, and quiet private areas for testing and evaluation. Additional office space may be designated for case management activities, conferencing, documentation, and educational presentations. Programs following more of a work-conditioning model usually require less space because work simulation is less emphasized. While work hardening often has permanent work-simulation stations, work conditioning often uses multipurpose adaptable stations and focuses more on using physical-conditioning equipment (Darphin, 1995).

Equipment Selection

As occupational rehabilitation programs continue to grow, new products are being developed to serve this specialized industry's needs. Some products are simple, functional, and inexpensive; others are very expensive and unnecessary. Decisions regarding the purchase of equipment should be based on the needs of the program's clients and the program's goals. Extremely expensive equipment is not required to return an injured worker to work.

For consistency and reproducibility, the equipment used for work-hardening and work-conditioning evaluations should be standardized within an organization. The organization must define and consistently use standard equipment for all types of testing (Saunders, 1995).

Types of equipment that are beneficial for programs include the following:

1. Work-simulation equipment that simulates real job activities. This equipment may include ladders, bricks, crates, tool boxes, circuit boards, work tables, and so on In many instances, workers use specialized tools and equipment. If so, it is most beneficial for these supplies to be brought to the program for the worker's use in rehabilitation. Programs that can justify cost and volume may choose to purchase computerized work-simulation equipment.
2. Aerobic or exercise equipment that facilitates physical conditioning includes treadmills, exercise bikes, stairclimbers, rowing machines, and an upper extremity ergometer.
3. Evaluation equipment may include standardized commercial products for evaluating strength and coordination, manual lifting, overall physical capacity, and work force. Products are also available for the evaluation of vocational abilities and aptitudes related to specific occupational categories.

Equipment should be user-friendly, durable, space-efficient, have a manufacturer's warranty, and be multitask capable. The work-simulation equipment should have face validity in the eyes of the user. In other words, it should simulate postures and movements of real-world functions. Clients should be able to recognize the transferability of physical and mental skills developed by the tasks performed in the programs as they relate to their own occupations.

Staffing

Staffing primarily depends on the client caseload and each program's components. The disciplines most commonly associated with occupational rehabilitation programs are occupational therapy, physical therapy, psychological/social services, and vocational services.

Adjunct services that deal with such issues as alcohol and drug dependency, nutrition, stress management, and medication reduction may be integrated into a program or referred as deemed necessary by the treating team. The client is a part of the team. Program plans are driven by the client's needs and are frequently and thoroughly reviewed.

Newly developing programs may initially hire an occupational or physical therapist to assist with program development. This professional may be responsible for all aspects of the program, from daily scheduling to program planning, client treatment, monitoring, and documentation.

As the program grows, additional staff may be hired, and the original therapist may assume a program directorship role. He or she would be in charge of supervising employees, participating in public relations activities, leading staff meetings, communicating with insurance representatives, and continuing the development of the program.

As a larger client base is acquired, a therapy assistant or trainer would prove to be a valuable member of the team. This person may be an occupational therapy assistant, physical therapy assistant, exercise physiologist, athletic trainer, or kinesiologist. She or he is invaluable in the role of overseer of day-to-day client care. An assistant or trainer is also instrumental in program development efforts.

The roles of different occupational rehabilitation therapies are vague and often overlap. The trend in occupational rehabilitation is toward a blending of duties (recognizing that no one profession can provide all the components of the various occupational rehabilitation programs) and promoting a philosophy of interdisciplinary cooperation (Saunders, 1995). More importantly, the professionals need to have the appropriate schooling, degrees, licenses, and certifications deemed applicable by their state laws and professional associations, with the addition of specialized training in the area of occupational rehabilitation.

Occupational rehabilitation programs tend to have therapists who are dedicated to their programs, not simultaneously seeing acute or general caseloads. These programs require good communications among a variety of players, including employers, insurers, families, physicians, attorneys, and other professionals. Therapists need to develop techniques to deal with the behavioral and physical issues facing injured workers. To work successfully with a team of professionals requires time and dedication on behalf of program personnel.

Program Components

Common components in occupational rehabilitation programs include, but are not limited to, work simulation, aerobic conditioning, strengthening exercises, and education.

Work simulation is usually based on the results of a job analysis or information obtained from the injured workers' job descriptions. Actual equipment obtained from the job site is sometimes incorporated into the injured workers' rehabilitation programs. An occupational rehabilitation program may begin with more emphasis on exercise but progressively add more work simulation activities.

Occupational rehabilitation programs are experiencing a trend toward shorter lengths of time between the client's date of injury and initial treatment. This change reduces the need for emphasis on physical conditioning. Still, a great majority of clients entering rehabilitation programs are aerobically deconditioned. Many programs build in an aerobic conditioning component to such clients' overall programs. Building in this component involves an initial cardiovascular screen to rule out inappropriate clients, communication with clients' physicians, and close monitoring of the clients' blood pressure and heart rate.

Strengthening exercises are developed based on the client's needs as determined by an initial assessment. Physical strength, as it relates to the client's required job functions, such as lifting, carrying, pushing, or pulling, is the focus. A strengthening program is developed in collaboration with the client. Many therapists provide initial instructions to clients about strengthening protocols and procedures. They then work on promoting client independence by posting plans where clients have easy access to them. Clients are expected to follow the written plans under the general supervision of the professional program staff.

An educational component to a rehabilitation program is developed to prevent reinjury and promote safe job performance. Clients are instructed on how to properly use their bodies to perform jobs safely. It is believed that their knowledge of health and disease will empower them to take more responsibility for their own health and apply the information learned. Educational topics depend upon the population served. The most common topics include back education, upper extremity education, and stress management.

Educational sessions are provided in group and individual sessions. Individual sessions focus on addressing the individual client's needs as they pertain to his unique situation or lifestyle. Clinics may develop their own literature for this purpose or use commercially available educational products.

PROGRAM OPERATIONS

Entrance Criteria

Entrance criteria varies among facilities. When work-hardening and work-conditioning programs were first conceptualized, specific entrance criteria was written for each. Examples of admission criteria for work-hardening programs included the following:

1. The client is unable to return to his job due to pain or dysfunction following injury.
2. The client must agree to participate in the program.
3. There is a reasonably good prognosis for improvement of employment capacity following participation in the program.
4. The client has a job-oriented goal.

The typical work-hardening client may have been out of work for over three months, had a compromised cardiovascular system, psychosocial deficits, and questionable employment prospects.

Work-conditioning admission criteria was quite similar to those of work hardening. The major difference was reflected in the client's concurrent ability to participate in productive activities or in a modified duty capacity while receiving rehabilitation services. Therefore, increasing the individual's level of functional abilities was emphasized.

Regardless of what element of the rehabilitation program is emphasized, the occupational rehabilitation professional needs to screen clients for any medical conditions that might prohibit them from participating in programs or resuming work. The issue of physician referral should be clarified. Some states allow evaluation and/or treatment of individuals without a physician's referral. However, often clients may present with unresolved medical complications that warrant communication between the physician and therapist, prior to evaluation to determine possible contraindications.

Today, primarily due to earlier intervention, occupational rehabilitation programs admit clients who are not as physically deconditioned or detached from the workplace. This change presents opportunities for programs to collaborate with employers and ultimately increases the potential for successful return-to-work outcomes.

As health care regulations and reimbursement changes occur, and programs continue to diversify and expand their practices, new client populations will be served. For example, cardiac rehabilitation clients and individuals with sports-related injuries are increasingly being seen in occupational rehabilitation programs. In some states, appropriately staffed occupational rehabilitation programs have become providers of vocational counseling, assessments, and placement services.

Intake

Interview

An intake interview is usually the clinician's first point of contact with the client. This interview presents an opportunity to establish rapport with the client and gather valuable information on medical and work history. Insight into what procedures have worked or failed in the past, as well as the client's beliefs or misperceptions about his or her condition, can be ascertained. It is important to obtain specific information related to job history, both pre- and postinjury. Equally important are details about how long the client has been off work or on light duty, how many times (and when) return-to-work efforts were tried, and the client's opinion of the reasons for their failure (Saunders, 1995).

Orientation

The therapist should thoroughly explain to the client the purpose of the program and its sequence of events, including the criteria for discontinuing a functional task and the need to put forth a sincere effort.

It is common for occupational rehabilitation programs to have written guidelines that indicate the rules and expectations of the program. These guidelines are reviewed with the client to clarify his or her expected performance and the program's delivery of services. This agreement is established to prevent conflict or misunderstandings. It usually is signed and treated as a contract between the client and the program.

Along with signing a written agreement, the therapist may also request that the client sign an authorization for release of information. This release is necessary in order to obtain information from the client's past and present health providers. A clients' rights list is another document often reviewed at this time.

Evaluation

An evaluation of a client's functional capacities is performed prior to any conditioning and/or work-related activities. Currently, programs lack a universally recommended method of evaluation. Controversy exists over which evaluation or its components yield the most accurate results. There are a number of commercially available evaluation packages on the market. Some rehabilitation programs prefer to devise their own evaluation systems. Differences in evaluation terminology also exist. *Baseline functional evaluation, functional capacity evaluation, physical capacity evaluation, work capacity assessment*, and *functional capacity assessment* are all terms used for evaluation, but each assessment may follow different procedures. Most leaders in the field share the opinion that obtaining work parameters through the functional approach, regardless of how it is labeled, appears to generate the most accurate results.

Although assessment may vary, certain basic requirements still remain constant. These requirements include using evaluators who have sound clinical knowledge, objective measuring tools to establish reliability and validity, and comprehensive, clear and logical report formats (Miller, 1991). (See Chapter 11 for details on the qualities and characteristics of functional capacity testing.)

The fundamental purpose of the initial evaluation is to become familiar with the client's current functional status, behaviors associated with work activity, potential latent symptom responses after activity, and body mechanics techniques. This information is compared with the client's job demands and goals for progress.

Establishing Goals

The client's motivation for participating in the program and returning to productive work are crucial to successful rehabilitation. Therefore, it is extremely important for the client to be actively involved in setting her or his own goals and being realistic about them. The therapist, in conjunction with the rehabilitation team, can assist the client in determining the appropriateness of the goals, revising them when necessary, and estimating the client's length of involvement in the program based on these goals. The results of the initial evaluation are used as a base for designing a client's treatment program.

The client's length of time in the program depends on his or her individualized treatment needs and the treatment protocols established by the program. Scheduling is done in collaboration with the client to enable the client to meet personal obligations. At one time, work-hardening clinics expected clients to participate in a program for up to eight hours per day, five days per week. This practice was viewed as expensive by insurance companies, and there was no scientific evidence to suggest that work-hardening services delivered results above and beyond what can be delivered more cheaply, quickly, and simply by conservative medical management and on-site return-to-work programs (Schwartz, 1993). Work-conditioning programs incorporated shorter days and still demonstrated success in returning clients to their jobs.

The current trend is to start the client in an occupational rehabilitation program for two hours per day, eventually progressing to four hours per day. To do so, clinicians need to devise highly focused and well-managed treatment plans. Such scheduling allows programs to accommodate more clients, provide more on-site services, and devote more attention to case management activities.

Progam Planning

Program planning requires a skilled clinician. It involves analysis and synthesis of previous care information with the results obtained from the initial client evaluation. The following variables are to be considered in the development of a treatment plan:

1. Previous care information
2. Initial evaluation results
3. Return-to-work job demands
4. Client's injury profile

With health care reimbursement activities focusing more on outcomes, occupational rehabilitation programs are striving for standardization in treatment approaches. This means that a program's approach and results are consistent from one client to another. Standardization allows programs to better predict outcomes.

Developing treatment protocols is difficult to do. It entails the integration of information from intake to discharge, while factoring in the processes of other disciplines. At the same time, there needs to be enough flexibility built into the protocols to be able to individualize programs to meet each client's specific needs. As difficult as this may seem, emphasis on critical pathways and outcomes generation warrants the need for occupational rehabilitation programs to become involved in protocol establishment.

Program Services

When administering a plan, it is important to follow a structured process that is guided by consistent standards and tailored to each client's needs. The services offered are dependent on the client's needs and ultimate goals.

Most programs start clients with warm-up activities involving stretching and exercise. This warm-up is followed by strengthening and job-simulation activities. Clients are selectively weaned from exercise activities until the majority of treatment time is devoted to job simulation.

Education is usually woven into the program. Educational needs vary with each individual. Information on risk factors that contribute to injury, proper use of the body to perform different job tasks, and prevention of reinjury are common educational components.

Occupational rehabilitation programs vary in the scope of services they offer. Services offered are usually determined by the size of the program, staffing, and other available resources. (An array of their services is listed in Table 14.2.)

Communication

Good communication among all parties involved needs to occur. It is particularly important to maintain close and frequent contact with the client's employer if the client's goal is to return to work. As the client progresses, an opportunity may arise for him to return to work on a part-time basis or in a modified duty position while continuing

**Table 14.2. Services Offered by
Occupational Rehabilitation Programs**

Individual graded work simulation
Baseline assessment of functional abilities
Job analysis (via client interview and/or on-site)
Education for injury prevention
Modification of workstation or tool design
Conditioning exercises
Stress management
Vocational assessment for job matching
Pain management
Preemployment/preplacement screening
Vocational exploration activities
Supported employment (e.g., job coaching)

rehabilitation. The work environment and peer interactions may assist in motivating the client toward productive employment.

Discharge

Discharge from an occupational rehabilitation program is usually the result of the combined input of the treatment team. The following are common criteria for discharge:

1. Client meets goals.
2. Client's progress has stopped or slowed to an imperceptible level.
3. Client has medical complications.
4. Client is noncompliant with the program.

Discharge documentation summarizes the client's participation in the program, outlining his or her activities and performance. It should clearly define the client's current functional activity abilities and ongoing needs. Some states have a standard form that the treating physician uses to indicate work abilities. This form is completed by the occupational rehabilitation program and signed by the physician. The summary should be discussed with the client and indicate whether the client is in agreement with the discharge recommendations.

PROGRAM EVALUATION

The program evaluation allows the administrators and managers to demonstrate that their program is achieving its goals. It is a systematic process that determines how effectively and efficiently improvements in a client's functional status have been achieved. Effectiveness is the extent to which a program's performance is congruent with its expectations. Efficiency is the relationship between an intervention's output and input. It involves measuring an intervention's effectiveness against the resources consumed (Hoffman-Grotting & Ralph, 1991).

A program evaluation system measures outcomes, progress, and the process of care delivery. This information is the basis on which decisions regarding performance, quality, and standards are made (King, 1993). According to the Commission on Accreditation of

Rehabilitation Facilities (CARF) (1995), there are four elements that must be included in a program evaluation system:

1. A purpose/mission statement for the organization
2. A program structure delineating all major programs and product lines
3. A system review mechanism
4. Management reports

More specifically, CARF requires occupational rehabilitation programs to provide an evaluation system documentating the following:

1. Progress toward functional, work-related goals
2. Frequency, duration, and costs of services
3. Work capability at discharge
4. Status of postdischarge functional, work-related abilities

In addition, work-specific occupational rehabilitation programs must collect information on the (a) percentage of persons returning to work, (b) receiving vocational services, (c) receiving other services, and (d) returning to their original jobs.

OUTCOMES STUDY

Analyzing outcomes is a complex task. Each client enters a program with different needs and desired outcomes. Furthermore, occupational rehabilitation programs provide individualized structured, graded, and work-oriented activities.

The problem of analyzing outcomes is multiplied when comparing programs. Occupational rehabilitation programs differ in size, staff, equipment, methods, and service.

External variables, such as policies on workers' compensation, disability benefits, and social security disability insurance, influence a client's motivation to return to work and his or her eligibility for services. Employer policies and procedures may influence return-to-work timelines for injured workers returning to their jobs. Other parties, such as the physician, insurance company personnel, attorney, therapist, and employee's family, may influence the client's rehabilitation.

Despite the complexities of outcomes analysis, consumers continue to demand outcomes studies to judge program effectiveness. Outcomes systems for occupational rehabilitation programs are available commercially. Companies selling these products often provide data management services or have an established comparative database. (Typical categories of data collection are identified in Table 14.3.) Quality of care is assessed via client satisfaction questionnaires. Follow-up services include telephone surveys at three-month, six-month, and one-year intervals.

SUMMARY

Occupational rehabilitation programs continue to be shaped by evolutions in the health care and insurance industries, employer demands, and employee needs. What was once a well-identified work-hardening or work-conditioning program is now an occupational rehabilitation program striving to creatively and effectively meet the needs of its customers.

Table 14.3. Categories of Information for Outcomes Data Collection

Age	Injury to admission time
Gender	Job attached to preinjury employer
Education	Time from discharge to return to work
Occupation	Length of time in program
Physical demand level of job prior to injury	Frequency of length of treatments
Primary diagnosis	Rehabilitation professionals involved
Referral source	Client outcome
Payment source	Physical demand level at completion of program
Activities performed	Cost of services

Case Study

Dan G, a 38-year-old male, worked as a metal worker for a large, metropolitan-based steel company for over three years. He was referred to an occupational rehabilitation program with a diagnosis of degenerative disc disease at L5 and S1 joints and lumbar strain.

Dan was injured while lifting heavy steel panels. He immediately experienced a sharp pain. The next day, Dan sought physician assistance for symptom relief of intense back pain. He identified his pain as a stabbing feeling in the back with pain radiating into the hip area.

Dan's social history showed that he lived with his wife and two children. He was independent in all daily living activities. He reported that he assisted with light chores around the home. Dan was able to drive a car for short stretches of up to one-half hour in duration with mild discomfort. He was unable to complete heavy yard work or car maintenance due to back pain. Dan anticipated being off of work until he was able to return to full duty. No modified job duties were reportedly available in his line of work.

Dan was initially referred to physical therapy and received modalities, a stretching program, strengthening exercises, and a home exercise program. Following two weeks of physical therapy, Dan began an occupational rehabilitation program to facilitate his safe return to full-duty work.

The occupational therapist completed an interview before the baseline evaluation was initiated. Dan reported a strong desire to return to full-duty work, meeting all demands of his job. During the interview, Dan described his job duties as heavy lifting at the waist and above shoulder height, pushing and pulling, kneeling, squatting, twisting, crouching, and walking across six-inch beams. To perform his job, he reported a need to frequently lift 50–55 pounds and carry it for from 1 to 20 feet. Dan used some tools, including a hammer, power drill, and steel cutters.

An on-site job analysis revealed positions of function in extreme ranges of motion for the arms and trunk flexion, forward reaching, and squatting positions.

The occupational therapist explained to Dan the purpose and services of the occupational rehabilitation program. The program's expectations of Dan were clearly identified. Dan reported a desire to return to work as soon as possible. He was cooperative and forthcoming with information to assist in the evaluation. The occupational therapist and physical therapist collaborated in administering the evaluation and writing the results.

Evaluation findings revealed that Dan demonstrated range-of-motion and strength limitations in lumbar flexion. He also demonstrated a light level of lifting ability.

The occupational therapist and physical therapist recommended a three-week rehabilitation program consisting of general strengthening of the abdominals, lumbar region, and upper extremities; endurance exercises; instruction in proper lifting techniques and use of body mechanics; and work simulation.

Dan was oriented to the program and signed a contract addressing his goals and mutually agreed-on expectations. He initially participated in the program for two hours per day. Dan progressed to three hours per day during his second week, and four hours per day in his third week. He recorded all of his exercises on daily work activity flowchart. Carrying weighted beams overhead and stair climbing while holding beams were eventually included in his rehabilitation program as work simulation activities. He was provided with education in proper body mechanics during the performance of work simulation activities.

Dan was discharged after successfully completing three weeks in occupational rehabilitation program. He was reevaluated by his physician and released with no restrictions.

Dan achieved the following goals:

1. Tolerate four hours of rehabilitation per day for a one-week period
2. Lift and carry 50–55 pounds at waist and above-shoulder heights for a distance of 500 feet
3. Complete stretching exercises independently
4. Demonstrate proper body mechanics during work simulation activities

A follow-up on Dan's status after resuming work for four weeks yielded a report of no physical limitations and only occasional soreness in the lumbar region following repetitive bending and reaching.

ACKNOWLEDGMENTS: The author wishes to thank Cathy Coughlin-Becker, a registered occupational therapist employed at St. Mary's Hospital, Ozaukee, Wisconsin, for her assistance in developing the case study. Photographs were provided by Dean Hanus, vice-president of Return to Work, Inc. Milwaukee, Wisconsin.

REFERENCES

Commission on Accreditation of Rehabilitation Facilities. (1988). *1988 standards manual for organizations serving people with disabilities.* Tucson, AZ: Author.

Commission on Accreditation of Rehabilitation Facilities. (1995, January). *1995 Standards for medical rehabilitation.* Tucson, AZ: Author.

Darphin, L. (1995). Work-hardening and work-conditioning perspectives. In S. Isernhagen (Ed.), *Comprehensive guide to work-injury management* (pp. 443–462). Gaithersburg, MD: Aspen.

Feuerstein, M. (1991). A multidisciplinary approach to prevention, evaluation, and management of work disability. *Journal of Occupational Rehabilitation, 1*(1), 5–12.

Gardner, J. (1987). Vocational rehabilitation: Lessons for employers. *Business and Health, 5*(20), 20–24.

Hazard, R., Matheson, L., Lehman, T., & Frymoyer, J. (1991). Rehabilitation of the patient with chronic low back pain. *Occupational low back pain: Assessment, treatment, and prevention.* St. Louis, MO: Mosby.

Helm-Williams, P. (1993, March). Industrial rehabilitation: Developing guidelines. *Magazine of PT,* 65–68.

Hoffman-Grotting, K., & Ralph, V. (1991). Enhancing the program's image and performance by comparing and using quality assurance and program evaluation information. *Occupational Therapy Practice, 2*(2), 16–25.

Key, G. (1996). Work conditioning and work hardening. in G. Key (Ed.), *Industrial therapy* (pp. 254–294). St. Louis, MO: Mosby.

King, P. (1993). Outcome analysis of work-hardening programs. *American Journal of Occupational Therapy, 47*(7), 595–603.

Matheson, L., Ogden, L., Violette, K., & Schultz, K. (1994). Work-hardening and work-conditioning interventions: Do they affect disability? *Physical Therapy, 74*(5), 471–492.

Miller, M. (1991). Functional assessments: A vital component of work injury management. *Work, 1*(3), 6–10.

Niemeyer, L., Foto, M., & Holmes-Enix, D. (1994). Implementing managed care in an industrial rehabilitation program. *Work, 4*(1), 2–8.

Niemeyer, L., Jacobs, K., Reynolds-Lynch, K., Bettencourt, C., & Lang, S. (1994). Work hardening: Past, present, and future—The work programs special interest section national work hardening outcome study. *American Journal of Occupational Therapy, 48*(8), 327–339.

Pati, G. (1985, October–December). Economics of rehabilitation in the workplace. *Journal of Rehabilitation,* 22–30.

Rundle, R. (1983, May 2). Move fast if you want to rehabilitate worker. *Business Insurance,* 10–12.

Saunders, R. (1995). Industrial rehabilitation: Techniques for success. Chaska, MN: The Saunders Group.

Scheer, S. (1990). *Multidisciplinary perspectives in vocational assessment of impaired workers.* Rockville, MD: Aspen.

Schwartz, R. (1993). Return-to-work programs. *Work, 3*(3), 2–8.

Shrey, D. (1995). Worksite disability management and industrial rehabilitation: An overview. In D. Shrey & M. Lacerte (Eds.), *Principles and practices of disability management* (pp. 3–53). Winter Park, FL: GR Press.

Simental, L. (1993, June 26). Managing the costs of managed care: Partnering. *Inland Employment Journal,* 81.

Smith, E. (1989). Ergonomics and the occupational therapist. In E. Hertfelder & C. Gwin (Eds.), *Work in progress* (pp. 127–156). Rockville, MD: American Occupational Therapy Association.

Weiler, P. (1986). *Permanent partial disability: Alternative models for compensation.* A report submitted to William Wrye, Minister of Labour, United Kingdom.

15

On-Site Therapy Programs

Anne K. Tramposh

In an era of shrinking health care dollars, the need has never been greater for on-site therapy programs. These programs meet two fundamental employers' needs: (1) high value for a lower overall cost of workers' compensation claims, and (2) a reduction of the incidence and severity of occupational injuries and illnesses. This chapter will explore the need for and the development of on-site therapy programs. Additionally, details regarding the types of services offered by on-site programs and associated financing and legal issues will be presented.

NEED FOR ON-SITE THERAPY

It is no secret that over the past decade rising workers' compensation costs have been a growing concern for many American companies. Surveys of human resource managers over the past ten years have consistently shown that workers' compensation management is one of the top five priorities these managers plan to address (Human Resources Magazine, 1995). Also, general medical and disability costs have been skyrocketing. Although medical inflation has fueled much of the increase, disability payments account for an equally high percentage of the overall cost of workers' compensation. The General Accounting Office (GAO) estimates that the number of workdays lost in industry due to disabling conditions nearly doubled between 1972 and 1992, topping 85 workdays per 100 employees (Business & Health, 1996).

Nationally, musculoskeletal injuries and illnesses account for the largest percentage of workers' compensation expenditures (Bureau of Labor Statistics, 1995). As costs have spiraled, medical and rehabilitation providers have mobilized to meet the challenge of containing these costs by developing innovative programs that address the specific needs of occupationally injured individuals. These programs have been offered primarily in outpatient clinical settings that provide on-site service options to companies.

Anne K. Tramposh • Advantage Health Systems, 8704 Bourgade, Lenexa, Kansas 66219.

Sourcebook of Occupational Rehabilitation, edited by Phyllis M. King. Plenum Press, New York, 1998.

Health care providers have demonstrated the effectiveness of work-oriented therapy programs in returning injured workers to work (Key, 1995; Mayer, Gatchel, Mayer, Kishino, Kelley, & Mooney, 1987; Miller, 1988). There are others, however, who question the maintenance of these results over an extended period of time (Baldwin, Johnson, & Butler, 1996). One thing is clear: Work-oriented therapy programs are more suited to the needs of employers than the traditional medical care model of treatment. They attempt to address the "nonmedical" aspects of cases, such as employee fear of reinjury and communication barriers between the employer and the employee, as well as the medical needs of injured workers. Support for these programs is evidenced by the fact that employers and insurers continue to turn to work-oriented therapy programs for the resolution of cases (Rogers, Winslow, & Higgins, 1993).

BENEFITS OF ON-SITE SERVICES

As occupational rehabilitation services continue to evolve, more and more companies are considering the adoption of on-site therapy services. There are a number of reasons for their attractiveness to employers: Overall cost reductions, psychosocial benefits, and improved quality of services are primary among them.

Overall Cost Reductions

Some of the reasons for compensation cost reduction related to on-site therapy services are obvious. On-site programs provide opportunities for employers to avoid a "fee-for-service" billing from health care providers. In a fee-for-service model, the therapist bills a fee for every service rendered. For example, if a modality such as electrical stimulation is used, the charge to the employer would be for that service. Alternatives to the fee-for-service model include a flat fee for all services, an hourly rate, or other billing methods. (Billing practices will be discussed in greater detail later in this chapter.)

There are also a number of less obvious cost factors. Costs associated with employee lost time contribute tremendously to the overall costs of workers' compensation cases. Lost-time reductions realized through on-site therapy services can yield significant savings without lowering actual medical costs. On-site therapy services reduce employee time away from work for therapy appointments. Close communication between the employees, health care provider, and employer facilitates the early return to work process. Care is less fragmented because on-site therapists have better access to the employer and employees, decreasing the likelihood of duplication of services and game playing. For example, workers' compensation cases frequently get "lost in the shuffle" between physicians and therapists. An on-site therapist is in a better position to monitor the entire case and prevent this phenomenon.

Psychosocial Benefits

It is well documented that once an employee leaves the worksite because of an injury, it is much easier for that employee to remain off work than to return to work (Kelsey & White, 1980). This condition is particularly true of longer lost-time cases. The primary reason that this situation occurs is because injured workers' lives are dramatically changed in terms of their schedules, their roles in their families, and their support systems. These changes produce psychosocial barriers to returning to work. These barriers can include fear, lack of motivation, secondary gain, and others.

On-site services reduce the likelihood of lost time. The therapist is in a position to assist in the placement of employees on restricted duty. Such placement reduces the occurrence of psychosocial barriers to returning to work in injured workers.

Other psychosocial benefits include opportunities for on-site therapists to get to know workers in their own settings, which improves the therapists' ability to effectively address the "whole patient" in a coordinated manner. For instance, it is well known that employees tend to trust an on-site occupational health nurse (Rogers, Winslow & Higgins, 1993) because the nurse has become integrated into the culture and understands the dynamics of the workplace. The same element of trust may be established with an on-site therapist who appreciates the employee and his or her environment.

Improved Quality of Services

As mentioned previously, on-site services are by design less fragmented than traditional medical and rehabilitative services. In the traditional medical model, employees are sent to multiple locations for services, and communication can be fragmented. In the on-site therapy model, many of the services are performed at the worksite. A more seamless continuum of care is provided, and injured workers can feel confident that the services they are receiving will be effective. By fully understanding the types of work performed by workers, on-site therapists can be more effective and efficient at placing employees on restricted duty assignments, which ultimately lead to improved productivity.

On-site therapy programs improve the overall quality of services by providing readily available rehabilitation services. As Galvin (1986) has so aptly stated, "to delay rehabilitation is to jeopardize rehabilitation." Better results are achieved with early referral than with late referral. Therapists will affirm that, in more traditional models of practice, referrals are often obtained late or not at all. In the on-site model, this tendency to receive services in a timely manner improves the overall effectiveness and quality of the care.

Finally, the on-site therapist is in the ideal position to ensure that prevention activities will take place, particularly with injured employees. Therapists who specialize in occupational rehabilitation are particularly concerned with the possibility of client reinjury. On-site therapists have access to the worksite, which puts them in a better position to monitor the injured employee's progress in a return-to-work situation and provide continued education and prevention.

DEVELOPMENT OF ON-SITE THERAPY PROGRAMS

The field of occupational rehabilitation is still in its infancy. Outpatient work-hardening programs were initiated in the late 1970s and early 1980s. By the late 1980s, the field of occupational rehabilitation was becoming more widely recognized. This was evidenced by attention to work-hardening guidelines, the development of work conditioning, and the addition of industrial rehabilitation topics to physical and occupational therapy academic programs. On-site therapy services in the United States have, for the most part, been an outgrowth of this expansion of services.

It is estimated that there are between 2,000 and 3,000 rehabilitation companies offering targeted industrial rehabilitation services. Approximately 35% of the revenue of outpatient physical therapy clinics is generated from workers' compensation claims. No similar estimate is available for outpatient occupational therapy clinics (personal communication, 1997).

Information is sparse in the literature regarding the extent of rehabilitation services in industry. This absence of information is partly due to the fact that outside their use by large companies, on-site therapy services are still quite rare. Even in the 1980s, when large numbers or providers were flocking to the field of occupational rehabilitation, major United States corporations did not have on-site therapy services. A 1985 survey of 400 large companies revealed that only 7% offered physical and/or vocational rehabilitation (Hochanadel & Conrad, 1993).

Although there appears to be no other study in the literature that compares with this 1985 survey, a 1995 survey of 686 company executives reported that 82% were utilizing some kind of "early return to work programs" as a strategy to reduce rising workers' compensation costs (Tillinghast-Towers Perrin, 1996). Although most of these executives' companies did not have on-site therapy, it appeared that the executives would have been receptive to this type of approach given their willingness to utilize early return to work principles.

PROGRAM PLANNING

Every company considering on-site therapy services has different needs. The on-site therapist needs to take the time to determine what these are prior to determining what specific services should be offered. Therefore, a needs analysis is warranted.

Needs Analysis

In order to determine a given company's specific needs for on-site therapy services, it is imperative that the therapist gather pertinent information. The type of information includes the following:

- Types of jobs in the company
- Workers' compensation history
- Programs currently in place
- The company's history of utilization of medical services
- Specific workers' compensation statutes that apply to the employer

The preferred way of gathering this information is by interviewing key personnel. Personnel typically interviewed include company executives, such as the owner, chief executive officer, chief financial officer, president, and so on; individuals with human resource responsibilities within the company, including safety mangers and health services department personnel—occupational health nurses, physicians, and so on; and supervisory personnel. These interviews will provide the on-site therapist with information on the types of services that are needed. The following type of information should be gathered in these interviews:

- History of the company's workers' compensation experience
- Programs the company has in place that relate to employee health and safety
- Nature of the jobs the employees perform

- Types of personnel the company has available to perform health and safety functions

For example, after interviewing key personnel, a therapist may determine that a company is receiving excellent rehabilitation services for its injured employees and identify a number of "killer jobs" that present a high incidence rate of injuries. In this case, the therapist identifies the need for prevention services, such as worksite analysis, job modification, and employee education, rather than rehabilitation services. Providing these prevention services would be of greater value to the employer than replacing currently effective rehabilitation services.

On the other hand, the therapist might find that the company has an excellent injury prevention program and simply lacks an effective and efficient injury management program. Then, greater emphasis on treatment services is needed.

Once a needs analysis is performed, the plan for specific services is drafted. Services typically fall into two areas: injury management and injury prevention.

Services

Injury Management

Injury management services include such traditional services as musculoskeletal evaluations, modalities, exercise programs, and education. In addition, many on-site therapists provide functional capacity evaluations, work conditioning, work hardening, worksite analysis, and job accommodation services. In some cases, a therapist may provide case management, serving as a liaison between the company, outside medical providers, and the insurance company.

There is tremendous variability in the scope of therapy services delivered to different companies due primarily to the rehabilitation providers' abilities to deliver specific services and the variability of the needs and capabilities of employers. In some situations, therapists are the only medical providers on-site. In other cases, they work closely with nurses and physicians and/or provide services in the company's in-house "fitness center," where exercise equipment is already available. Some companies have limited resources and severe space constraints that challenge therapists to be flexible and creative in their delivery of services.

Injury Prevention

An area that is frequently overlooked by on-site therapists is injury prevention. There is some overlap in prevention and treatment services. For example, in an effective injury management program, worksite analysis is used to match employee capabilities with job requirements. It can also be performed in an injury prevention program to identify the risk factors potentiating injury. Likewise, job accommodation or job modification is practiced in an injury management program to allow an injured worker to safely return to work. In an injury prevention program, job modification is applied to a broader employee population to reduce health risk factors. Employee education is also included in injury management practice to train injured employees to prevent reinjury. Employee education is included in injury prevention services for the general worker population to minimize the risk of on-the-job injuries.

Other aspects of prevention may include proactive health surveillance and/or the use of employee symptom surveys. Many industries are plagued by injuries that are cumulative in nature. Often, the key to successful intervention is in early identification of these disorders. Proactive testing and symptom surveys provide a means for early detection of possible disorders.

When putting together a prevention program, the development of a local occupational health network is a key consideration. This activity consists of reviewing past cases, looking for trends in injury management, and selecting providers who consistently demonstrate sound medical and rehabilitative practices. it is wise to undertake this activity in cooperation with the company's insurance carrier. The carrier has information on past claim histories with different providers that will assist the therapist in making good selection decisions.

It should be noted that some states are "employee choice" states. In other words, the employer cannot choose where the employees go for medical care under the workers' compensation law. In these states, the development of a local network becomes more of an educational service provided by the company for the local medical community. The time spent on these educational activities pays dividends in the long run through the improvement of the care received by company employees. The company's educational activities regarding the types of injuries experienced by its employees open the lines of communication between the company and the local medical community. In addition, these activities assist physicians in upgrading their skills in the evaluation and management of these specific injuries. Educational activities to consider include the following:

- A facility tour with information on the company's prevention and/or injury management programs
- Cosponsorship with a local medical school of a continuing medical education program
- A dinner event with a guest speaker who is a recognized expert in the treatment of injuries and illnesses experienced by company employees

As noted, prevention activities are a frequently overlooked area of opportunity for on-site therapists. Services such as worksite analysis, employee education, job modification, health surveillance, and assistance with development of the local occupational health network can provide employers with greatly needed tools for reducing their workers' compensation costs.

Referral Issues

In states with direct access, the referral requirement issue does not exist, as long as the therapist's activities are within the scope of practice defined by the state practice acts. In nondirect access states, the issue becomes more compelling. There are many situations in an on-site setting in which the need for a referral is questionable. For example, what if therapists are providing prevention services and are asked to adjust individual workstations? Do they need physician referrals? In some nondirect access states, this situation would not necessitate a referral because the therapist is dealing with a "healthy" individual. In other states, it does not matter whether the individual is "healthy," the therapist must have a referral to legally perform a workstation adjustment.

Before undertaking an on-site practice, the provider should contact the individual state about an interpretation of which activities necessitate a referral and which do not.

Most state boards are very cooperative in issuing opinions on specific activities. It is better that a practitioner have their information in advance rather than endangering his or her license.

Staffing Concerns

Many companies believe that "not just any therapist will do." The on-site therapist is expected to be an expert. Therapists with little experience have less credibility with employers. In general, the more experience a therapist has in the field of occupational rehabilitation, the more confidence employers will have in her or him.

There are several human resource issues unique to the industrial setting. In many on-site practices, individual therapists are somewhat isolated from other "medical personnel." The day-to-day dilemmas facing these therapists may be difficult to manage without peer interaction.

Additionally, the primary business of the company is not health care. Therefore, management tends not to understand all of the health-related issues. Often therapists find themselves in difficult positions when management wishes to compromise on health care issues that medical professionals hold dear. For example, medical personnel in industry frequently are asked to discuss confidential medical histories with management personnel. Although this is illegal, company managers frequently feel they have a right to this information. These types of pressures present challenges to on-site therapists.

A company delivering on-site therapy services must meet efficiency "challenges." In many on-site situations, just one therapist is needed to staff a program. Such licensed personnel must be available; lower cost personnel such as assistants and aides cannot be used as effectively. Additionally, clinics in industry are not generally as efficient from a "patient-flow" perspective. Many services that are delivered on-site are necessarily one-on-one services. Therefore, the number of employees that an individual therapist will see in one day tends to be much lower than in a traditional outpatient clinic.

Equipment and Space

The types of injuries incurred will vary with the type of business. Industries with heavy labor demands will tend to incur back, shoulder, and knee injuries, whereas lighter manufacturing, such as workbench assembly, may have a preponderance of upper extremity cumulative trauma disorders. These factors will dictate the types of therapy equipment and space requirements needed.

The on-site therapy clinic will require space and equipment to evaluate the musculoskeletal structures involved and the employees' functional abilities as they relate to the specific physical demands of their jobs. Likewise, the clinic should be equipped with tools to evaluate the work that employees perform. (Table 15.1 lists different types of equipment for evaluation and/or treatment purposes.) At a minimum, an isolated area should be provided for employee confidentiality and privacy. A treatment table is necessary for evaluating musculoskeletal concerns.

Some functional evaluation equipment may be used in the treatment process as well. Physical agent modalities and specific exercise equipment should be considered on a case-by-case basis, depending upon the types of injuries encountered.

One principle that is essential in occupational rehabilitation, whether on-site or in an outpatient clinic, is the focus on function. Although the promotion of tissue healing

**Table 15.1. Types of Equipment Considered
for Evaluation and/or Treatment of Injuries**

Body parts	Primary physical demands (indicated by employer's job descriptions)	Examples of evaluation/treatment equipment to consider
Back/neck	Sit Stand Walk Kneel Lift/carry Push/pull Reach Climb Balance Stoop Squat	Assembly or similar activities performed when sitting, standing, kneeling, etc. (actual job activity preferred) Ladder Balance beam Lifting evaluation station Brick stack Nail/peg board
Upper extremities	Lift/carry Push/pull Reach Climb Dexterity Coordination Grip/pinch	Stationary vertical ladder Lifting station Brick stack Nail/peg board Dexterity/coordination evaluation equipment (i.e., Purdue Pegboard, Crawford Small Parts, etc.) Grip/pinch dynamometers
Lower extremities	Stand Walk Kneel Lift/carry Climb Balance Squat	Lifting station Ladder Brick stack Balance beam Assembly or similar activities performed when sitting, standing, kneeling, etc. (actual job activity preferred)

and improvement of range of motion and strength, and other rehabilitation goals should be kept in mind, the primary responsibility of the occupational rehabilitation provider is to improve function. Additionally, the therapist must focus on providing employees with the tools to manage their own health as a part of the educational component of the program.

When considering these responsibilities, less rehabilitation equipment rather than more is often indicated. The on-site therapist's own creativity and ability to use existing tools and workstations as "therapy equipment" is of primary importance. Like the home health environment, where a lot of equipment cannot and should not be carried into a patient's home, the on-site therapy clinic should use resources already available in the workplace. This does not mean that the therapy clinic should be devoid of traditional therapy equipment. It simply means that care should be taken to avoid overuse of tools unfamiliar to the employees in the workplace. Some on-site providers do use portable equipment, such as portable ultrasound machines and weight sets, that can be moved when needed and used at multiple locations.

In planning for the needs of an on-site clinic, the therapist must determine now to best utilize the available space. Space devoted exclusively to educational programs is important, but there may be other areas of the business that can be used for education. For example, creative scheduling of available conference rooms or break rooms may be an option.

FINANCING

Financial issues in an on-site therapy service include start-up and equipment costs and billing considerations. Although each company situation may be somewhat unique, the manager of the prospective on-site therapy service should give careful consideration to how these more general issues will be addressed prior to entering the marketplace. Having explored options in advance, the therapy provider will be better prepared to deal with these financial issues during contract negotiations.

Reimbursement for Services

There are several ways to bill for on-site services: hourly rate, salary, fee for service, or contract pricing. Each of these methods has advantages and disadvantages to the client—the employer—and the practitioner.

Hourly Rate

Different hourly rates can be charged for different types of services or different types of personnel. For example, services that can be delivered by an assistant can be billed at a lower hourly rate, whether or not an assistant actually performs the services. Similarly, evaluation services might be charged at a higher rate because a higher paid individual is needed to perform these services.

An hourly rate has the advantage of being simple. The practitioner simply charges a negotiated rate for the hours of services delivered on-site. Payment for additional hours spent working on employer projects can also be negotiated. This can include time spent on documentation, travel time, and so on. Another advantage for the on-site therapist is that all services are billable, including prevention services that can be difficult to build into a fee-for-service arrangement.

One disadvantage for the employer is that unless the number of hours are initially specified, the budget is unpredictable. Another disadvantage for an insured employer (as opposed to a self-insured employer) is that insurance reimbursement for evaluation and treatment services may be difficult to obtain.

Salary

Another popular financial arrangement for on-site therapy programs is an employer–employee relationship. This relationship is the one favored by large employers that have an established on-site medical department staffed with physicians, therapists, occupational health nurses, and assistants. The advantage to the employer is that the budget is predictable, the costs of services tend to be lower (assuming that the therapists are well utilized), and the employer becomes "the therapy provider" for insurance reimbursement purposes. The insurance reimburses the employer in the same way that it does a traditional provider. Many such employers are self-insured, so there is no insurance reimbursement in the traditional sense. An additional advantage for the employer is "built-in" expertise for prevention services.

One advantage for the employer becomes a disadvantage for the therapist. Typically, therapists are paid at a lower rate by employers that they would receive as independent contractors. However, many therapists prefer to be employees of a large company because such jobs are typically more secure than independent contractor relationships.

Another advantage of the employer–employee relationship is that the therapist can devote his or her full attention to one employer. Therapists who are employed by a number of different clients have less time to devote to any one of them. This lack of time translates into less familiarity with all aspects of an individual workplace.

Fee for Service

In the fee-for-service arrangement, the therapist bills the employer (or the insurance company) for services actually rendered, as if the employees were receiving services in an outpatient clinic. The advantage for the therapist is that standard fee-for-service prices are utilized. This may be (but is not necessarily) a higher rate than the typical negotiated hourly rate. However, the danger in this type of arrangement is that there may be no mechanism for billing for "prevention" or other activities, such as case meetings or consultation with an individual regarding workstation adjustment, unless previously specified.

The disadvantage for the employer in a fee-for-service system is that the fees are higher than an hourly rate or salary arrangement. However, the advantage is that the employer tends to get a lot of "freebies." It is harder for the therapist to charge for some activities, such as assisting well individuals with workstation adjustments, meeting with supervisors, and so on. Another advantage for the employer is that typically an insurance company pays the bills directly to the therapist, and the employer basically gets the services with no outlay of cash. If the employer is self-insured, this is of course, not the case.

Contract Price

The therapist who uses contract pricing specifies the services that will be delivered and offers them at set prices. This approach is a "value-based" approach for the therapist and the employer. In other words, the therapist can show the employer how to achieve a certain amount of savings in the area of workers' compensation costs and can price the services based on that value to the customer, rather than on the actual services to be delivered. The therapist takes the risk that more services might be needed to achieve the results promised. The reward for the therapist is that contract pricing can be much higher than traditional pricing.

In a contract price arrangement, the advantage for the employer is that the costs will be known. Also, contract pricing gives the employer a more visible means of knowing if the investment in on-site therapy services will provide a return on investment that is greater than their expenditures. If the results are not as expected, the therapist is responsible for providing additional services to reach the intended targets—without additional expense to the employer. The disadvantage to the employer is that the total cost probably will be higher than it might have been under another billing arrangement.

LEGAL ISSUES

As in more traditional medical settings, the on-site therapist should be aware of potential areas of liability. Many of the risks of liability are the same as in traditional practice. However, several additional areas should be considered.

Malpractice versus Errors and Omissions Coverage

Traditional malpractice insurance covers a therapist for areas of practice that are considered "standard practice," including treatment services that are governed by state practice acts and most prevention activities. However, there are potential areas of weakness in traditional malpractice coverage for the on-site therapist. For example, if a therapist serves on a company's safety committee, standard malpractice insurance may not cover every item that the committee discusses. Areas where the duties of a nurse and therapist overlap also may not be covered.

These are gray areas that are not specifically defined in malpractice policies. Before assuming that these issues are covered, it is wise to address all potential areas of concern with an underwriter from the insurance company proposing coverage. Gray areas can be clarified in advance by describing scenarios in which someone may sue and asking for the underwriter's written opinion on whether each proposed event would be covered. Additionally, insurance company underwriters may be provided with a rehabilitation company's brochures describing its specific services. After reviewing company literature, an underwriter will be in a better position to evaluate potential loopholes in coverage.

Another type of coverage to explore is "errors and omissions coverage." This type of coverage is designed for "consultants" and serves to supplement the weak areas in traditional malpractice insurance. The drawback of this type of insurance is that it is typically very expensive. Therapists have reported that this type of coverage can cost as much as ten times the price of malpractice coverage. Again, providing the insurance underwriter with examples of the types of risks foreseen will help to guard against inadequate insurance coverage for the practitioner. Any full-service insurance broker can provide information on this type of policy.

Workers' Compensation and Other Insurance

If an on-site therapist works for a company as a salaried employee, it is the company's responsibility to provide him to her with workers' compensation and general liability insurance. If however, the therapist works on contract or for a therapy agency, workers' compensation and general liability insurance coverage will not be provided by the company. If a therapy agency provides this coverage for its employees in a clinic, this coverage will extend to employees outside of the clinic as well. However, it is essential that the insurance company be kept informed of the locations at which the company routinely provides services.

Licensure in Other States

Some on-site practices service companies in multiple locations. If a therapist provides direct services in a given state, it is clear that he must have a license in that state (if there is state licensure) to perform those services. The gray area involves "supervision." If a therapist supervises an individual in another state, does the supervisor need a license in that state? The answer depends on the type of supervision offered. If the supervision does not involve direct assistance with individual cases, the answer may be no. However, if the supervisor is asked to consult on a specific case, a license may be needed because the individual may be considered to be "practicing physical or occupational therapy" by assisting in the evaluation and treatment planning in the case. Again, whether a license is required would depend on the specific state's definition of what is considered the "practice of physical or occupational therapy."

CONCLUSION

On-site therapy services are proving to be highly effective in controlling the high costs of workers' compensation. Therapists in these settings are in a unique position to influence an employee's ability to return to work quickly. Additionally, the situation lends itself to early intervention and prevention efforts. Services offered vary from company to company, but often include traditional evaluation and treatment services, which are supplemented by work hardening, work conditioning, case management, and prevention services, such as worksite analysis, employee education, and job modification.

Although on-site programs are somewhat unique, they offer new challenges, and the rewards of helping companies gain control of their workers' compensation problems are great. At a time when private inpatient and outpatient therapy visits are decreasing, the opportunities in industry remain unlimited.

ACKNOWLEDGMENTS. Special thanks to the following individuals for providing specific information on their on-site therapy services: Neal Wachholtz, Excel PT, Omaha, Nebraska; Sylvia Davila, Hand Rehabilitation of San Antonio, San Antonio, Texas; and Lorie Ebenkamp, Off-Site PT, St. Joseph Medical Center, Wichita, Kansas.

REFERENCES

Baldwin, M., Johnson, W., & Butler, R. (1996). The error of using return-to-work to measure the outcomes of health care. *American Journal of Industrial Medicine*, *29*, 632–641.

Business and health. (1996, October). *Copy Editor*, *14*, 75.

Galvin, D. (1986). Employer-based disability management and rehabilitation program. *Annual Review of Rehabilitation*.

Hochanadel, C. D., & Conrad, D. E. (1993). Evolution of an on-site industrial physical therapy program. *Journal of Occupational Medicine*, *35*(10), 1011–1016.

Human Resources Magazine. (1995, March). HRM update. *HR Magazine*, *40*(3), 16.

Kelsey, J. L., & White, A. A. III. (1980). Epidemiology and the impact of low back pain. *Spine*, *5*, 133–134.

Key, G. L. (1995). The impact of industrial therapy. In G. L. Key (Ed.), *Industrial therapy* (pp. 31–41). St. Louis, MO: Mosby.

Mayer, T., Gatchel, H., Mayer, H., Kishino, N., Keeley, J., & Mooney, V. (1987). A positive two-year study of functional restoration in industrial low back injury. *Journal of the American Medical Association*, *258*(13), 1763–1767.

Miller, M. (1988). Cost savings in four cases. In S. Isernhagen (Ed.), *Work injury management and prevention* (pp. 181–183). Gaithersburg, MD: Aspen.

Rogers, B., Winslow, B., & Higgins, S. (1993). Employee satisfaction with occupational health services: Results of a survey. *AAOHN*, *41*(2), 58–64.

Tillinghast-Towers Perrin (1996). Reality testing: Assessing the performance of workers' compensation cost management initiatives. *Biennial Survey of Public and Private Sector U.S. Employers*. Author.

U.S. Department of Labor, Bureau of Labor Statistics. (1995). *Annual report*. Washington DC: U.S. Government Printing Office.

16

Job Modification/ Accommodation and Assistive Technology

Roger O. Smith and Edward F. Ellingson

Job modification, accommodation, and assistive technology interventions (JMAATIs) subscribe to preventative ergonomic principles and acknowledge the need for worker training. They concentrate on individualizing workstations and work environments to create a custom match between a job and a worker.

Typically, JMAATIs assist two types of workers. The first type is the worker who has recently been injured and is returning to the workplace. The second type is the worker who has a chronic disability and requires a specialized intervention to find and keep a new job.

JMAATIs are provided by individuals who have a background of knowledge and skill in disability diagnoses, functional impairments due to disabilities, traditional rehabilitation processes, assistive technology applications, fundamentals of ergonomics, and engineering principles. This breadth and depth of knowledge and skills has customarily required advanced training and experience in JMAATIs. It is common for JMAATIs to be provided by professionals who call themselves "assistive technology specialists."

This chapter on JMAATIs serves three primary purposes. First, it provides an introduction to job modification, job accommodation, and assistive technology interventions. Second, it highlights the importance of preventative, rehabilitative, and accommodation perspectives in ergonomic practice. Third, this chapter stresses the utility of aspects of universal design in ergonomic job design, so all workers can be integrated into the workplace without requiring special accommodations.

Roger O. Smith • Occupational Therapy Program, University of Wisconsin–Milwaukee, Milwaukee, Wisconsin 53201. **Edward F. Ellingson** • Zerrecon Inc., 1549 North 51st Street, Milwaukee, Wisconsin 53208.

Sourcebook of Occupational Rehabilitation, edited by Phyllis M. King. Plenum Press, New York, 1998.

ASSISTIVE TECHNOLOGY AND JOB ACCOMMODATION DEFINITIONS

Job accommodation is the broad term used to describe types of changes made to help a person with disabilities become or remain employed. Job modification and assistive technology both can be a part of the job accommodation process. *Assistive technology* is specific to devices and their applications, while *job modification* is characterized by hardware changes to the machines and tools that are part of the job. Because job modification and assistive technology may be required as part of a complete job accommodation solution, these terms are used together. In fact, experts in job accommodation often find themselves needing to become assistive technology experts, and visa versa. In this chapter, these terms are used somewhat interchangeably.

Assistive technology has been defined by the federal government and is present in several legislative acts related to people with disabilities. These definitions are broad and encompassing. They were initially defined in the Technology-Related Assistance for Individuals with Disabilities Act of 1988 (PL 100-407).

According to the act,

> an assistive technology device is any item, piece of equipment or product system, whether acquired commercially off the shelf, modified, or customized, that is used to increase, maintain, or improve functional capabilities of individuals with disabilities.

These products range from devices that allow a worker to independently manage his or her personal needs at work to augmentative communication systems that enable a person who cannot talk to communicate with others at work. Database search headings from a representative search of the 1997 AbleData database of assistive technology products show an overall scope of the types of devices in the field. (See appendix A.)

The act defines an assistive technology service as

> any service that directly assists an individual with a disability in the selection, acquisition, or the use of an assistive technology device. Evaluations, purchasing, leasing, selecting, designing, fitting, customizing, adapting, applying, maintaining, repairing, or replacing assistive technologies are part of the services.

Understanding the significance of this dual definition is essential to understanding the nature of JMAATI service provision. In 1985, Barry Rodgers, of the University of Wisconsin-Madison, published a seminal paper on the process of providing assistive technology services. Basically, he described the process of assistive technology service provision. He sketched 19 steps needed to successfully provide assistive technology devices to people with disabilities. (See Figure 16.1.) His description is significant because only one of the nineteen steps pertained to the selection of the devices. The remaining 18 dealt with the need for services surrounding the products: for example, the complete evaluation of the individual with a disability, the review or the array of appropriate assistive technology devices available from which to choose, the procurement of funding for the device, the fitting and installation of the devices when they arrive, the reassessment process to assure appropriateness, and the maintenance of the devices when they break down. Rodgers basically dismantled the storefront consumer shopping model for delivering assistive technology devices. Although Rodgers (1985) highlighted the obvious need for the consumer to be integrally involved, the assistive technology professional had an ethical role to provide the full spectrum of services and to customize the services as needed for the assistive technology recipient.

1. Identify the student and the environments where assistive technology would benefit.

2. Assess particular needs of individual and systems available.

3. Select and acquire components of system.

4. Make modifications for compatibility of all components.

5. Assemble the system.

6. Mount the system.

7. Fit the system to user's particular needs.

8. Select methods for training.

9. Train the user basics of system.

10. Train people in the user's environment.

11. Provide ongoing training.

12. Set up an on-call system for problems.

13. Set up a preventive maintenance program.

14. Set-up a repair strategy and provide repairs PRN.

15. Upgrade the system as upgrades are available.

16. Reevaluate the effectiveness of the system.

17. Obtain feedback from the user on effectiveness.

18. Provide an improved system as the technology advances.

19. Provide a new system as user's needs change.

Figure 16.1. Barry Rodgers's 19 steps of the assistive technology service delivery. *Source*: B. L. Rogers (1985), *A Future Perspective on the Holistic Use of Technology for People with Disabilities*. Madison, WI: Trace R&D Center.

Early legislation interchanged the terms *rehabilitation engineering* with *assistive technology*. Several federal laws, including the Americans with Disabilities Act (ADA) (PL 101-336), the Rehabilitation Act Amendments (PL 99-506), and the Individuals with Disabilities Education Act (IDEA) (101-476), require the application of rehabilitation engineering or assistive technology as necessary to provide equal opportunity for people with disabilities. Probably the most well known requirement is the ADA's establishment of "job accommodation" as an important and necessary consideration in the employment of people with disabilities. Section 103 (5) of Title I calls for "reasonable accommodation" to allow a potential worker with a disability to perform the "essential functions" of a job.

Job accommodation is a term that was first well defined as a part of the ADA. It applies to job applicants who have a disability, employees who have a disability, or employees who acquire a disability while on the job. Concerning this last group, an injured employee who has progressed through treatment, seems to have plateaued in regaining function, and is not yet able to return to his previous job should be considered to have a disability and is subject to the "reasonable accommodation" provision of the ADA.

HISTORICAL BACKGROUND

Although federal legislation firmly established job accommodation and the application of assistive technology as a national mandate in 1990, these concepts date back many years. Informal developments using JMAATIs have been plentiful and widespread. A well-known example is the Teletype machine, the TTY. Deaf people found that they could communicate over telephone lines very effectively by typing messages back and forth on TTYs. These devices were readily available at relatively low cost. Although the initial Teletype machine is no longer produced and has become obsolete, deaf people still communicate using this technique. A market has developed for devices using the TTY technique, specifically designed for deaf users. This design sufficiently changed so that TTYs became TDDs, telecommunication devices for the deaf. These commercial devices have features for specific use by deaf people and are marketed as such. Most recently, TTYs or TDDs are now called a more generic TT for text telephone. Even newer communication techniques that provide many options for communications for people who are deaf are available, including intercomputer communication via E-mail or fax machines. TTs, however, are "real-time" communication and remain an essential assistive technology by accessing common telephone lines for people who are deaf to communicate.

Other early job accommodation interventions for people with disabilities were geared toward the individual. People observed their friends, family members, or co-workers struggling because of a disability and made changes to help them. These interventions were typically simple, such as adding a step, changing a handle, widening a door opening, incorporating a magnifying lens, or specifying someone else to do particular tasks. Some were more complex, such as adding speech synthesis to a computer for a blind computer-user or for a person who could not speak. Today, speech synthesis is in its third or fourth development generation and, remarkably, intelligibility has approached the sound of everyday human speech. Applying this JMAATI, however, requires choosing a speech synthesizer from an array of dozens of options of which only a few might fit the particular needs of the individual. In fact, there are currently more than 23,000 assistive technology devices cataloged in Abledata, a federally sponsored database of such devices. Multiply this number by the combinations available in instances when numerous devices are helpful, add the application strategies that accompany any JMAATI, and you have a very complex process. In less than two decades, JMAATI options have exploded from a few hundred to countless numbers of devices and strategies.

The concept of utilizing devices and technical assistance to help people with disabilities was more formally established with the formation of two rehabilitation engineering centers by the U.S. Department of Health, Education, and Welfare in 1971. Three more centers were added in 1972. Today the National Institute on Disability and Rehabilitation Research funds about 15 rehabilitation engineering and research centers (RERCs). Each center focuses on a topic related to assistive technology and disability. Most of these RERCs are highly important to occupational rehabilitation. The following, in fact, have vocational goals as primary components of their research mission.

- Adaptive Computers and Information Systems
- Low back pain
- Modifications to worksites and educational settings

- Rehabilitation robotics
- Rehabilitation technology services in vocational rehabilitation

In addition, there are several RERCs that disseminate current information and develop products that are relevant to occupational rehabilitation, but they do not espouse a primary mission toward the work setting. These include RERCs on the following topics:

- Augmentative and alternative communication
- Hearing enhancement and assistive devices
- Personal licensed transportation for disabled
- Prosthetics and orthotics
- Technology for blindness and visual impairments
- Technology evaluation and transfer
- Technology to improve wheelchair mobility

Also, several membership organizations have developed over the past two decades, highlighting the interest in assistive technology applications, including the International Society of Augmentative and Alternative Communication, the Technology Special Interest Section of the American Occupational Therapy Association, and the Rehabilitation Engineering and Assistive Technology Society of North America (RESNA). RESNA's 20 Special Interest Groups (SIGs) encompass the breadth of specialties in assistive technology. Twelve SIGs include assistive technology applications specific to occupational rehabilitation (see Table 16.1).

The Job Accommodation Network (JAN) was formed in 1984 by the President's Committee on Employment of People with Disabilities. It was expanded in 1991 to provide public access information to businesses and services that were required to comply with the ADA. The mission of JAN is to assist in the hiring, retraining, retaining, or advancing persons with disabilities by providing accommodation information. JAN is a

Table 16.1. RESNA Special Interest Groups (SIGs) 1997

SIG-01	Service Delivery and Public Policy*
SIG-02	Personal Transportation*
SIG-03	Augmentative and Alternative Communication*
SIG-04	Dysphagia: Feeding, Swallowing, and Saliva Control
SIG-05	Quantitative Functional Assessment*
SIG-06	Special Education
SIG-07	Technology Transfer
SIG-08	Sensory Loss and Technology*
SIG-09	Wheeled Mobility and Seating*
SIG-10	Electrical Stimulation
SIG-11	Computer Applications*
SIG-12	Rural Rehabilitation*
SIG-13	Assistive Robotics and Mechatronics*
SIG-14	Job Accommodation*
SIG-15	Information Networking
SIG-16	Gerontology
SIG-17	International Appropriate Technology
SIG-18	Tech Act
SIG-19	Universal Access*
SIG-20	Cognitive Disabilities and Technologies*

*Include assistance technology application specific to occupational rehabilitation.

no-cost central resource for information on relevant options concerning job accommodations. It purports to have advised on over 100,000 such accommodations.

ASSISTIVE TECHNOLOGY THEORY

There are several assistive technology application theories that are relevant to occupational rehabilitation. The Human-Environment Technology Interface (HETI) model (Smith, 1991) incorporates classical ergonomic theory. The Six Approaches to Disability accommodation highlights the methods used by people with disabilities to be successful at work and identifies how traditional rehabilitation and assistive technology fit into the formula (Smith, Benge, & Hall, 1994). The Parallel Interventions approach (Angelo & Smith, 1989) emphasizes the strength of combining training and assistive technology interventions. The Human Activity Assistive Technology (HAAT) model (Cook & Hussey, 1995) places JMAATIs in the context of activity. The balance theory (Smith & Sainfort, 1989) places the interventions within the whole work environment.

Human-Environment Technology Interface (HETI) Model

Chapanis described a fundamental human interface model in human factors engineering in 1976. He portrayed a cycle that included sensing; information processing and control on the human side of the cycle; controls, operations, and displays on the machine side of the cycle. This perspective has been regularly cited in human factors textbooks (McCormick & Sander, 1982). Bridging this model to assistive technology, the Human-Environment Technology Interface (HETI) model has been suggested as one way to consider the implementation of assistive technology for people with disabilities (Smith, 1991). (Figure 16.2 displays this model.)

The HETI model is divided into top and bottom parts. The top section depicts three aspects of the human, sensory, cognitive, and motor functions. This figure suggests that when a person has impairments in any of these areas, the functional cycle is interrupted, and some type of medical or rehabilitation treatment may be required. For example, if someone was losing eyesight, surgery to resolve the visual problem may be indicated. On the other hand, surgery or other rehabilitation training programs, such as eye-muscle education, may not be of help. In these cases, an assistive technology, such as corrective lenses in the form of eyeglasses, contact lenses, or both, might be applied.

The bottom half of the HETI model highlights not only assistive technology applications as they relate directly to the individual with a disability, but adaptations in the environment as primary contributors to restoring function. For example, if an individual with vision loss was not sufficiently assisted by eyeglasses, the visual impairment would result in many functional problems across life functions, including in the workplace. If the individual worked at a computer workstation, the HETI model would suggest that the computer was not stable to produce information usable to the operator. Thus, it is the computer, not the individual who needs the accommodation in this instance. Some alternate output would be required to bring the computer system up to its functional capability. Magnifiers, screen enlargement software, or voice output are among the assistive technology alternatives that might be considered to improve the computer workstation output interface.

This classical human factors cycle points out that the accommodation process may

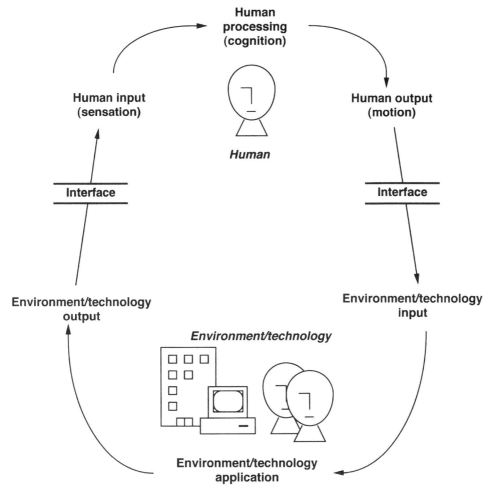

Figure 16.2.   Human environment-technology interface model. *Source*: R. O. Smith (1991), "Technological Approaches to Performance Enhancement," *Occupational Therapy: Overcoming Human Performance Deficits*, edited by C. Christiansen & C. Baum. Thorofare, NJ: Slack Publishers. Reprinted with permission.

be one that changes the person or the machine interface to enable the best match between the person and the work environment.

Six Approaches to Disability Accommodation

The HETI model highlights the need for an intervention to consider approaches that change the person and change the work environment. In occupational therapy, a multiple-option approach (Christiansen, 1991; Smith, 1991) that builds on the idea that intervention can be oriented to remediate the person or adapt the environment is often described. Most interventions can be classified into one of six approaches. In fact, many mismatches between a worker with a disability and the job are due to poor choices among the six intervention options. (Figure 16.3 illustrates this point.) Although the

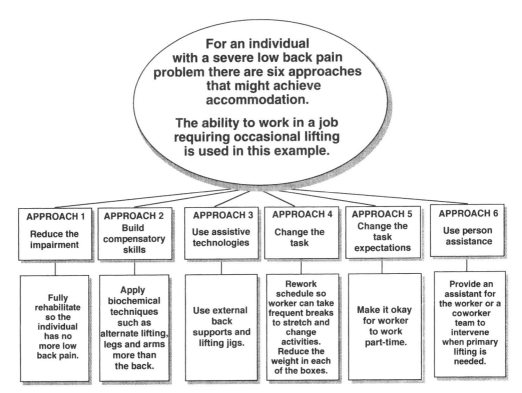

Figure 16.3. Six rehabilitation intervention approaches.

first two intervention types tend to be classical rehabilitation/education models, the remainder are types of accommodation. Understanding each is a key to successful job accommodation.

Parallel Interventions

The parallel inventions model (Figure 16.4) suggests that not only are there many approaches to accommodating a worker in the job, but also the strategy may enlist more than one approach at the same time. The Parallel Interventions concept suggests that people can develop skills that make a given assistive technology device outdated. Although use of an assistive technology device may be correct for a person's skill level at a given time, ongoing rehabilitation may indicate a less obtrusive or a more powerful assistive technology device at a later date. The significance of this concept is that assistive technology devices should be considered temporary. Workers' abilities in any job can develop and change over time.

The Human Activity Assistive Technology (HAAT) Model

Cook and Hussey (1995) suggested that there are four major components of applying assistive technology: the human, the activity, the assistive technology, and the context. Applying this model to the workplace, the human components are the intrinsic abilities

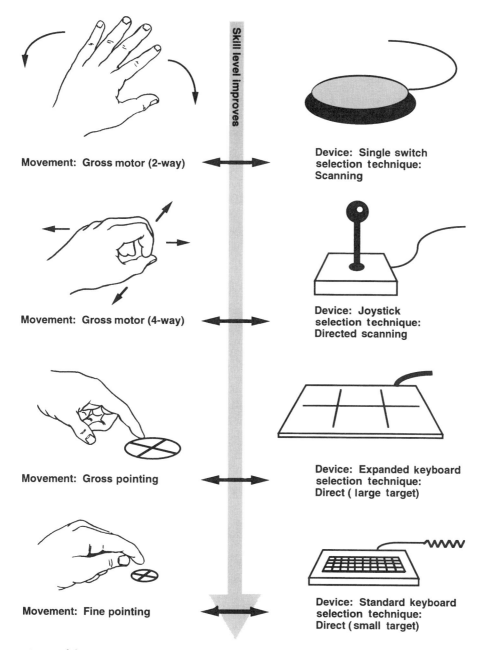

Figure 16.4. Model of parallel interventions. *Source*: Smith (1991). Reprinted with permission.

of the worker in the situation. This worker is placed in a specific work activity. The assistive technologies are the tools that are available to the worker. The human, the work activity, and the assistive technologies are all placed in the context of the setting, the social expectations, the cultural factors, and the physical environment.

Cook and Hussey explained that the size of the human and assistive technology resource components may vary over time or when the location changes. In a given setting, an activity such as communicating with others may bring a limited set of human resources that requires a substantial assistive technology contribution. In another setting, the human resources may result in more effective communication. Thus, the assistive technology requirements may be comparatively smaller.

This change over time is consistent with parallel systems thinking. As time progresses, a person's abilities and needs change. As a person becomes more or less effective using intrinsic resources, different sets of assistive technology intervention may be needed.

The Balance Theory

Many work theories have been promoted in human factors engineering. The balance theory, described by Smith and Sainfort (1989), is particularly related to JMAATIs. The balance theory submits that the individual is in the center of four aspects of the work context: the physical environment, the activity, the organization, and the technology. The theory is unique not because it holds that the four components and the person are central, but because of the overt discussion of the balance between the available resources being the key to a functional worker. Smith and Sainfort relay a casual expectation that any worksite will have areas of deficit. One job may have strong organizational support or the latest in technology, but it may not have a well-tuned physical environment. For example, temperature conditions may be too erratic and suboptimal for daily comfort. Or, the tasks of the job may be very difficult or stressful. Smith and Sainfort presented research to suggest that the positive aspects of a workplace can compensate for weak areas and result in a productive situation.

ASSISTIVE TECHNOLOGY APPLICATIONS

Job accommodation can vary from no-cost simple projects to extremely complex and costly projects that require the work of skilled professionals. If it involves adding special tools or devices or changing the existing machines or tools in some way, then it is also called "job modification." Projects in job accommodation are typically categorized as follows:

No Cost. These accommodations are usually procedural changes. Allowing a person to work part-time or to have a two-hour lunch period are examples of such an accommodation.

Simple. Projects that involve the purchase and use of standard commercial items to solve problems exemplify simple accommodations. Utilizing a commercial magnifier-light unit is a good example of a simple project. Some easily implemented projects with custom fabrication may likewise be considered simple.

Extensive. These projects require complex equipment and/or modifications, including combining these modifications with simple and no-cost accommodations. This project usually involves modifying the workstation or environment. For example, making all the changes necessary to enable a person in a wheelchair to do all aspects of a job that was originally intended for a worker in a standing position would most likely involve extensive effort.

Products Used for Accommodation

There are a wide variety of commercial products available to assist with job accommodation. In order to help any given client, it is important to know generally what these products are, how they can help an individual, and where they can be obtained. These products run a continuum, but it is useful to consider them in three categories:

Assistive Technology Specialty Products

This product category is usually associated with disability accommodation. It covers relatively common devices found in catalogs, such as reachers, one-handed brooms, voice output communication systems, magnifiers, and voice recognition computer systems. It also includes more specialized devices, items with such a specific market that they are more elusive. Examples of these specialized devices are one-handed computer keyboards, refreshable braille computer displays, mouthsticks with interchangeable tool attachments, powered lazy-Susan workstations, and environmental control units (ECUs) that operate by switch selection and scanning.

One way to learn about these products is through Abledata, a database of products intended for people with disabilities. It now includes over 23,000 items and lists almost 2,600 companies that sell these products. Abledata information is available as a CD database that you purchase and run on your computer (Trace R&D Center, 608-263-2309), via telephone (AbleData 800-227-0216), or on the World Wide Web (http://www.abledata.com/ or http://trace.wisc.edu/tcel/).

Commercial Mass-Produced Assistive Technology Products

If a person with a hand injury cannot operate a certain latch, it is very likely that an easier-to-operate latch can be found in a local hardware store or in a hardware catalog. This example is one of standard commercial products being used as assistive technology devices. The knowledge and creativity of the professional are the important part of this application. There are no lists to peruse to identify these potential problem-solving techniques. Successful strategies used in locating these types of products include brainstorming with others, reviewing published case studies, maintaining a vigilant watch over new products, and browsing gift catalogs and hardware and tool stores regularly. Although the cost of maintaining an effective up-to-date mental database of these types of assistive technology options may be high, the cost of the purchased items is usually relatively low.

Assistive Technology Products Available in Specialty and Mass Markets

There are a few products that are available in the mass market and also marketed as specialty devices. An example of this is the X-10 series of products for controlling lights, appliances, and other electrical devices in the home. These products are widely marketed through specialty catalogs and stores for the security and convenience they offer; they have been picked up by large distributors such as Sears and RadioShack. They are also utilized by assistive technology suppliers for the advantages they offer to people with disabilities. They are often bundled with other assistive technology devices, such as integrated environmental control or communication systems, to increase their utility.

Table 16.2. Examples of Common Work Limitations before Accommodations and JMAATI Implications

Areas of impairments	Functional limitations without accommodation	Common reasons	JMAATI examples	Accommodation implications
Low vision	Cannot use visually detailed information.	Traumatic injury, retinopathy, cataracts, aging.	Computer screen magnifiers, (printed material) magnifiers, high-intensity lighting.	Gestalt of large drawings or other panoramic information takes longer for individual to obtain.
Blindness: Field cut	Misses information in part of work area.	Stroke.	Mirrors, selective positioning of materials.	Similar to low vision, plus with stroke may also need to accommodate spatial-perceptual cognitive impairment.
Blindness: Severe/total	Cannot use visual information.	Congenital blindness, traumatic injury, retinopathy.	Computer screen readers, optical character recognition, printed text readers, auditory and tactile messaging and signage.	Graphical information and handwriting continues to be inaccessible without verbal descriptions. Significant training required.
Hard of hearing	Cannot discriminate or use detailed auditory information.	Traumatic injury, aging.	Adjustable sound, visual messaging and signaling.	Alert, feedforward and feedback information is provided auditorially. This will often be overlooked without careful task analysis.
Deaf	Cannot use auditory information.	Congenital deafness, traumatic injury.	Visual messaging and signaling.	Many multimedia audio tracks do not have captioning available yet.
Reading impairment	Cannot use text information easily or at all.	Learning disabilities, mental retardation, stroke, brain injury, English as a second language.	Provide auditory and pictorial messaging (reception and expression), allow sufficient time for reading	Pictorial messaging may not be consistent with verbal. Pictorial messaging may require training.
Short attention span	Cannot sustain work tasks.	Attention deficit disorder (ADD).	Break up task into segments, change pace of tasks. Consider alternate information media sources.	May not be able to perform complex or lengthy activities. Type of media used for information can make significant difference.
Problem-solving impairment	May not make effective decisions in novel situations.	Mental retardation, mental health disorders, brain injury.	Reduce problem-solving complexity, use decision charts, provide call system for assistance.	Often need to determine if difficulty is due to lack of problem identification versus poor problem solving per se.

Limitation	Description	Associated conditions	Solutions	Notes
Poor memory	May not learn new tasks easily.	Mental retardation, Alzheimer's, brain injury, substance abuse disorders.	Provide sufficient training, use pedagogical techniques, use cognitive prostheses, such as checklists or personal information managers.	Making the work environment routine may be the key to success.
Poor time organization	May not be timely on tasks.	Mental health disorders, substance abuse disorders, head injury, Alzheimer's.	Use cognitive prostheses, such as calendars, schedule sheets, timers, alarm watches, personal information managers.	Accommodation may require involvement of individual's family and other support people.
Slow cognitive processing	May be slow at tasks.	Mental health disorders, head injury, mental retardation.	Avoid tasks dependent on fast reaction times, create feedforward signals, increase routine of tasks.	Careful task analysis may be required and innovative alternatives specific to the tasks.
Lack of coordination	May have difficulty selecting, manipulating, or controlling objects.	Cerebral palsy, stroke, multiple sclerosis, Parkinson's.	Provide control substitutes to allow use of existing motor capabilities, such as scanning systems or presets; use control adaptations, such as "slow keys" on a keyboard.	Need to be aware of the range of alternative control methods.
Limitations of reach/movement	May be unable to obtain or place objects.	Spinal cord injury, low back pain, multiple sclerosis, cerebral palsy, amputation, peripheral nerve injuries, other musculoskeletal injuries, shortness or tall height.	Redesign workstation layout, mechanize material handling, divide job tasks.	Need to reduce mobility requirements of tasks using smaller and more efficient work envelopes.
Limitations of speed	May be able to achieve tasks, but only slowly.	Head injury, cerebral palsy, low back pain.	Redesign workstation layout for efficiency, mechanize material handling, divide job tasks.	May result in two fully automated tasks instead of one less-automated task.
Limitations of strength	May be unable to lift or move objects.	Spinal cord injury, low back pain, other musculoskeletal injuries.	Redesign workstation layout to optimize capabilities and positioning of individual, reduce size/weight of material packages, mechanize material handling.	Integration of mechanization and worker tasks becomes key.
Limitations of endurance/activity tolerance	May be unable to perform lengthy or repetitive tasks.	Repetitive motion injuries, such as carpal tunnel syndrome; spinal cord injury, low back pain, other musculoskeletal injuries.	Orthotics, workstation redesign, rest periods, change of activities, reduce size/weight of materials, mechanize material handling.	Situation can be aggravated without provision of adequate physiological healing.

Classes of Accommodations

Job accommodation is undertaken using a very individualized approach, matching the person's abilities/disabilities with the constraints of the job. Even though each project is unique, experience has shown that there are similarities between projects. These similarities are based on the nature of the disabling condition and the functional outcome desired. The following discussion provides an overview of JMAATIs by the functional areas they address. Table 16.2 offers a summary of accommodations that can be made based on areas of impairment.

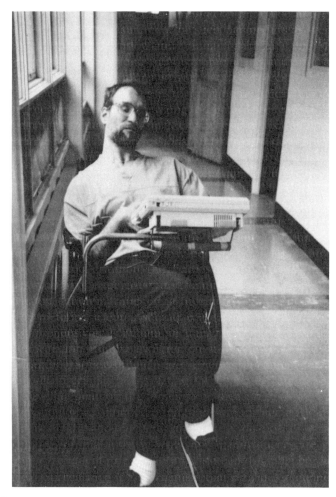

Figure 16.5. (a). User of an augmentative communication device. This device has a touch screen for selection and voice output. It is mounted to the wheelchair with a commercial mounting bracket. (b). Close-up view of the touch panel. This panel has a dynamic display. Selection of messaging units available can programmed to automatically change.

Accessibility

Accessibility covers the items, devices, or modifications necessary to open the physical plant—workstations, restrooms, lunchroom and food services, and training areas—to a person with a disability. A major part of accessibility is providing sufficient space and ramps or lifts so that a wheelchair-user can move in and out of all of the necessary areas. Title III of the ADA Final Rule includes design information on standards for accessible design. Other issues covered in this standard are visual alarms (for people who are deaf), railings and grab bars, raised and braille-embossed signage, detectable warnings, and text telephones.

Communication Enhancement

A person who needs an "augmentative communication device" probably uses it for all communication, including work-related interaction with co-workers. (Figure 16.5a,b shows a typical device and its attachment to a wheelchair.) An employer might be requested to allow the use of such a device for communication. Augmentative communication is not usually regarded as an occupational rehabilitation issue, but often telecommunication is essential to job duties. For example, a deaf employee may need a TT and a

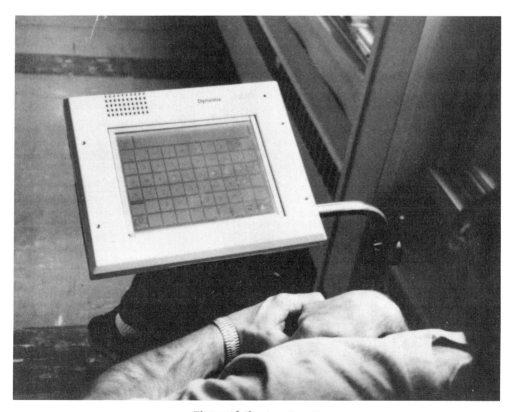

Figure 16.5b   *(continued)*

separate phone line. An interpreter for the deaf may be required for certain training opportunities. Training information on audio cassettes may need to be transcribed.

Mobility and Specialty Seating

As with augmentative communication, this area of assistive technology is a "stand-alone" specialty. In fact, in the assistive technology field, this is the largest specialty area. Often, a person who needs a wheelchair and special seating will already have her or his personal mobility and seating equipment from previous rehabilitation involvement. Although this is not commonly regarded as an occupational rehabilitation issue, it is essential to understand the consequences of appropriate wheeled mobility and seating in the workplace. The worker in a wheelchair, or one using another ambulation device such as a cane or walker, will probably request relevant accommodations so that he or she can use it in the workplace. This request would generally be addressed by the accessibility issues covered earlier.

However, two types of situations move beyond the general accessibility issue. First, the worker may not have been properly evaluated for seating, positioning, and mobility. For whatever reason, the worker may not have been involved in a rehabilitation program in which effective mobility and seating services were provided. For example, canes, walkers, and wheelchairs are often available from a local pharmacy. A person discovering the need for such a device may simply purchase one on his or her own. In this circumstance, it is not uncommon for the individual to purchase a less-than-optimal device. When this occurs in the workplace, the individual should be urged to acquire a proper assessment of his seating, positioning, or mobility needs from a credentialed professional.

Second, even when an individual may have the perfect assistive technology for her or his personal daily use, the individual's job performance can sometimes be substantially improved with specialty seating, positioning, or mobility aids, including pneumatic tires for a wheelchair-based worker with outdoor jobs duties, a stand-up wheelchair for assembly line duties, heavier batteries for power wheelchair users who have jobs in locations with many inclines, or adapted walkers for carrying materials.

General Workstation Seating and Positioning

There are numerous devices available that assist people with back pain and musculoskeletal injuries. Ergonomic chairs with a wide range of adjustments are available. These chairs allow an individual to vary the seating position considerably and still be comfortable. These chairs can also accommodate individuals with substantially different body proportions. (Figure 16.6 shows a person using such a chair, plus other typical adaptations.) Sit-stand stools give a person support, yet allow him or her to be at a position close to standing. Adjustable height desks can allow a person to work in both sitting and standing positions. An array of computer workstation positioning guidelines have been published (Eastman Kodak Company, 1983; Grandjean, 1985; Hermenau, 1995), although almost no data that document the success of these devices, particularly for people with existing disabilities, are available.

Computer Access

An increasing number of service sector jobs require the use of computers. Computer-based jobs seem like a good match for people with disabilities because the physical

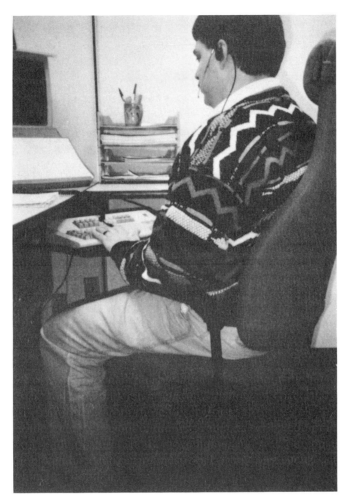

Figure 16.6. Chair modifications for a person with low back pain. He has an ergonomic chair, an adjustable keyboard support, a slant board for holding papers in front of the monitor, and a headset for telephone work.

requirements are quite low. A computer-based job does not have significant lifting restrictions, strength limitations, or mobility limitations. Unfortunately, disabled workers may have difficulty using standard computers because of sensory limitations or physical impairments. Fortunately, there are products that allow alternative input to and output from computers. Representative technologies in each of these categories are described below.

Alternative Input. Computer users can have problems with the keyboard, the mouse, or both. Alternative keyboards include keyboards that have large keys or adapted layouts for the keys, and special angled hand placements. There are one-handed keyboards, virtual keyboards you can point to on the monitor, and even keyboards you can place in your mouth. There are also alternatives to the mouse available for moving the cursor or pointer. Trackballs and touchpads are on the mass market, as are joysticks used

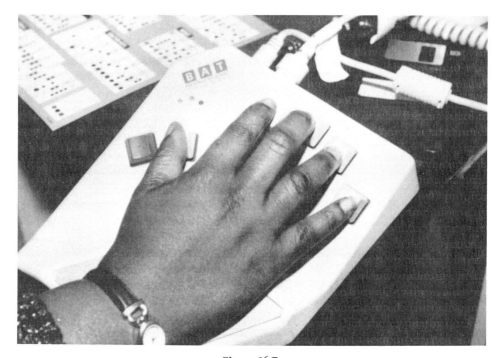

Figure 16.7a

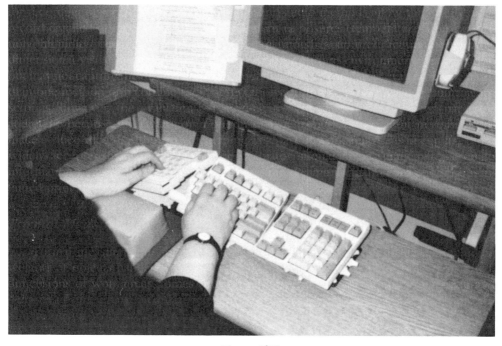

Figure 16.7b

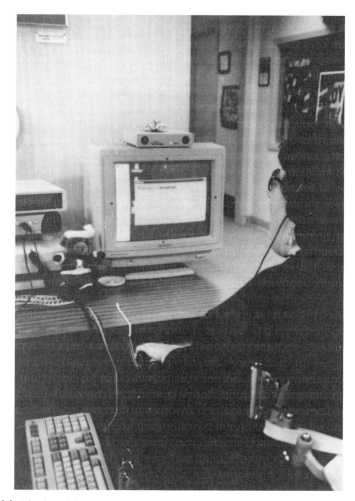

Figure 16.7. **(a)**. A keyboard for use with one hand. All of the characters can be selected with this keyboard, but the user must press combinations of keys at the same time, a technique called *chording*. **(b)**. A split, adjustable keyboard. The three separate sections can be independently adjusted through a wide range of positions. **(c)**. This computer user controls the cursor through head movement and a reflector mounted on her glasses. She also has a small button switch under her left thumb that is a replacement for the left "mouse button."

with the lips/jaw, head-mounted pointers, and voice-controlled mice, as special alternatives. (The person shown in Figure 16.7c is using a head-mounted pointing system.)

Software modifications solve many specific computer control problems. The "sticky keys" software technology allows individuals who only have one finger or use a headstick to type to successfully strike "chords" of keys, which usually require the simultaneous pressing of two or three keys (like control-alt-delete). This solution sequences the key strokes and causes the computer to react as if they were all pressed at once. For example, if the shift key is pressed, the next key is automatically shifted to uppercase. After you strike the desired key, the function automatically returns to the unshifted mode. Another commonly used software keyboard adaptation has been designed for people with poor hand coordination. "Slow keys" holds the keystroke until the key is pressed for an extended length of time. For example, if someone had such poor coordination that he or she frequently hit unwanted keys, slow keys could ignore a keystroke until a key was deliberately held down.

Currently, these features are included with most computers. Windows 95 includes "accessibility" options. Similar features have been available for Windows 3.1 and MS DOS. In the Macintosh operating system, the option is called "Easy Access."

Alterntive Output. People who are blind or vision impaired have the most difficulty dealing with computer output information. Several key techniques assist people with visual impairments.

Many people with vision impairments can still see objects if they are large enough. Several manufacturers distribute screen enlargement software that magnifies computer-generated text and graphics. Lenses are also available that can be positioned in front of the screen to provide low-level magnification for people with mild impairments.

If a person has no useful vision, or if screen enlarging is too slow, screen-reader techniques seem to be the best option. In its simplest form, a text reader "reads" documents by sending entire texts of a computer file to a speech synthesizer. This option can work very well for someone who can see, but lacks the endurance to read for long periods of time. A full-featured screen reader, however, has many more capabilities. Such a screen reader will read the command options of a program; provide cursor placement feedback; read text by word, line, sentence, or paragraph; and adjust the rate of reading. (An individual who is proficient in using a screen reader can increase the rate of speech synthesis so that is becomes incomprehensible to anyone but individuals who are practiced.)

For someone who is blind, the preferred computer output source might be a braille display rather than speech output. This is especially true for users who are also hearing impaired or deaf. Computer-generated text can be converted to the braille system of raised dots and embossed on heavy paper. It can also be converted to raised dots through a refreshable braille display (see Figure 16.8a,b).

Sensory Enhancements

Two senses, hearing and sight, can be enhanced through amplification or magnification techniques. If any of the other senses—taste, smell, or touch—are impaired they can only be compensated for with the remaining senses. Low vision, blindness, hearing impairment, and deafness each have unique accommodation options.

Low Vision. Vision can be enhanced by using magnification and special lighting techniques. Assistive devices include special eyeglasses, telescopes, magnifying lenses, closed-circuit television, special frequency lighting, and color filters. The user typically benefits from magnified targeted objects that are brightly lit without glare, set in front of a dark, glare-free background. Several adjustable "task" lights positioned for the specific activity are usually required to accomplish this.

Blind. When magnification and special lighting are not sufficient, then a total compensatory approach must be taken. This approach typically relies on the senses of hearing and touch, often integrated with a computer. Such computer systems include a scanner that converts paper documents to electronic text by using an optical character recognition (OCR) program. Electronic text can then be read with a screen-reader program and a voice synthesizer or printed in a braille format. There are also devices that combine these functions in one package to make it easier for a blind person to use. OCR technology continues to work best with printed text, the technology for recognizing handwriting is not yet practical. Special devices are available with a text-to-speech converter and speech output or tactile braille output. (Figure 16.8c shows a portable "note-taker" device for braille [keyed] input and presentation on a refreshable braille display.)

Hearing Impaired.   The standard enhancement for impaired hearing is sound amplification using hearing aids. In cases in which hearing aids do not provide sufficient enhancement to meet the functional needs, it may be necessary to utilize techniques and devices normally used with people who are deaf.

Real-time adaptations are required for people who cannot hear voice communications from others but need to obtain this information in a compensatory sensory mode as it is being generated. This is usually accomplished using a visual format (e.g., interpreters of American Sign Language). An interpreter hears the spoken word and translates it to signs that the deaf person can see and understand. Some messages can be typed rather than spoken (on a TT), allowing the receiver to read the typed message.

In other situations, the transformation can be delayed. For example, when using a training session video, accommodation may necessitate that the dialog be recorded, transcribed, and dubbed at a later time. This procedure has obvious advantages over real-time communication during which an interpreter may need to be present for training sessions with live speakers or for meetings.

A deaf person may not be able to hear a doorbell, a fire alarm, or other important signals. There are devices that detect a high sound level, such as a doorbell, and produce a signal. The signal is usually a flash of light, but it could also be a buzzer in a pagerlike device. The user could keep this device on her or his person and respond appropriately when the vibration is sensed.

These techniques are very common for individuals who are blind or deaf. These individuals are likely to be familiar with these types of accommodations, or they know where local resources are readily available. However, it is essential to recognize that the employer may need to be the expert, as the occasional blind or deaf worker may not be aware of these types of accommodations. Thus, the responsibility cannot be placed fully on the worker.

Cognitive Enhancements

Some people have a difficult time mentally processing the various tasks and requirements of a job. They might be poor spellers or become easily distracted. Cognitive enhancements are not commonly used, but there is much interest in this area. New developments in assistive technology in the area of cognitive prosthetics are expected in the near future.

Spelling checkers and grammar checkers available on computers are good examples of cognitive enhancements. It might be considered a reasonable accommodation to allow someone to use a spelling checker to help compensate for a learning disability. Adding a voice synthesizer and a screen reader program to a computer can also be helpful for some individuals who need to review and edit text but have dyslexia.

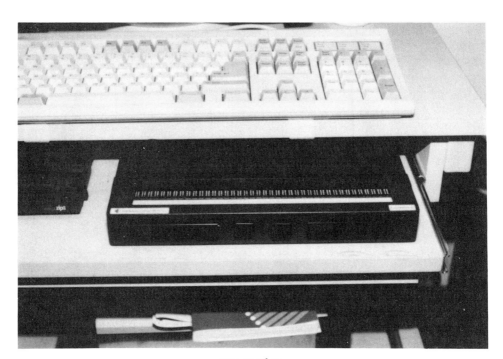

Figure 16.8a

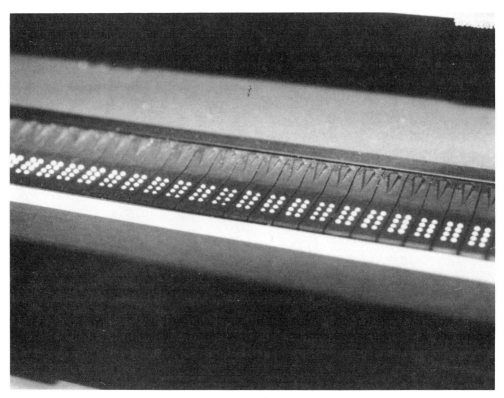

Figure 16.8b

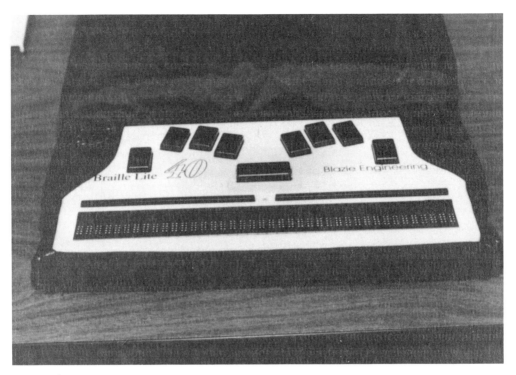

Figure 16.8. **(a)**. A refreshable braille display is mounted under the standard keyboard of this computer workstation. This display is used in conjunction with a screen-reader program and will display in braille whatever is highlighted on the screen. **(b)**. A close-up view of the electromechanical "pins" that pop up to form the braille letters and codes. There are eight pins per cell and 40 cells on this particular unit. **(c)**. A portable "note-taker" device with braille keys for input and a refreshable braille display for output. Photos provided courtesy of the Center for Deaf-Blind Persons, Inc., Milwaukee, Wisconsin.

A number of cognitive enhancements in the workplace are low-tech but effective. Examples include a carefully designed assembly line that can make it difficult to assemble components in the wrong order, a recorded message of instructions that can be played if a worker has not completed an assembly within an allocated number of minutes, pocket alarms or cell telephones that can be used to obtain immediate help, and handheld information managers, such as schedulers, that can be of substantial assistance to those with cognitive impairments. Sometimes these devices are categorized as cognitive prostheses or cognitive orthoses.

Power Tools and Material Handling Aids

A person with an injury or disability may have lifting restrictions, but he or she otherwise may be able to do a job. Most manufacturing plants use mechanical lifting devices for the heavier items but have workers lifting and carrying the lighter ones. Allowing a worker to use existing mechanical lifting devices for lighter items would be considered an accommodation. When mechanical lifting devices are not available, and the lifting requirement exceeds a worker's restriction, then it may be necessary to identify and purchase an appropriate device. There are a variety of industrial, health care, and personal lifting assistive devices available from respected distributors.

Machine or Workstation Modification

The workstation is frequently the focus of JMAATIs. The workstation is where many interventions are interfaced into a working accommodation system. The accessibility of the workstation is the key and it may not have been covered when reviewing the general accessibility of the building. For example, a wheelchair user requires sufficient maneuvering space, while a lower limb amputee needs special steps with less rise on each. (Figure 16.9 shows a custom workstation in construction that allows a wheelchair user access to the keyboard, files, books, and other desk items necessary to do a standard office job.)

The second concern is the method of operation. Specific job tasks, such as pushing buttons, pulling levers, turning knobs, and grasping and pulling material, need to be adapted for the given worker. Modifying handles, levers, and other operator controls allows a match of the ability (disability) of the worker and to the function of the machine. If the amount of force necessary to perform a task is too high, it may be possible to extend handles so the operator will have more leverage, and thus, be able to exert the necessary force. If a worker cannot pull, it may be possible to change the design of the handle so that a push force is required. These adaptations may be required for interfacing computer monitor controls, volume controls, or mechanical control panels.

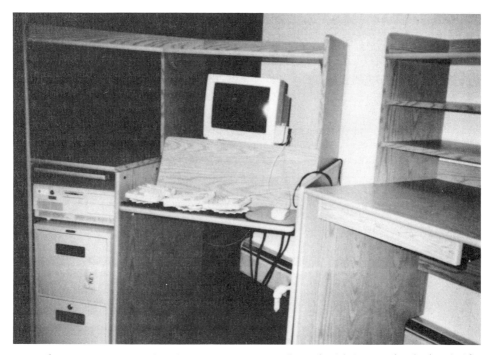

Figure 16.9. A custom-designed workstation in construction for a wheelchair user who also has significant reaching restrictions. Office space is utilized to place everything that the user needs within a comfortable reaching distance.

For individuals with very substantial physical limitations, converting the controls to power (electric, hydraulic, pneumatic) operation is a sensible accommodation. If it is not possible to extend levers or otherwise obtain a mechanical advantage for the worker, it may be necessary to add power to the process so that the operator force requirement is reduced. If the actual lifting force is provided by an electric linear actuator, then the operator needs only to control a switch to engage the actuator. Often extensive job or machine redesign is required to eliminate problem operations for an individual with a disability.

The modifications required for an individual can take different forms and may be essentially unique for them. (Figure 16.10 depicts a receiving chair as part of a computer workstation adapted for a woman who needs to keep her legs at heart level for three hours per day and yet be productive.)

THE JMAATI TEAM

Success of JMAATIs is dependent on a number of factors:

1. Knowledge of the client's abilities/disabilities
2. Medical knowledge regarding the client's disabilities
3. Knowledge of the job, including the importance of specific tasks

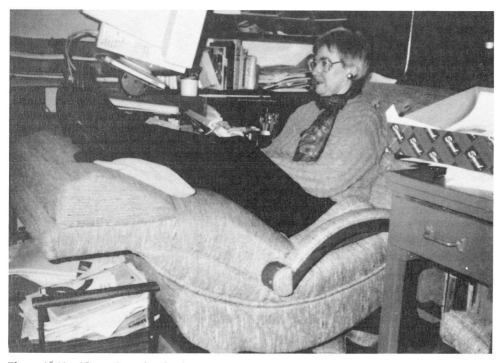

Figure 16.10. This recliner chair has been modified so that it can bring the user's legs up to heart level. The computer workstation has been modified so that the user can rotate a monitor and keyboard to the front and work three hours per day from this position. The mouse is on the original desk surface, and the user can reach it with the right hand without further workstation modifications.

4. Knowledge of laws and issues regarding employment, insurance, and worker's compensation
5. Knowledge of the equipment used on the job, including options and alternatives
6. Knowledge of commercially available products that are frequently used to help people with disabilities, and how to use those products effectively
7. Knowledge of custom adaptations generally appropriate to the client and the tasks, and the ability to implement those adaptations

Only the rare JMAATI expert can have sufficient knowledge of all factors that might be important. Thus, the composition of the team and competence of the team members are essential. Sometimes the team is formed early in the JMAATI process. Frequently, however, the team starts out small and grows in response to problems or concerns that develop.

Often, the team begins as the client and one person from the human resources department. The human resource person may become the team leader or may bring in another person to become team leader. Typically, the next team member is a case manager, vocational rehabilitation counselor, or disability management specialist.

The team at this stage must decide how to expand to bring in the expertise they feel is necessary. This expertise could be found in any of a large number of people, whether they be in-house staff or consultants from outside the organization. It could range from an orthopedic surgeon to a furniture upholsterer. A doctor, rehabilitation therapist, and/or a work area supervisor may very likely be included.

Core Team

To achieve an effective job accommodation for a worker with a disability, team membership is likely to include the following individuals:

Worker with a Disability

Workers have knowledge of their own abilities/limitations and of the job or jobs under consideration. Workers often have knowledge of adaptations or techniques that work for them or for other people with similar disabilities. The ADA mandates a strong role for the person with the disability. The worker must request reasonable accommodation and identify needs regarding the disability. This person must be consulted regarding proposed accommodations.

Human Resource Specialist

The human resource specialists have knowledge of all of the jobs open or potentially open and the general requirements of each. They should be knowledgeable about the ADA. If not, an ADA specialist should become part of the team.

ADA Specialist

This expert has knowledge of the ADA and its procedures and mandates. He or she not only knows the law and recent judgments but also the ADA Accessibility Guidelines (ADAAG) in detail. This includes knowing where the ADAAG fall short.

Rehabilitation Counselor or Case Manager

Counselors or case managers should already be involved with the worker with a disability and his or her rehabilitation. They understand how the worker's recovery will continue, and the specific activities that the worker will find difficult. One of these persons often is the team leader.

Possible Additional Team Members (Outside Consultants)

Assistive Technology Specialist in JMAATIs

The assistive technology specialist should have knowledge of commercial devices available to help people with disabilities and know generally how to install and use these devices. The assistive technology specialist should also have a broad understanding of disability and human performance.

This is a relatively new field and people from a variety of backgrounds work under this general title. In order to insure quality service delivery to clients, RESNA instituted an Assistive Technology Practitioner (ATP) credential starting in early 1997. The person who has this certification must have a documented background in the rehabilitation field. If "extensive" modifications are to be considered, people with specific expertise need to be added to the team.

Occupational Therapist or Physical Therapist

Often, at least one of the traditional rehabilitation therapists is already involved with the worker's rehabilitation program, and he or she is therefore easily accessible for additional involvement. The therapist should be able to help the team solve problems and make certain that recommended solutions match the worker's abilities.

Engineer (Plant Engineers, Production Engineers, Industrial Engineers)

Modifications of machinery often require consulting an engineer to consider fully the concept and implementation. Essentially, all states in the United States and all provinces in Canada require engineers to be registered or licensed before they can legally offer services to the public. A credential labeled Professional Engineer (P.E. or P. Eng.) is the usual designation. Engineers have specialty areas in which they practice, such as mechanical, civil, industrial, chemical, or electrical. A large company is very likely to have engineers on staff to design the equipment used in factorylike production. They have the skills necessary to make custom adaptations to machines. There is usually no requirement for these "in-house" engineers to be registered or even have an engineering education. These people are normally responsible for certain machines and work areas. Usually, no modifications can be made in equipment without the support and permission of plant management.

Rehabilitation Engineer

An engineer who has expertise in working with people with disabilities and JMAATI is called a rehabilitation engineer. The background of individuals calling themselves rehabilitation engineers varies considerably. Currently, there is no credentialing program in place for assurance of the quality of such a professional. In the late 1990s, efforts are being made to create a credentialing program.

Rehabilitation Engineering Technologist

A rehabilitation engineering technologist would normally have a technical background in computer programming, industrial design, mechanical design, or engineering, for example, plus experience working with people with disabilities. She or he may have a similar background and capabilities as a rehabilitation engineer but lacks some component that could quality her or him as a PE. In the late 1990s, efforts are being made to create this credentialing as well.

Ergonomist

Generally, ergonomists have an understanding of the average variations among humans in regards to size, strength, work capacity, vision acuity, and other factors. They are familiar with products and techniques used to match work tasks with as broad a portion of the population as possible. The Human Factors and Ergonomics Society supports the credentialing of ergonomists.

Technicians

Larger companies usually have a variety of support personnel (machinist, repair technician, shop and maintenance personnel) who accomplish many of the tasks needed to be done to accommodate a worker. These tasks might involve installing commercial equipment, assembling purchased items that are shipped "knocked down," or building positioning items, such as a custom support for a phone.

Safety Supervisor

A safety specialist can often function as an in-house ergonomist. He or she is usually familiar with the equipment that is available to help workers and may be able to help problem-solve for a worker with a disability on an individual basis.

TIMING OF JMAATI PROJECTS

The timing of JMAATI services can be a significant issue, particularly if extensive accommodation is involved. Some of the factors that relate to the proper timing of JMAATIs are discussed in the following sections.

Scheduling

Setting up the initial meetings is not usually a problem except that all of the team members need to be present. Scheduling a time that all team members can meet may be a challenge.

Obtaining Commercial Devices

Many of the common assistive technology and commercial devices are normally stocked at the factory or distribution centers and can be delivered in just a few days. The more specialized devices may be built to order or are only produced once or twice a year. In such cases, the delivery time could very likely be a matter of weeks to months. Obtaining a shipping estimate before ordering is helpful if timing is a serious issue.

Custom Design and Fabrication

Customizing devices tends to take a relatively long time from start to finish. The engineer needs to complete the design and order parts and special materials. The design information is then turned over to a shop for fabrication, where a project backlog could cause extensive delays. If the shop is a separate organization, your project could actually get bumped from the promised schedule if another customer has priority.

Trials

When trial use is needed, some devices may need to be ordered or fabricated. Thus, equipment trials may actually double the overall implementation time of the project. Sometimes, it is preferable to perform a trial simulation with alternative devices to reduce potential delays.

Training

Even after equipment is on hand, it is of no value until the person knows how to use it effectively. Some assistive technology devices are simple to operate, but some require extensive training. For example, a person may require 30–40 hours of practice on a computer voice input system before reaching proficiency.

RESOURCES ON ASSISTIVE TECHNOLOGY

The field of assistive technology is in its infancy and is developing rapidly. Only a few years ago, no assistive technology textbooks were available. Today, dozens of "do-it-yourself" books, reference guides, assistive technology manuals, periodicals, databases, academic-oriented textbooks, and training programs are on the market. (Appendix B lists some of the classical print resources.)

Several assistive-technology-related organizations publish journals to disseminate the latest research and applied practice articles (*Assistive Technology* by RESNA, *Rehabilitation Engineering* by IEEE [Institute of Electrical and Electronics Engineers], *Rehabilitation Research & Development* by the Veterans Administration). Additionally, there are journals and magazines by mainstream publishers that focus on assistive technology content (*Technology & Disability* and *Team Rehabilitation Report*). The most prolific numbers of publications are in the form of newsletters. In the late 1980s, the technology assistance federal legislation stimulated programs in the United States to coordinate assistive technology services. Most of these programs developed newsletters as a method of sharing of assistive technology information.

A major conference providing a rich resource on this topic is the annual RESNA meeting. The types of presentations and affiliated opportunities for networking related to job accommodation and disability are illustrated by some of the papers from past meetings. Grant, Kozole, Sax, Smaby, and Tung (1994) presented on the use of assistive technology in job development, and Gunderson and Mendelson (1997) presented on the usability of the WWW for people with visual impairments. Huffman and Loy (1997) highlighted the use of a split keyboard for cumulative trauma disorders, while Lown (1997) examined employers hiring assistive technology users. Mallik and Stinson (1994) presented on the partnerships of business and rehabilitation perspectives.

The assistive technology field has also adopted modern information media approaches. Electronic resources include several CD databases, numerous web sites, and countless E-mail groups and listserves, providing interaction among users of assistive technology information. Web searches can quickly locate many of these newest resources (Smith, 1996).

Another resource that is often overlooked but should be held in tentative status is the assistive technology supplier (ATS). Qualified assistive technology suppliers often have some of the best ideas about the products they distribute. The cautionary remark is that too often suppliers only know the products they carry well. Therefore, it is more likely that they may miss an effective alternative assistive technology device or technique if one lies outside of their product line.

FUTURE TRENDS

Although the assistive technology field is relatively young (25 years), most indications are for project growth. In the next 10 years, this area of specialty will likely look much different. A few of the areas of projected maturation are posed here.

As in many fields, assistive technology is undergoing scrutiny in the age of accountability. Consequently, effort is being expended to develop better outcome assessment instruments and indicators for intervention. The 1997 RESNA Annual Conference Program was packed with quality assurance and outcome related sessions. Over the next decade, it is anticipated that there will be much more data available that identifies when assistive technology as an intervention is warranted, and how JMAATI compares to other types of interventions in occupational rehabilitation.

We will likely see an increase in teaming and the use of assistive technology specialists. As the recognition of the needs of JMAATIs is better understood, integration of the assistive technology specialists into the occupational rehabilitation team process will become more common. Part of this process will include the discovery of not only the general benefits of assistive technology but also the benefits of the specialties within JMAATIs. While at first professionals in related professions will increase their expertise in JMAATIs through in-service training workshops and conferences, they will later discover that additional, more formal training in JMAATIs is needed. To respond to the increasing needs for training, knowledge, and skills in JMAATI, more and more colleges and universities will begin teaching courses and developing full curricula in this field.

A general increasing societal awareness of assistive technology and its potential will continue. The ADA has increased the viability of assistive technology in accommodating the needs of people with disabilities. For example, universal disability signage has now become commonplace in public locations. Adaptations such as automatic doors are overt accommodations the public sees on a daily basis. Furthermore, as public figures increase the social acceptance of having a disability and using assistive technology (Christopher Reeve, Jim Brady, Bill Clinton), society will increasingly understand the needs for accommodations and the application of assistive technology. These public stories accumulate.

Lastly, the designs of jobs, job sites, products, and inventions of any type will form a new paradigm. Once, designers and engineers thought the population had a normal curve of abilities. They designed for the majority or average. In the 1990s, more and more discussion has suggested that the curve may not be as peaked as we once thought. Aging patterns in the United States indicate that in the next century the population will skew toward becoming older, with an increase in disabilities and the need for accommodations (Vanderheiden, 1990). Furthermore, the concept of "us" able-bodied and "them" with disabilities is eroding. New terminology, such as *temporarily able-bodied* (TAB) or *currently regarded as able-bodied* (CRAB), highlights the shift in thinking that we are all in the same population pool. From a design standpoint, there will be a movement away from having design thresholds and absolute specifications. We will move toward a strategy that assumes a more flat population distribution that promotes the up-front design of all places, products, and systems to be maximally accommodating for the widest range of people's abilities and disabilities.

CASE STUDY: ANITA

Anita sustained a back injury at work and subsequently underwent two surgeries and months of physical therapy. When she reached a healing plateau, her doctor released her to return to work with some very severe restrictions; a 10-lb lifting limit, only minimal rotation of the spine, the need to change position at will, and the need to take frequent breaks at her own (variable) schedule, up to 20 minutes every hour.

She was employed at a small company whose president handled all administrative functions and was active in the day-to-day operations of the plant. He was her contact person and represented the company in the entire process of medical care and return to work.

A case manager for this client represented the worker's compensation insurance. The case manager was extremely knowledgeable regarding medical rehabilitation but did not fully understand the employee's job or potential job modifications.

Anita tried to return to work on three separate occasions, but her efforts were not successful. She claimed, "They didn't provide the accommodation that I needed." The employer stated, "Everything that we asked her to do was within her restrictions." It was obvious that a new plan needed to be implemented. The case manager recommended that the client obtain help from the state vocational rehabilitation office and made an official referral. The employer hired an attorney who specialized in worker's compensation and ADA issues.

The vocational rehabilitation (VR) counselor was willing to pursue a variety of job options, but the client wanted to resolve this particular job before considering other jobs possibilities. Was it possible for this client to do this job or not? The counselor requested a rehabilitation engineer consultant to work with the team. The vocational rehabilitation counselor referred the client for a functional capacity evaluation (FCE) at a local rehabilitation center, and then learned about her job through job descriptions, discussion with the employer, and on-site visits.

The rehabilitation engineer studied relevant documents (job description, FCE, medical reports) and went to the employing company for an on-site evaluation. The engineer met with the VR counselor, Anita, the company president, the supervisor of the particular job under consideration, and the person responsible for setups in the shop. One problem that Anita identified was that a back-twisting motion was required to manipulate certain larger parts on the assembly line. This problem was presented to the area supervisor with questions about the product mix and the frequency of using the problem parts. The supervisor volunteered that an accommodation could be made for the client because she did not need to be assigned to work with these particular parts. There were a variety of assembly tasks that used smaller, more easily manipulated parts.

In a similar manner, Anita was asked to review all of the tasks of the job and identify problems. Each of these problems was analyzed to determine the mechanism of body stress in the injured area. Plus, further brainstorming was encouraged for the whole team. The rehabilitation engineer functioned as the team leader, solicited meaningful dialogue from all others, recorded data, and synthesized information in a meaningful plan.

The rehabilitation engineer issued a report that described the client and the problems that were identified at this evaluation. The report discussed the alternative approaches that were considered and depicted the pros and cons for each alternative. The team's comments and ideas were synthesized and specific recommendations were made.

The report recommended that a trial that utilized a variety of techniques to reduce the stress on Anita's back be conducted. The following recommendations were made:

1. Restrict the part size Anita was required to handle to $6'' \times 6''$ or smaller.
2. Provide a workbench with a top surface height of $43''$ for working in a standing position. The suggestion was to purchase a powered adjustable-height table. Literature (from several suppliers of this type of equipment) was attached. Not all prices were included, so it was necessary to work with the dealers to obtain quotes. The employer was told that the size of the table and the height range should be determined and then price quotes obtained. The dealers needed to quote from the same specification, and the table should be purchased from the low bidder. Total cost was anticipated to be around $2000.
3. Purchase an adjustable-height foot stool with adjustment up to $14''$ high. Cost for this stool was expected to be about $65.
4. Explore "lift and tilt" positioning devices. Literature on this type of product was attached, but it was necessary to study the materials more closely before actually ordering or custom building them. It was estimated that adjustable units that would place the material in the desired position for Anita would cost about $500.
5. Explore special seating. An improved seating unit such as a kneeling chair or a chair with back support was recommended. This could potentially be better for Anita's back than the simple stools available in the shop.
6. Consider accommodating other needs. Specifically, the client would need to take more and longer breaks than other employees, per her doctor's restriction. She also would need a rest location. Anita would not be able to handle large, rigid parts. She would need to be allowed to work on small parts or flexible materials so that reaching with her left arm and twisting her back were not required.

Trial with Mock-Ups

Anita's employer arranged a special workstation to help determine if she could tolerate the work after all of the requested modifications were in place. Two work benches were provided, one at the proper height for sitting and working, and the other set at 43″ good height for her to work at while standing. Several chairs, stools, and foot stools were also provided so that Anita could work in a variety of positions. She could change positions as often as she wanted and, after experimenting with some of these devices, she identified four comfortable working positions.

Material that met the size requirement was selected for this trial, as was the lightest of the products generally available. All items were positioned according to Anita's request, using devices made for this purpose by the set-up supervisor. Anita directed the arrangement of the work and all of the items in the workstation.

Resolution of the Original Job

After Anita was satisfied that the modified workstation provided all of the accommodation she needed, a test was conducted. Anita terminated the test after 50 minutes, reporting that she was in severe pain. She seemed to be honestly surprised that she could not work longer.

In addition to the pain she experienced, Anita was deeply affected by the realization that she could not go back to her old job.

Identifying a New Career

Anita worked with her VR counselor to identify other career opportunities that would be more realistic for her. The VR counselor had her work with a career counselor and placement specialist. There were several career objectives that seemed realistic, but they all required good computer skills, something she was lacking.

Anita also worked with her physical therapist and doctor to identify a better chair for her. A chair with a contoured back was identified. This chair was purchased and the rehabilitation engineer, working under direction of the physical therapist and doctor, removed a small amount of foam to reduce the pressure on the injured area of Anita's back. An upholstery shop was hired to recover the back rest.

Anita started taking a computer class. She could make it through the one-hour instruction period by alternating between sitting and standing. She could even walk around the back of the room. Anita had extreme difficulty working in the computer lab.

She found that she needed a break after the class ended before beginning the hands-on session in the computer lab. Anita used her chair in the computer lab, but it was not set up to allow her to stand up and work, so she needed to take a break every 15 minutes to walk around. This did not work well in the lab because students thought her temporarily empty station was available for use.

In order to solve these problems, a complete computer workstation was purchased for Anita. She tried a spring-balanced workstation first, but the forces required to adjust it were too high for her. A power adjustable workstation was selected that would allow her to work in both sitting and standing positions. The computer was purchased following the recommendations of the computer class instructor.

Project Resolution

Anita has been employed for over three months as an insurance claims investigator and reports satisfaction with her work. She is still in a probationary period, but her reviews have been good. She works flexible hours, about 20 hours per week. Anita works out of her home and networks with her employer's computer. She only travels to the office about once a week for meetings or to review hard-copy information. She continues to alternate between sitting and standing positions when working on the computer, and takes breaks 2 to 4 times per day.

APPENDIX: OVERALL SCOPE OF ABLEDATA WITH EXAMPLE SEARCH

===
Action: Topic selected for search: Mouthstick with interchangeable tools
===

Result:

Main Menu	
ARCHITECTURAL ELEMENT	1678
COMMUNICATION	*2521*
COMPUTERS	3374
CONTROLS	974
EDUCATIONAL MANAGEMENT	2371
HOME MANAGEMENT	1232
ORTHOTICS	886
PERSONAL CARE	4621
PROSTHETICS	62
RECREATION	1592
SEATING	1452
SENSORY DISABILITIES	3247
THERAPEUTIC AIDS	2631
TRANSPORTAION	486
UNIVERSAL	2355
VOCATIONAL MANAGEMENT	622
WALKING	864
WHEELED MOBILITY	1918

➢ **Action: Click on COMMUNICATION**

Result:

Communication Menu	
ALTERNATIVE AND AUGMENTATIVE COMMUNICATION	721
HEADWANDS	29
MOUTHSTICKS	*38*
READING	610
SIGNAL SYSTEMS	248
TELEPHONES	502
TYPING	56
WRITING	317

➢ **Action: Click on MOUTHSTICKS**

Result:

Mouthsticks Menu	
mouthstick	10
mouthstick control of cursor control device	2
mouthstick holder	5
mouthstick kit	*4*
optical mouthstick holder	0
optical pointer	17

➢ **Action: Click on mouthstick kit**

Result:

Mouthstick Kit Menu
1:ARROW MOUTHSTICK KIT (MODEL BK6004)
2: CLORAN ORAL TELESCOPING ORTHOSIS
3: HEYER-ABADIE MODULAR MOUTHSTICK
4: MOUTHSTICK KIT (MODEL 31000)

➢ **Action: Click on HEYER-ABADIE MODULAR MOUTHSTICK**

Result:

Product Entry

Product Name: HEYER-ABADIE MODULAR MOUTHSTICK

Generic Name: MOUTHSTICK KIT, MOUTHSTICK

Description: *(Picture Available).*
The Heyer-Abadie Modular Mouthstick is a mouthstick kit and mouthstick designed for professional use. The mouthstick has a V-shaped mouthpiece for a comfortable, firm grip. The all metal telescoping mouthstick can be used with a variety of mouthstick bodies. OPTIONS: Various mouthstick bodies and tip attachments are available. WEIGHT: 2.2 ounces.

Pricing (approximate): 477.00 to 99.95, AUG 1993

Contact Information:
Extensions for Independence
555 Saturn Blvd., #B-368
San Diego, CA 92154
619-423-7709

➢ **Action: Click on Picture Available**

Result:

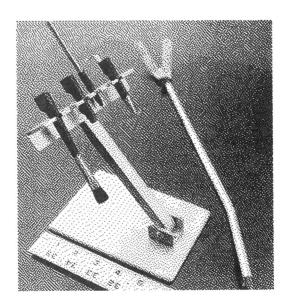

REFERENCES

Angelo, J., & Smith, R. O. (1989). The critical role of occupational therapy in augmentative communication services. In *Technology Review '89* (pp. 49–54). Rockville, MD: American Occupational Therapy Association.

Chapanis, A. (1976). Engineering psychology. In M. D. Dunnette (Ed.), *Handbook of industrial and organizational psychology*. Chicago: Rand McNally.

Christiansen, C. (1991). Occupational therapy: Intervention for life performance. In C. Christiansen & C. Baum (Eds.), *Occupational therapy: Overcoming human performance deficits* (pp. 2–43). Thorofare, NJ: Slack Publishers.

Cook, M., & Hussey, S. M. (1995). *Assistive technologies: Principles and practice*. St. Louis, MO: Mosby.

Eastman Kodak Company. (1983). Ergonomic design for people at work (Vol. 1). New York: Van Nostrand Reinhold.

Grandjean, E. (1985). *Fitting the task to the man: An ergonomic approach*. Philadelphia, PA: Taylor Francis.

Grant, J., Kozole, K., Sax, C., Smaby, N., & Tung, D. (1994). The successful integration of assistive technology and job development for an individual with a disability: A case study. *Proceedings of the RESNA 1994 Annual Conference*, 492–494.

Gunderson, J., & Mendelson, R. (1997). Usability of World Wide Web browsers by persons with visual impairments. *Proceedings of the RESNA 1997 Annual Conference*, 330–332.

Hermenau, D. C. (1995). Seating. In K. Jacobs & C. M. Bettencourt (Eds.), *Ergonomics for therapists* (pp. 137–155). Boston, MA: Butterworth-Heinemann.

Huffman, D. L., & Loy, B. A. (1997). Effects of split keyboard use on cumulative trauma disorders. *Proceedings of the RESNA 1997 Annual Conference*, 431–433.

Job Accommodation Network (JAN) (1991). West Virginia University. P.O. Box 6080, Morgantown, WV 26506-6080.

Lown, N. F. (1997). Employers who hire assistive technology users: A case study. *Proceedings of the RESNA 1997 Annual Conference*, 17–19.

Mallik, K., & Stinson, D. (1994). Business and rehabilitation: A partnership of worksite accommodation. *Proceedings of the RESNA 1994 Annual Conference*, 486.

McCormick, E. J., & Sanders, M. S. (1982). *Human factors in engineering and design*. New York: McGraw-Hill.

Rodgers, B. L. (1985). *A future perspective on the holistic use of technology for people with disabilities*. Madison, WI: Trace R&D Center.

Smith, M. J., & Sainfort, P. C. (1989). A balance theory of job design for stress reduction. *International Journal of Industrial Ergonomics, 4*, 67–79.

Smith, R. O. (1991). Technological approaches to performance enhancement. In C. Christiansen & C. Baum (Eds.), *Occupational therapy: Overcoming human performance deficits* (pp. 746–786). Thorofare, NJ: Slack Publishers.

Smith, R. O., Benge, M., & Hall, M. (1994). Technology for self-care. In C. Christiansen (Ed.), *Ways of living: Self-care management for people with special needs* (pp. 379–422). Rockville, MD: American Occupational Therapy Association.

Technology-Related Assistance for Individuals with Disabilities Act of 1988, Public Law No. 100–407, 29 U.S.C.A. 2201 *et seq.*

Vanderheiden, G. C. (1990). Thirty-something million: Should they be exceptions? *Human Factors, 32*, 383–396.

CLASSICAL TEXTS COVERING THE ASSISTIVE TECHNOLOGY FIELD

Angelo, J. (1997). *Assistive technology for rehabilitation therapists*. Philadelphia, PA: F. A. Davis.

Charlebois-Marois, C. (1985). *Everybody's technology: A sharing of ideas in augmentative communication*. Montreal, Canada: Charlecom.

Church, G., & Glennen, S. (1992). *The handbook of assistive technology*. San Diego, CA: Singular Press.

Cook, M., & Hussey, S. M. (1995). *Assistive technologies: Principles and practice*. St. Louis, MO: Mosby.

Cromwell, F. S. (Ed.). (1986). *Computer applications in occupational therapy*. New York: Haworth Press.

Enders, A. (1990). *Assistive technology sourcebook*. Arlington, VA: RESNA.

Flippo, K. F., Inge, K. J., & Barcus, J. M. (1995). *Assistive technology: A resource for school, work, and community*. Baltimore, MD: Paul H. Brookes Publishing.

Hedman, G. (1990). *Rehabilitation technology*. Binghamton, NY: Haworth Press.

Lane, J. P., & Mann, W. C. (1991). *Assistive technology for persons with disabilities: The role of occupational therapy*. Rockville, MD: American Occupational Therapy Association.

Leslie, J. H., & Smith, R. V. (1990). *Rehabilitation engineering*. Boca Raton, FL: CRC Press.

Webster, J. G., Cook, A. M., Tompkins, W. J., & Vanderheiden, G. C. (1985). *Electronic devices for rehabilitation*. New York: Wiley.

17

Case Management

Sally Maki

You have likely heard the term *case management* used in one or more contexts. Not since the inception of managed care, however, has there been such a coordinated effort to expand an area of practice. The growth of case management in health care has created vast opportunities for those who understand and are able to apply its concepts.

Interestingly enough, case management is not a profession. It is an area of practice within a profession. Nurses, vocational specialists, social workers, therapists, discharge planners, and rehabilitation counselors are among those who perform case management. Their goal is to achieve a successful, cost-effective method to return clients to work. To achieve this goal, the professional must be knowledgeable about all available resources and act as a liaison between interested parties.

DEFINITION OF CASE MANAGEMENT

There are a variety of definitions of case management. The most widely used definition is the one established by the Case Management Society of America (CMSA). This nonprofit organization was established in 1989 as the official body that governs case management and sets national standards. In the booklet, *Standards of Practice for Case Management*, CMSA defines case management as "a collaborative process which assesses, plans, implements, coordinates, monitors and evaluates options and services to meet an individuals health needs through communication and available resources to promote quality cost effective outcomes" (Case Management Society of America, 1995, p. 8). Case management can also be defined as an ever-changing process through which the coordination of functional rehabilitative services results in a return to work and/or vocational independence. This more specific definition would apply to occupational rehabilitation.

Sally Maki • NovaCare Outpatient Rehabilitation, 260 East Highland Avenue, Milwaukee, Wisconsin 53202.

Sourcebook of Occupational Rehabilitation, edited by Phyllis M. King. Plenum Press, New York, 1998.

THE CASE MANAGEMENT PROFESSIONAL

Case management is performed by a diverse group of skilled and experienced health care professionals, including nurses, vocational specialists, social workers, therapists, discharge planners, rehabilitation counselors, and many others. A certification exam has been developed by the Commission for Case Manager Certification (CCMC) to monitor professional conduct and provide standards of practice to those who perform case management functions.

The certification process demands that the individual performing case management be able to perform the following components independently:

- Assessment
- Planning
- Implementation
- Coordination
- Monitoring
- Evaluation

Eligibility to sit for the certification exam consists of the following criteria:

- Currently licensed or certified professional in good standing
- Able to document a minimum of 12 months of acceptable full-time case management experience or its equivalency under the supervision of a certified case manager

or

- Able to document 24 months of acceptable full-time case management experience

or

- Able to document 12 months of acceptable full-time supervision experience, supervising activities of individuals who provide direct case management services

(These requirements are based on those found in the booklet published by the Commission for Case Management Certification, Case Management Society of America, 1995.)

The professional who successfully passes the certification exam receives the title of certified case manager (CCM). Many professionals who perform case management pursue the CCM certification to distinguish themselves as experienced professionals who have passed a comprehensive written exam. Certified or not, a successful case manager must be skilled in communication, diplomacy, and relationship building. He or she must demonstrate skill in identifying cost-effective resources and make appropriate referrals to promote case closure.

Currently, nurses are the greatest number of professionals performing case management. CMSA indicates that 56.6% of its members are registered nurses. Closely linked with other health care providers, nurses often obtain timely information on clients more easily than does a claims administrator or an employer. Their relationships with employees/patients have historically been perceived as more supportive than those of claims adjusters or employers. Although nurses seem to have more credibility with providers, other health care professionals have taken on case manager responsibilities as well. Regardless of the practitioner's discipline, keeping multiple players (employee, employer, physicians, claims administrator, etc.) focused and working together for a common cause is the ultimate challenge faced by all who assume the case management role.

THE EVOLUTION OF CASE MANAGEMENT

Case management services were developed out of the need to control and reduce costs associated with work-related injuries and expedite employees' return to work. Up until the early 1980s, workers' compensation costs were relatively low. Injury care was typically managed by the industrial nurse or company benefits clerk. Often, injury claims were denied as noncompensable under workers' compensation. Due to the fact that workers' compensation benefits were nearly identical to those of the worker's sickness and accident benefits, there were no pressures from the employee to pursue a workers' compensation claim.

Simultaneously, the dynamics of health care were beginning to change rapidly. Suddenly, medical costs were skyrocketing, and weekly workers' compensation benefits were on the rise, surpassing sickness and accident benefits. Job security was becoming a thing of the past. As time went on, other significant changes occurred that continued the upward spiral of workers' compensation costs and claims. These changes included the following:

- A significantly older work force (fewer people retiring at an early age)
- People working harder and faster (Easy jobs earned through seniority disappeared, and production rates increased to compete with foreign markets.)
- A broadening of work-related injuries and diagnoses deemed compensable under workers' compensation laws with cumulative disorders (i.e., tendonitis and carpal tunnel syndrome) now recognized as being work related
- High replacement labor costs (As benefits costs and wages quickly rose, so did the speed with which the injured worker who was off work was replaced.)
- Shifting of costs from the medical claim to the workers' compensation claim in order to achieve 100% coverage (versus using one's own health insurance to avoid paying high deductibles, copayments, and benefit limits)
- Increased fraud and abuse as workers justified the filing of a claim as an earned benefit (Often workers in high-risk or high-seniority jobs saw a need to receive benefits they never used and to which they were entitled.)
- Rising litigation and appeals for workers' compensation claims

All these factors resulted in uncontrolled claims and costs. As a rule, workers' compensation lost time, known as total temporary disability (TTD), and worker replacement costs represent a significant expenditure to employers. These costs are higher than the medical fees associated with the injury. According to Helen Knight (1997), the indemnity–medical ratio can be as high as 3 to 1, depending on the type of work performed.

THE CIRCLE OF PLAYERS

There are typically four players involved in early workers' compensation case: the injured employee, the employer, the insurance carrier, and the physician. Each player has

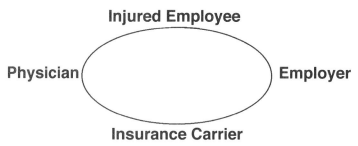

Figure 17.1. The circle of players.

a different perspective on the injury. These players often resemble an unbreakable circle (as seen in Figure 17.1) because their roles and return-to-work goals are often clouded by a lack of communication with and mistrust of each other. What follows is a representation of the perspectives of each player.

The Injured Worker

An injured worker may feel that workers' compensation is an entitlement, a right earned by seniority, which the employer should pay for without question. The employee may be fearful or angry that an accident that caused an injury occurred. He or she may fear a lack of job security or become angry over experiencing pain as a result of the injury. The injured worker may feel that it is the employer's responsibility to facilitate a successful return to work. Animosity on either side at this point may facilitate a breakdown in the lines of communication.

The Employer

The employer, depending on the sequence of events, may see the accident as a result of an unsafe employee act or inattentive employee work habits. Feelings of resentment or suspicion toward the injured worker may develop. If this happens, the employer may feel as though the responsibility for the successful return to work of the employee rests in the hands of the insurance carrier. Communication between the injured worker and the employer often stops at this point.

The Insurance Carrier

The insurance carrier, on receiving the injury claim, has two primary responsibilities: The carrier must set up an employee file and reimburse that employee for lost wages. Weekly benefits must be paid within a predetermined time, depending on state statutes. The claims adjuster sees his or her role as administrative, with return-to-work responsibility shifting to the physician. If a delay of benefits occurs, communication with the injured worker continues to be compromised and communication continues to be a problem.

The Physician

The physician considers his or her number one priority to be the well-being of the injured worker. Return-to-work considerations are discussed between physician and patient. Often, because an employer doesn't communicate with the physician, delays may occur in getting the employee back to work. An employer may set up a return-to-work program or temporary alternate duty that would allow the employee to go back to work. However, if the physician has not been informed, further delays may occur. The employer and the insurance carrier may consider themselves left out of the return-to-work process if communication between them does not occur. Animosity between all players may continue, and efforts toward returning the injured employee to work may dissolve.

At this point, case management can be very effective in opening the lines of communication between players. The case manager can assist and act as a liaison to all parties. Following the guidelines of case management; the case manager will facilitate a win-win situation for the injured worker, the employer, the insurance carrier, and the physician. Acting as an advocate, the case manager can provide suggestions for quality cost-effective medical services, investigate alternative return-to-work options, and intervene when communication barriers between the players exist.

The players in workers' compensation are also known as clients. Perhaps nowhere in health care is the client as undefined or ambiguous as in the occupational rehabilitation arena. There is often more than one client served in occupational rehabilitation case management. Regardless of how many people are involved in a claim or case, the injured worker should always be regarded as the primary client. That does not mean, however, that other clients or customers are not important. Other participants involved in a work injury case who may be regarded as clients are the employer, the physician, the insurance carrier (or the claims adjuster), the rehabilitation nurse, the vocational counselor, and/or an attorney.

TYPES OF CASE MANAGEMENT

Case management and the coordination of health care may take different forms, based on employer and insurance carrier preferences. The employer and the workers' compensation insurance carrier may have an agreement with an independent case management firm to assist in case resolution. Or, the insurance carrier may assign its own in-house case manager to the claim when it is received. The case management process may take place in the field or over the telephone.

Field Case Management

Field case management takes place either outside or inside the workplace. When a claim translates into a lost time case, a case manager may be assigned. Rarely is a medical-only claim in need of case management. The case manager personally meets with the injured worker and maintains ongoing face-to-face contact. This contact includes participation in physician visits and therapy appointments, visiting the worksite with the injured worker, and coordinating return-to-work options with the employer. When severe injuries occur, the case manager may immediately be sent to the hospital to initiate the case management process.

In-House or Telephonic Case Management

In-house or telephonic case management involves coordinating return-to-work services over the phone. The information that the case manager obtains is the same as in field case management, however, no on-site or in-person calls are made. Often times, computerized case management programs are used to document, track, and remind the case manager of upcoming client appointments. These calls are essential for case managers when handling injury claims and facilitating early return-to-work for injured employees. Currently, many insurance institutions utilize telephonic case management as a more productive and cost-effective means to managing workers' compensation claims.

ECONOMIC BENEFITS OF CASE MANAGEMENT

Case management and rehabilitation services have realized substantial savings for employers by managing medical claims. The Health Insurance Association of America (HIAA) has reported that for every dollar insurance carriers spend on medical rehabilitation and case management programs, they average a 30 to 1 return on investment. In their most recent survey, as reported in the *Work Injury Management Digest*, HIAA reported the actual return-on-the dollar ratios of individual responding carriers ranged from $4 to $75 (Devlin, 1996, p. 3).

A survey of 52 insurance carriers of various sizes yielded the following return-on-investment averages for the years 1991–1993:

$32 for $1 in 1991
$29 for $1 in 1992
$28 for $1 in 1993

However, in a recent article in the *Workers' Compensation Managed Care Newsletter*, a representative of CNA Insurance indicated that case management involvement in workers' compensation claims has only resulted in a 20% savings ("Changes Coming in Workers' Compensation Industry," 1997). The 20% savings was realized when nurses, who specialized in case management and had five years of workers' compensation experience, managed the claims. These nurses also spent a majority of their time communicating with all the players.

MEASURING OUTCOMES

Measuring case management outcomes is challenging. Is it even possible to measure the effects of case management intervention? Outcome data in rehabilitation is often collected by comparing nonmanaged claims against case-managed claims. However, a number of other variables, such as incidence, extent of injury, and labor–management relations, remain uncontrolled. Another uncontrolled variable is the time of entry of case management into the process. Some insurance carriers assign case management on receipt of a claim. Some initiate case management only if the case involves lost time. Other carriers assign case management as late as from 30 to 60 days following an incident. Occasionally, case management is implemented only after an injury is deemed catastrophic, although most carriers now see the value of early intervention. Regardless of when case management is assigned, the health care and insurance communities continue to watch and collect outcome data to determine the cost-effectiveness of the practice.

COMMON PRACTICES

An intake interview usually starts the case management process. The intake form identifies the basic information to be obtained during an initial meeting with the injured worker. (Figure 17.2 provides an example of an intake form.) Although forms vary among case management firms and insurance carriers, the information collected to start the case management process is similar.

Rationale for Intake Questions

Questions 1–3. Self-explanatory.

Question 4. What is the date of injury and the last date worked? This question looks for consistency of information. The date of injury should coincide with the employer's, physician's, and insurance carrier's documentation. The same holds true for the last date worked.

Question 5. What is the client's marital status, and does he or she have children? If so, what are their ages? This question looks beyond marital status and children in school. The case manager is gathering information on the financial status of the injured worker and family. Will the injured worker be supported by a full- or part-time working spouse? Will the workers' compensation check be enough to support the family, or will the tax-free workers' compensation check actually be additional income? Will day care be stopped and the injured worker assume this responsibility, thus eliminating day care expenses? If the workers' compensation income becomes greater than the working paycheck, is there sufficient incentive to return to work?

Question 6. What alternate work activities are you involved in? When asking about alternate work activities, the case manager is looking for a possible correlation between the injury and other frequently performed home activities. For instance, is the injured worker an avid knitter or home computer operator? How do these activities relate to a workers' compensation claim for carpal tunnel syndrome? Is the injured with a knee injury an active winter skier or snowboarder?

Question 7. What is the description of the injury as given by the injured worker? Again, this question is looking for consistency of information between the various parties involved. Perhaps the injured worker is now angry about the injury, and because of a resultant loss of income has become resentful toward the employer. Does he feel the injury was the employer's fault and, therefore, feels no self-responsibility in the return to work process? What barrier will this attitude to be returning to work?

Question 8. Which extremity is dominant? This question is important when specific return-to-work restrictions are written. "No use of the injured hand" will be a difficulty if the job demands fine motor skills. Identifying appropriate jobs for the injured worker to enable her or him to return to work early will contribute to a successful outcome.

Question 9. How would you rate your pain on a scale of 0 to 10? This question quantifies the worker's pain by using a numerical scale. Zero indicates no pain, while a

1. Name _____

2. Address _____

3. Phone _____

4. Date of Accident (DOA)_____   Last Date Worked (LDW) _____

5. Marital Status _____ Children (ages) _____

6. Alternate work activities (i.e., side jobs, hobbies, sports)

7. Description of injury as described by injured worker

8. Which extremity is dominant (if upper extremity injury)?

9. Current symptoms and rated 0–10 scale

10. Injured worker's barriers for returning to work (i.e., needs restricted duty versus full duty, or wants to be pain free in order to return to work)

11. Past medical history, including allergies, past surgeries, past worker's compensation injuries, motor vehicle injuries, etc.

12. Current habits (i.e., smoking, alcohol use, other drug use)

13. Worker's description of current work experience

14. Description of past employment experiences and reasons for leaving (i.e., seasonal layoff, downsizing, or discharge)

15. What does the injured worker see as a successful resolution to his/her injury?

Figure 17.2. Case management intake form.

score of 10 warrants immediate medical intervention. Observe the worker during each meeting to determine congruency between what is reported and what is demonstrated. For example, if the injured worker with a back injury describes a pain level of 10 but does not physically exhibit pain behavior compatible with this rating, then the provider may want to further investigate the reason for this discrepancy. This may identify the existence of problem pain behaviors which may impede the recovery process and early return to work efforts.

Question 10. What are barriers in returning the injured worker to work? This question ascertains the injured worker's return-to-work goals. Are they realistic and achievable? Is the injured worker open to temporary light duty return-to-work options? If so, this should be immediately explored with the physician and employer. If his or her return to work is expressed by the worker as being contingent on the absence of pain, the physician and employer should be notified. Once aware of this pain-focused behavior, the physician and employer may desire to change the approach to the worker's care. For instance, ordering therapy that is functionally focused will be more successful than therapy based on modalities, which often addresses subjective pain complaints. Helping the injured worker understand the importance of functional return-to-work goals must be discussed as soon as possible.

Question 11. What is your past medical history? For instance, does the injured worker have allergies, and what other injuries on or off the job have occurred? If the patient suffers from allergies, this needs to be addressed, especially if he or she is working in an environment that may contribute to the current injury or illness. Identifying previous workers' compensation or personal injuries is very important. This information will help identify any correlation between the current injury and a preexisting condition. This information may be considered by the physician when the case is ready for closure, and final disability ratings are given.

Question 12. Is the injured worker aware of the effects of various habits from a medical perspective? For instance, smoking slows the healing process of any surgical procedure, and drug use has an adverse effect on successful return-to-work and employment opportunities.

Question 13. Getting the worker's description of his or her job and what physical demands it takes is essential. Understanding the employee's (worker's) perception of the job demonstrates that his or her input is valued and will be taken into consideration when return-to-work plans take place. The case manager should also get a job description from the employer. If one is not available, the case manager may want to perform one with the employee present. This process will assist the physician in determining return-to-work dates and appropriate restrictions.

Question 14. What are the injured worker's past experiences? (Often times these past experiences, which may include past injuries, contribute to the current claim.) What return-to-work opportunities will be accepted? It is more likely that the injured worker who is satisfied with his or her job will be more open to early return to work then the injured worker who hates the supervisor or employer. Current job satisfaction plays an intricate part in the return-to-work process. The case manager must be aware of this issue.

Question 15. What is the injured worker's return-to-work goal? The answer to this question is key to successful case management. The case manager needs to be aware of how her or her liaison position can help all parties achieve a successful return-to-work outcome.

CASE STUDY

Scenario: Lost Time Back Injury

Week 1. Jim is hurt in a manufacturing plant while lifting a part from the assembly line. He immediately reports the injury to his supervisor. Complaining of back pain, Jim is unable to continue working and asks to go home. The next morning, Jim experiences stiffness and soreness in his lower back and feels unable to report to work. He calls his physician and is given an appointment for four days after the injury. On evaluation, Jim is told by his physician that he has a lumbar strain. He is given a referral for three weeks of physical therapy. The doctor asks Jim about returning to work. Jim states that he has too much pain, and that his job involves heavy lifting and repetitive work. The physician writes an order for Jim to remain off work indefinitely. Jim is to see the physician again in three weeks. The physician's receptionist gives Jim the name of the nearby hospital therapy department and asks him to call for an appointment.

Week 2. Jim calls to schedule therapy and is given an appointment for the following week. Jim is now 18 days postinjury.

Week 3. After Jim's initial therapy evaluation, he is told to come in three times a week for therapy. The treatment goals established are to have Jim pain free and able to return to his job.

Week 4. Jim misses two therapy appointments. He calls in to cancel therapy the first time, stating he is having too much pain to drive his car. He calls into cancel therapy a second time because he has to take his child to the doctor.

Week 5. Jim returns to the physician one week after therapy was initiated. He states he is no better. The physician again asks Jim if he can return to work. Jim states he still has too much pain. The doctor writes another order to continue therapy services.

Week 6. Jim misses another therapy appointment, stating he had another commitment that he forgot about.

Week 7. Jim reports to the therapist that his pain has lessened, but he feels he would be unable to perform his regular heavy-lifting job. He misses two more therapy appointments.

Week 8. Jim again is seen by the physician. The physician verbalizes his concern to Jim that he has missed many therapy appointments and perhaps a return to work in a light-duty capacity is appropriate. Jim states that there is no light duty available. The doctor writes an order for light duty and continuation of therapy. Jim takes the new order to work. Jim's employer, not sure of what the order for light duty means in terms of real work, calls the workers' compensation carrier. A case manager is assigned.

The following are a few case management strategies that could have been implemented earlier to reduce lost-time days, and thus reduce total temporary disability benefits.

1. Ask Jim if he would like to be seen by a physician within 24 hours of his injury. A case manager should have several resources available that accommodate urgent appointments. Should Jim have agreed to see another physician, four days of lost time might have been eliminated.
2. Ask the employer to identify alternate duty jobs with lighter or no lifting requirements. All lost-time days may have been eliminated had Jim and the physician known these accommodations were feasible options.

3. Ask the employer to accommodate Jim with an alternate duty job on a part-time basis, 2, 4, or 6 hours per day.

4. Inform the physician of the company's ability to accommodate Jim in any capacity, honoring any restrictions.

5. Ask the physician if a therapy referral could be made to a more responsive provider. In this case, four days of total temporary disability could possibly have been avoided.

OBSTACLES

As is true of any profession, there are always obstacles to case management that make the achievement of goals a challenge. In occupational rehabilitation case management, there is often more than one client. The injured worker's interests must be considered along with the other players. Multiple customers sometimes raise issues of ethics and professional burn-out.

The question of what is most appropriate in health care practice is asked every day by case managers. Providing quality, cost-effective treatment, coupled with timely return-to-work goals, can present a dilemma. For instance, if the employer and the insurance carrier request early return to work to contain costs, and the injured worker desires to be pain free prior to returning to work, the case manager must work with both parties to resolve these issues.

Guidance on ethical questions is provided by the Commission for Case Managers (1995). The commission has developed a Code of Professional Conduct for Case Managers, with disciplinary rules, procedures, and penalties. Adopted in November 1996, it has since been used as a reference for case managers.

Trying to satisfy multiple customers may lead to burn-out. It becomes difficult to repeatedly focus on issues that all parties are not satisfied with, especially when they are in conflict. The case manager is challenged to try to remain as objective as possible. To do this, the case manager must explain to all parties that the goal of case management is to achieve a successful return to work in a cost-effective and efficient manner. Achievement of this goal involves the following:

- Developing a trusting relationship with the injured worker, the employer, the insurance carrier, and the health care providers
- Taking a consistent approach to working with all parties
- Maintaining personal integrity with every case
- Understanding that not all parties may be satisfied with the timing or the outcome of the case

Recognizing the obstacles or frustrations associated with a case, and networking with other case managers to find solutions or additional resources enables the case manager to better define approaches to effective case management.

CUSTOMER SERVICE

Case management in occupational rehabilitation serves to meet the needs of clients through intensive communication and interaction. Customer service is the cornerstone of its foundation. It is impossible to successfully resolve a case without applying the following principles of good customer service.

1. Always return *all* phone calls and messages. A case manager will earn more respect by consistently performing this one simple task.
2. Be on time, *every* time. Tardiness shows a lack of respect for the other person's time.
3. Respect the client. He wants and needs the case manager's attention to his or her issues.
4. Case managers should always do what they say they are going to do. If not, they become part of the problem.
5. Case management and case managers have developed a high professionalism. They should act it and practice it.
6. Promise less and deliver more.

MANAGED CARE VERSUS OCCUPATIONAL REHABILITATION CASE MANAGEMENT

Although case management in the managed-care setting has become quite sophisticated, occupational rehabilitation case management is still in its infancy. (Table 17.1 describes some of the differences between managed care case management and occupational rehabilitation case management.)

Protocols and management processes have been developed to reduce costs and maximize services in managed care. In the occupational rehabilitation arena, case management still must deal with challenging workers' compensation statutes. The occupational rehabilitation case manager should look forward to continuing changes as medical costs and lost-time costs are reduced. Employers are becoming more sensitive to the demands of their stockholders. To ensure that profits increase, costs in all areas will need to be managed. New case management strategies will need to be developed. These strategies will be aimed at (a) developing provider relationships with those who are willing to help reduce their costs for services; (b) working with each employer to prevent injuries and develop early return-to-work programs; and (c) monitoring and tracking outcomes.

CONCLUSION

Case management has developed into an important process that is designed to positively impact the outcome of each work-injury case. In occupational rehabilitation,

Table 17.1. Differences between Managed Care Case Management and Occupational Rehabilitation Case Management

Managed care case management	Occupational rehabilitation case management
Benefits are plan driven.	Benefits are injured-worker driven.
Coverage limited to plan.	No coverage limits.
Premiums and co-pays.	100% medical coverage.

case management is now demonstrating its ability to keep communication lines open. The ultimate goals of a successful return to work or vocational independence will be to reduce workers' compensation premium rates. The dollars saved will show up in the outcome data currently being collected.

REFERENCES

Case Management Society of America. (1995). *CMSA standards of practice for case management guidebook.* Rolling Meadows, IL: Author.

Changes coming in workers' comp industry. (1997, April). *Workers' Comp Managed Care, 4,* 5-6.

Commission for Case Managers. (1995, November). *Code of professional conduct for case managers.* Rolling Meadows, IL: Author.

Devlin, P. (1996). Insurance carriers discover that rehabilitation case management generates substantial savings. *Work Injury Management, 5,* 3.

Knight, H. (1997, January-February). 24-hour care today. *The Case Manager, 8,* 39.

18

Vocational Rehabilitation

Robert E. Breslin

Vocational rehabilitation counseling is a specialized form of counseling that originated in the United States in response to a series of federal mandates designed to promote the independence and vocational functioning of individuals with disabilities. After 75 years of existence, rehabilitation counseling is well established as a distinct profession and has expanded beyond the United States to become internationally recognized as an area of professional practice.

The rehabilitation counseling model combines three distinct theoretical models to assist individuals with disabilities in the development and implementation of individualized plans to attain maximum independence in daily living and vocational function (Williamson, 1965). The rehabilitation counselor utilizes the medical model to understand the disabling impairment and evaluate the appropriateness of curative or restorative interventions. The vocational guidance model is used to guide individuals with disabilities through a process of vocational exploration and goal development. Finally, the mental health model is employed to address issues of personal adjustment to disability.

THE HISTORY OF VOCATIONAL REHABILITATION

Origins of Vocational Rehabilitation

Rehabilitation counseling possesses the unique distinction of being the only profession established by an act of the United States Congress (Wright, 1980). In 1954, Congress mandated and funded the development of university-based graduate programs for pre-employment training of vocational rehabilitation counselors. The same legislation established research foundations for vocational rehabilitation, which had the effect of expanding the unique body of knowledge associated with vocational rehabilitation practice.

Robert E. Breslin • Center for Occupational Health, University of Cincinnati Medical Center, Cincinnati, Ohio 45267-0458.

Sourcebook of Occupational Rehabilitation, edited by Phyllis M. King. Plenum Press, New York, 1998.

Although vocational rehabilitation personnel have functioned within the state–federal system of vocational rehabilitation since the passage of the Smith-Fess Civilian Rehabilitation Act of 1920, and in spite of early recognition by the federal rehabilitation agency of the primary importance of counseling as a prerequisite for the development of vocational rehabilitation and training plans, rehabilitation counseling had not existed as a distinctly separate professional discipline outside of the state–federal agency structure until the passage of the 1954 legislation (Public Law 565 of the 83rd Congress).

The Rehabilitation of Individuals with Disabilities: A Brief History

The history of vocational rehabilitation, although relatively short, is complicated by its symbiotic relationship with the ongoing development of federal legislation regarding veterans affairs, economic security, public education, civil rights, and public health throughout the twentieth century. More complete histories of the vocational rehabilitation movement can be found in several texts designed to orient entering rehabilitation counseling graduate students to the historical development of rehabilitation counseling. (Several of these works are cited in the reference section to this chapter.) The following summary is intended to provide a modicum of historical context for those unfamiliar with the development of the vocational rehabilitation counseling profession.

The Rehabilitation of War Veterans

Not unlike the history of trauma medicine, the history of vocational rehabilitation in the United States has been inextricably linked to the aftermath of war. The first national pension was established in 1776 to provide compensation to soldiers and sailors of the American Revolution who lost the ability to earn a living due to physical disabilities resulting from military service. This concept of federal responsibility to compensate military veterans for economic loss resulting from service-connected disability has remained a central tenet of veterans benefits in the United States until the present time.

The Civil War

After the Civil War, Congress took several significant steps to expand the scope of federal responsibility to assist military veterans in readjusting to civilian economic self-sufficiency. Union veterans received preferential consideration when applying for federal civil service employment. Military service time was also counted toward the residency requirement to make homesteading claims in western states and territories.

The First World War

Following the turn of the century, the federal role in the vocational rehabilitation of veterans accelerated greatly. Even prior to the entrance of the United States into the Great War, the War Risk Insurance Act provided vocational rehabilitation and training by the federal government to veterans with permanent, war-related disabilities. This act also chartered the Federal Board of Vocational Education to coordinate the provision of vocational education and rehabilitation in the various states.

In 1918, Congress passed the Soldiers' Rehabilitation Act. This law charged the Federal Board of Vocational Education with responsibility for providing vocational rehabilitation to any veteran with a disability who qualified for compensation under the War Risk Insurance Act. For the first time, Congress had acknowledged a federal obligation to provide veterans with disabilities more than financial compensation for their losses. The legislative process that preceded the passage of the Soldiers' Rehabilitation Act was notable for another reason. The equity of excluding citizens with disabilities unrelated to military service from eligibility for vocational rehabilitation and training was questioned and vigorously debated. This debate led, in 1920, to legislation that extended eligibility for vocational rehabilitation services under the direction of the Federal Board of Vocational Education to eligible civilians, laying the groudwork for the state–federal vocational rehabilitation program.

From the Second World War to the Present

The Servicemen's Readjustment Act of 1944, commonly referred to as the G.I. Bill of Rights, had a profound impact on the vocational education and rehabilitation in the period after the Second World War. The G.I. Bill provided tuition support for veterans and required the government to participate in numerous contractual relationships with technical schools, colleges and universities, and professional schools. In its implementation, the G.I. Bill recognized the primary importance of vocational assessment and counseling for all veterans who sought education and vocational training. An unprecedented number of staff were trained to assist veterans to identify vocational goals and select appropriate training and educational programs. Related legislation extended rehabilitation services to the severely disabled veterans who were served by the Veterans Administration in its hospital system.

Educational and rehabilitative assistance similar to that found in the G.I. Bill was extended to veterans of the Korean War and Vietnam War eras. In 1962, the Veterans Rehabilitation Program was established as a permanent program, available to all veterans with disabilities.

Early State–Federal Rehabilitation Programs

As previously noted, the question of the expansion of vocational rehabilitation programs to the civilian population arose during the development of the Soldiers' Rehabilitation Act of 1918. In 1920, Congress passed the Smith-Fess Civilian Rehabilitation Act, or Vocational Rehabilitation Act, which charged the Federal Board of Vocational Education with the responsibility to administer a grant-in-aid program for states that agreed to collaborate in an effort to provide vocational training and rehabilitation to eligible individuals with disabilities. Prior to the passage of this law, only 8 of the 48 states had any form of vocational rehabilitation program in operation. By 1930, 44 of the 48 states had developed a vocational rehabilitation program in response to the availability of federal matching grants-in-aid.

In 1935, the Social Security Act significantly expanded the level of federal support for the vocational rehabilitation program. More importantly, the mandate for a federal role in the vocational rehabilitation of individuals with disabilities was embedded in an immensely important and popular piece of legislation designed to provide basic economic security for all Americans, regardless of disability status.

In 1943, the Vocational Rehabilitation Act was amended to extend eligibility for services to individuals with emotional and intellectual disabilities. The available services for eligible individuals were also expanded to include physical and medical restoration services provided that they could be expected to increase the probability of vocational success. The 1943 amendments removed the federal vocational rehabilitation agency from under the administrative control of the Office of Education, allowing for significant experimentation and innovation at the federal and state agency levels, particularly in the areas of rehabilitation counseling and case management.

As previously described, legislation in 1954 provided funding to develop graduate training programs for preemployment preparation of vocational rehabilitation counselors and established an ongoing system of funding for rehabilitation related research.

In 1973, Congress enacted the Rehabilitation Act. The passage of this act was significant for several reasons. Two previous versions of this bill had been vetoed by President Nixon in October, 1972 and March, 1973. The passage of an amended version in the face of continued hostility from the executive branch demonstrated the strength of the Congressional support garnered by the vocational rehabilitation program over the years. Additionally, the Rehabilitation Act of 1973 was significant in that it addressed the issue of workplace accessibility and the requirement that employers provide accommodations to qualified individuals with disabilities to allow them to work (Havranak, 1993). Finally, and perhaps most importantly from the perspective of the development of vocational rehabilitation programs targeted toward individuals with work injuries and occupational illnesses, the 1973 act directed state agencies to prioritize individuals with severe disabilities without regard to their prognosis for employment.

THE STATE–FEDERAL VOCATIONAL REHABILITATION PROGRAM

The Federal Rehabilitation Agency

The state-federal system of vocational rehabilitation has existed since its inception in 1920 as a partnership between the federal rehabilitation agency and the various state agencies. The federal agency has undergone several name changes and been assigned to various federal government departments in its more than 70 years of existence. Since 1979, the federal agency, known as the Rehabilitation Services Administration (RSA), has been located in the U.S. Department of Education's Office of Special Education and Rehabilitation Services. The RSA develops the federal regulations that implement rehabilitation-related legislation enacted by Congress and monitors the compliance of state agencies to those regulations. Additionally, the RSA manages the grant-in-aid program that provides funding for the provision of vocational rehabilitation services.

The State Vocational Rehabilitation Agency

The state vocational rehabilitation agencies are responsible for the provision of vocational rehabilitation services to eligible individuals residing within their respective states. State agencies submit a plan to the federal agency, outlining the structure of their programs, and detailing how they will comply with federal mandates and regulations in order to meet the goals of Congress and qualify for federal matching funds. The federal government, through the RSA, provides funding in the form of grant-in-aids equivalent to 80% of the state's expenditures on vocational rehabilitation.

State agencies vary to a degree in their organization, administrative location within state government, and even name. In general, the agencies are responsible for providing case management and vocational rehabilitation services to individuals who qualify for services under the eligibility criteria set by Congress. These services are provided in the context of a case management system in which various stages in the rehabilitation process are assigned status codes. This standardized system has allowed for meaningful program evaluation based on client outcomes and the case management process.

OCCUPATIONAL INJURIES AND VOCATIONAL REHABILITATION

The State–Federal Role

Individuals with industrial injuries and occupational illnesses have been a significant consumer population served by the state–federal vocational rehabilitation program since its inception. One of the earliest studies of rehabilitation outcomes, published by the Federal Board for Vocational Education in 1928, reported that 53.6% of vocational rehabilitation clients served by the state–federal program had disabilities attributable to employment accidents. Indeed, the incidence of industrial injury during the early twentieth century was a significant impetus for the expansion of vocational rehabilitation eligibility beyond military veterans to the civilian population.

Workers' Compensation and Vocational Rehabilitation

In 1911, the first workers' compensation law to withstand court challenges to its constitutionality was enacted. In all, 10 states passed some form of workers' compensation legislation that year. By 1948, all states had passed a workers' compensation law. The enactment of the workers' compensation system changed the nature of the employer–employee relationship with regard to work-related injuries and accidents. Although there are significant differences between the various state and federal workers' compensation laws covering the nation's workers, there are some common elements. Workers' compensation laws essentially acknowledge that the employer is liable for accidents, injuries, and illnesses arising from the course of employment without regard to issues of negligence or fault. Employers are responsible to provide a predetermined level of wage replacement as well as reasonable and necessary medical and restorative services. In return, the employer is protected from civil litigation and the associated risk of costly legal proceedings and more substantial penalties by the exclusive remedy provisions of workers' compensation law.

A secondary, but intentional, effect of the enactment of workers' compensation laws was to increase the financial interest of employers in safety and health activities. Workers' compensation laws generally provide temporary wage replacement during periods when an injured worker is unable to work because of the work-related disability. As a consequence, employers and insurers perceive an economic interest in avoiding unnecessarily long periods of convalescence. Likewise, most workers' compensation systems are designed to indemnify the injured worker from economic loss associated with permanent and total disability, that is, work-related disability that results in an inability to continue to earn a living. These standard provisions of workers' compensation law served as an incentive for the development of vocational rehabilitation programs and services targeted at workers' compensation and other disability insurance claimants.

The Emergence of Private-Sector Rehabilitation

During the 1970s, the insurance and employer communities began to focus increased attention on the cost of providing workers' compensation insurance. Most of the rise in these costs was the result of increases in wage replacement costs rather than increases in medical costs. These increases in the cost of indemnifying injured workers against wage loss could be attributed to expansion of the wage replacement benefit and increased lost time as the result of occupational injuries and illnesses.

Prior to 1970, the majority of injured-worker rehabilitation took place within the state–federal rehabilitation system. The stage agencies, however, did not prioritize the rehabilitation of workers' compensation claimants or conceptualize the rehabilitation of injured workers in ways that differed from that of other eligible individuals with disabilities. In fact, the Rehabilitation Act of 1973 directed the state agencies to prioritize the provision of services to those individuals with the most severe impairments and charged the state agencies with a broad responsibility for the habilitation and rehabilitation of these individuals. In this environment, it is not surprising that insurers and employers did not view the state–federal program as a sufficient resource for the provision of vocational rehabilitation services to workers' compensation claimants who were unable to return to their former employment.

It was during this period that private-sector vocational rehabilitation services emerged in the marketplace, targeting the population of workers' compensation claimants with vocational handicaps and identifying insurers and employers as customers and sources of funding. This proprietary system of vocational rehabilitation service delivery was rapidly embraced by the workers' compensation insurance industry. Several large workers' compensation carriers developed rehabilitation companies as subsidiaries of their insurance businesses during the late 1970s.

The passage of workers' compensation reforms in California in 1975 mandated the provision of vocational rehabilitation to workers' compensation claimants under certain circumstances (Deneen & Hessellund, 1981; Matkin, 1985). Because of the size of California's labor force, this reform had the effect of greatly accelerating the accumulation of insurance rehabilitation experience, and California became a model for private-sector rehabilitation practice in much of the rest of the country. The California reforms also influenced the development of workers' compensation reform legislation in the rest of the country. Over half of the 50 states had enacted some sort of vocational rehabilitation benefits in their workers' compensation statutes by 1983 (Worrall & Butler, 1986).

This trend, combined with slow growth in the funding of the state–federal rehabilitation program, resulted in rapid expansion of the field of private-sector rehabilitation. It should be noted that the provision of vocational rehabilitation services by for-profit agencies was extremely controversial. There was a strong orientation toward the mission of state and federal rehabilitation programs embedded in the education, research, funding, and professional socialization of the rehabilitation counselor. The introduction of a profit motive was viewed with suspicion by most rehabilitation agency personnel and rehabilitation educators (McMahon, 1979). Of particular concern was the impact of the profit motive and involvement in the litigious workers' compensation arena on the ethical foundations of the rehabilitation counseling profession. State agencies also experienced an exodus of credentialed and seasoned personnel as the result of increased opportunity in the private sector (Havranak, 1993). Although private-sector rehabilitation has been a growing and increasingly accepted employment setting for rehabilitation counselors for over 20 years, these tensions are still present to some degree.

Scope of Professional Role

Jacques (1970) observed that the role of the rehabilitation counselor is unique among counseling professions because it demands the active involvement of the counselor in the elimination or circumvention of the barriers to employment and independent living that confront clients with disabilities. In this sense, the rehabilitation counselor's role differs from the interpersonal therapeutic role of other counselors. The rehabilitation counselor's responsibility extends beyond the promotion of the client's psychological adjustment to disability. Wherever possible the rehabilitation counselor is obligated to assist the client in eliminating barriers to the fullest possible use of his or her abilities, whether those barriers be physical, psychological, environmental, or societal. This implies a broader focus than is typical of the counseling role, that is, to include the community and employment environment in which the client seeks to live and work.

The Tertiary Level of Disability Prevention

Hershenson (1990) borrowed a theoretical model from the field of public health to elaborate on the unique aspect of the rehabilitation counselor's role in the rehabilitation of individuals with disabilities. He described primary, secondary, and tertiary levels of disability prevention and suggested that the majority of rehabilitation counseling interventions appropriately occur at the tertiary level.

In this model, primary disability prevention strategies are those designed to prevent the occurrence of disability and/or minimize the impact of disability-producing events. Interventions typically are aimed at large populations and focus on eliminating risk by changing the behavior of individuals and/or changing elements of the environment. Examples of primary-level interventions designed to prevent disability by changing behavior would be educational campaigns to promote seat-belt use, alert drivers to the dangers of drinking and driving, and promote safe sex practices. Regulations requiring the use of safety equipment in the workplace or the installation of air bags in new cars would be examples of primary disability prevention strategies that seek to prevent disability by modifying the environment. Ergonomic engineering controls and industrial hygiene programs are primary-level disability strategies commonly associated with occupational rehabilitation.

Secondary-level disability prevention focuses on the individual with a disability and seeks to prevent or ameliorate functional disability by repairing or removing the impairment or condition responsible for the disability. Most medical-model interventions fall within this level of disability prevention, as does traditional mental health and psychological treatment. Much of what is understood to comprise rehabilitation in contemporary society would be classified as secondary-level disability prevention, including rehabilitation medicine, physical therapy, speech therapy, psychology, and most occupational therapy. These medical-model and allied health interventions are directed at the patient and seek to improve function by removing the pathology.

The third, or tertiary, level of disability prevention encompasses much of the work of the rehabilitation counselor. Tertiary-level interventions place equal focus on the individual with a disability and the environment in which the individual desires to function more effectively. This dual focus allows the rehabilitation counselor to consider the modification of environmental demands when matching a client to a work or living environment. In this model, rehabilitation planning can and should consider interventions to remove attitudinal, legal, architectural, and ergonomic barriers to the client's successful functioning in the community or workplace. This orientation provides the rehabilitation client with greater flexibility when considering vocational and independent living options and increases the likelihood of a successful outcome. When viewed within this theoretical framework, the rehabilitation client is no longer limited to the functional level at which he or she "plateaus" following the completion of secondary-level disability prevention activities.

Outcome Orientation

Rehabilitation counseling is unique among contemporary mental health and allied health professions as the result of its historical emphasis on outcome over process. As previously described, the vocational rehabilitation profession developed within the state–federal vocational rehabilitation system. The express purpose of Congress in establishing and maintaining the state–federal system has been to promote employment and economic independence among individuals with disabilities. The system at all levels, federal agency, state agency, and individual counselor/case manager, has been evaluated and funded based on the number of successful case closures demonstrated. This focus on job placement and retention as the primary measure of program quality and professional performance has profoundly influenced the development of the emerging rehabilitation counseling profession, shaping its educational, personnel, administration, and research priorities.

The Vocational Rehabilitation Process

Bitter (1979) identified three significant, related components of the vocational rehabilitation process: goal orientation, individualization, and sequential service delivery. Goal orientation refers to the identification of vocational and independent living goals to be achieved by the rehabilitation client. The attainment of these goals has always served as the primary measure of success of the rehabilitation plan. It is this concept of goal orientation that gives the vocational rehabilitation profession its unique outcome orientation.

Individualization is the result of collaboration between the rehabilitation client and the rehabilitation counselor to develop a plan that is specific to the needs of the individual client. In the state–federal vocational rehabilitation system, this collaborative planning is formalized in the development of the Individualized Written Rehabilitation Program, which must be signed by both the client and the rehabilitation counselor. Many workers' compensation systems mandate that similar plans be developed. Accepted vocational rehabilitation practice dictates that an individualized plan be developed regardless of the administrative requirements of the system in which the counselor functions. This individualized plan is a primary mechanism insuring professional accountability of the vocational rehabilitation counselor.

Sequential service delivery refers to the process of providing or coordinating appropriate services as they are needed for the successful implementation of the rehabilitation plan in a timely and efficient manner. This component of the vocational rehabilitation process is more commonly referred to as case management; it is a particularly important aspect of vocational rehabilitation practice in the public-sector and private-sector programs.

Bitter's description of the vocational rehabilitation process was developed with the public-sector vocational rehabilitation program as a model. It is essentially the same process utilized in workers' compensation or industrial rehabilitation. Several comparisons of case management practice and service delivery between public- and private-sector rehabilitation agencies have found that private-sector rehabilitation differs from public-sector rehabilitation more in terms of the emphasis placed on certain services than in the provision of services that are unique to the insurance rehabilitation setting (Deneen & Hessulhund, 1981; Matkin, 1985; Organist, 1979; Shrey, 1979). Diamond and Petkas (1979) identified timeliness of service delivery and personalization of case management services to be the primary elements of private-sector rehabilitation practice. They further indicated that insurance rehabilitation was shorter term in focus, prioritizing the identification of transferable skills and job placement, while the state–federal program was more oriented to diagnostic evaluations and long-term vocational and educational plans. An overview of the vocational rehabilitation functions most commonly utilized in the rehabilitation of individuals with industrial illnesses or occupational diseases within the workers' compensation and disability insurance environment follows.

REHABILITATION COUNSELOR FUNCTIONS IN OCCUPATIONAL REHABILITATION

Matkin (1982) surveyed members of the National Association of Rehabilitation Professionals in the private sector and identified 29 distinct functions provided by the respondents. Of these 29 functions, the vast majority of insurance rehabilitation practitioners, over 70%, reported that they performed 10 of these functions, while fewer than half of the respondents performed the other 19. These 10 functions, in order of frequency, were vocational counseling, job analysis, job placement, job development, case monitoring and follow-up, labor market surveying, vocational evaluation, medical case management, vocational testimony, and job-restructuring consultation. This list supports the contention that vocational rehabilitation services provided in the private-sector insurance environment tend to be focused more specifically on vocational rather than independent living or educational goals, and that the rehabilitation-planning process in insurance rehabilitation is directed toward short-term resolution of vocational problems as opposed to the longer term orientation of the state–federal rehabilitation program.

Vocational Counseling

As identified by Matkin in his 1982 survey, vocational counseling remains a primary function of vocational rehabilitation counselors working in the insurance rehabilitation environment. Wright (1980) has stated that counseling is "inherent" in vocational rehabilitation. He suggested that clients will have difficulty benefiting from the provision of other services if the counseling relationship does not act as a catalyst for decision making and change. The rehabilitation-counseling process is one which allows the injured worker to assess his or her strengths and limitations relative to the world of work following the occurrence of disability. Rehabilitation counseling involves the injured worker in the process of assessment and plan development, insuring that the individualization of the rehabilitation plan takes place.

Rehabilitation counseling requires that the rehabilitation counselor be familiar with theories of vocational development and choice as well as with the world of work. Occupational information is utilized to help the client to identify vocational options, and the counseling process facilitates decision making and plan development.

Vocational Assessment

Vocational assessment refers to the process of identifying the injured worker's vocational assets and liabilities to make a determination regarding vocational prognosis and, if indicated, begin the process of rehabilitating planning. As an integral component of vocational counseling, vocational assessment is an ongoing process that continues over the course of the rehabilitation-counseling relationship. Vocational assessment utilizes a variety of data from many sources (Miller, 1980). Objective data from formal assessments, medical and vocational, are utilized to establish current or expected levels of capability. Job analysis data and aggregate occupational information regarding the demands of particular jobs or classes of jobs are used to identify skills that have been developed in the client's previous work life to formulate potential job goals that are consistent with the client's aptitudes, interests, educational and skill background, and functional capabilities. The goal of the rehabilitation counselor in workers' compensation is generally to return the injured worker to a level of vocational functioning that is as close as possible to his or her preinjury skill level in the least possible amount of time. This goal is the result of limitations on the responsibility of the insurer/employer and of best-practice research in cost-effectiveness and outcome (Chiet, 1961; Matkin, 1981; Welch, 1979).

Job Analysis

The most common form of vocational evaluation utilized by the vocational rehabilitation counselor in the insurance rehabilitation environment is job analysis. As described by the U.S. Department of Labor (1991), job analysis is the systematic study of a specific job in terms of the worker's relationship to worker functions, work fields, machines, tools, equipment and work aids utilized, materials, and subject matter or services produced, as well as the worker attributes that contribute to successful performance of job functions. Job analysis information is compared with the characteristics of the individual worker in order to identify appropriate jobs, isolate limitations that must be addressed to facilitate job placement, and identify barriers to employment that exist in the environment and must be accommodated through administrative or engineering controls.

Aggregate job analysis information that summarizes job demands and worker characteristics is also the basis for the most important occupational information utilized by the rehabilitation counselor in the assessment and vocational-counseling process. By assisting the injured worker in effectively utilizing occupational information to predict appropriate jobs, the rehabilitation counselor attempts to promote the best job "fit" possible to promote safe and successful job placement and job retention.

Transferability of Skills

Job analysis data from a work history is utilized to identify jobs that are related to an injured workers' previously successful employment in terms of demands, work fields, or worker characteristics. There are currently a number of computerized systems available that allow the sophisticated consumer of occupational information to search the U.S. Department of Labor database with profiles of a client's worker characteristics. All of these systems are based in large part on the pioneering work done by McCroskey, Wattenbarger, Fields, and Sink (1979) in the development of the *Vocational Diagnosis and Assessment of Residual Employability*. The issue of transferability of skills is crucial in the workers' compensation rehabilitation environment because of the emphasis placed on setting job goals that are related to the individual's preinjury employment. Transferability of skills is often a pivotal factor when making vocational disability determinations for the purposes of disability insurance retirement or when assessing economic damages in civil litigation.

Job Development and Placement

A return to work is the stated goal of virtually every occupational rehabilitation case that is referred to vocational rehabilitation. Job placement and development services are those services that support the rehabilitation client in seeking and securing appropriate employment once a vocational goal has been established. These services may include interview training, resumé preparation, employer consultation, on-the-job training program development, and job-lead identification. Rehabilitation counselors and job placement specialists utilize a variety of techniques to assist clients in obtaining interviews and job offers, depending on the individual needs of the injured worker. Job placement activity has been prioritized in the area of workers' compensation and disability insurance rehabilitation due to a perceived positive relationship between job placement, case resolution, and cost avoidance.

Case Management

As noted earlier in this chapter, rehabilitation practice in the state–federal rehabilitation agencies is structured into a series of "status codes," which describe the rehabilitation client's position in the vocational rehabilitation process at any given time. It is this professional commitment to case planning and counselor accountability that, in combination with the focus on vocational outcome, has been largely responsible for the recruitment of vocational rehabilitation counselors into the area of workers' compensation rehabilitation. Case management has been widely cited as a mechanism for controlling cost in workers' compensation (Weed & Lewis, 1994).

Matkin and Wallace (1985) divided the insurance case management process into four functions: evaluation, planning, medical care coordination, and vocational service coordination. All of these functions have fallen under the professional purview of the vocational rehabilitation counselor in the state–federal system. This familiarity with disability case management methodology initially resulted in the recruitment of large numbers of vocational rehabilitation counselors into the private sector in specialized areas of rehabilitation practice, including industrial or occupational rehabilitation, traumatic brain injury rehabilitation, spinal cord injury rehabilitation, and life-care planning (Havranak, 1993). Nurses, social workers and other professionals have also moved into case management positions in large numbers.

There has been a recent movement among many case managers to develop a case management profession. Professional societies and organizations have been created to provide education and training to case managers. Several interdisciplinary national certifications exist that purport to demonstrate that the holder possesses some minimal standard of qualification as a case manager. Although this movement has gained widespread initial support, it remains to be seen whether case management will attain the status of profession. At present, the primary professional identity of the vocational rehabilitation counselor remains that of the Certified Rehabilitation Counselor (CRC).

FUTURE TRENDS FOR VOCATIONAL REHABILITATION COUNSELING

Several societal trends would appear to be acting to place the profession of rehabilitation counseling in a state of dynamic change. As described earlier, economic, political, and cultural forces have historically shaped and driven the development of rehabilitation counseling. As we approach the twenty-first century, U.S. society faces a daunting array of challenges in all of those spheres. Some of the changes have been predicted and analyzed. Others, such as the potential impact of quantum changes in technology, can only serve as a source for speculation. Certain specific forces, however, have already begun to have an effect on the practice of vocational rehabilitation in the insurance industry.

The Question of Cost Benefit

Vocational and medical rehabilitation have been seen for several decades as commonsense solutions to the expensive problem of work-related injury. In recent years, however, the rehabilitation industry has come under increasing attack over the issue of whether the benefit of the provision of rehabilitation services outweighs the added cost of providing those services (Gardner, 1994). This question, although a complicated one to assess, is central to the survival of rehabilitation benefits in occupational rehabilitation. Although this question legitimately concerns all professionals providing rehabilitation to injured workers, it is of special importance to the rehabilitation counselor. Workers' compensation insurance has been the primary funding source that has allowed vocational rehabilitation counselors to move from the public to the private sector. Traditional health insurers have little or no liability to replace lost wages or incentive to increase vocational functioning. It is, therefore, incumbent on all rehabilitation counselors in the field of industrial rehabilitation to develop research-based, best-practice care models that will maximize the cost benefit of services provided in the workers' compensation and disability insurance areas and demonstrate the cost-effectiveness of vocational rehabilitation.

Managed Care

The term *managed care* refers to a whole group of strategies and approaches to insurance coverage that are being utilized to bring down the costs of health care (Clifton, 1995). Because of long-standing employee and organized labor hostility to the concept of employer choice of the medical provider in a potentially litigious situation, workers' compensation has, until recently, not been subject to extensive managed care reform. As of this writing, state workers' compensation laws are rapidly being amended to allow more employer influence in the choice of the medical provider. Several large states, including Ohio, Florida, New Jersey, and Connecticut, are undergoing massive overhauls of their workers' compensation systems to allow for managed care and, potentially, fully integrated health and accident and workers' compensation insurance benefits.

This change in direction represents a challenge and an opportunity for the vocational rehabilitation profession. It can be assumed that employers and their insurance carriers will continue to have the responsibility for replacing wages in the workers' compensation system, even if medical care is delivered in a managed care environment. Given the pressure to bring down health care and insurance costs, there will be a strong financial incentive for managed care providers to collect and analyze data regarding rehabilitation costs and outcomes. Managed care may, therefore, provide a second chance for insurance rehabilitation practitioners to manage their practices in a way that provides added value rather than simply adding cost to the management of workers' compensation claims. The return of the worker with a disability to competitive employment in the most efficient manner possible remains an enormous opportunity for cost avoidance in the workers' compensation industry. Conversely, if vocational rehabilitation does not convincingly demonstrate its usefulness in returning injured workers to employment, managed care has the potential to result in the elimination of vocational rehabilitation as a benefit in workers' compensation programs.

The Americans with Disabilities Act of 1991

The Americans with Disabilities Act is clearly the most significant development in the legislative history of vocational rehabilitation since the Rehabilitation Act of 1974. The ADA has shifted a significant portion of the burden of preventing employment discrimination from the individual with a disability and the federal government to the society as a whole (Breslin & Olsheski, 1996). The reasonable accommodation provisions of Title I of the act provide support to the occupational rehabilitation professional attempting to negotiate job modifications that were not present in occupational rehabilitation prior to 1991 (Kornblau & Ellexson, 1995). Heightened awareness of the potential for job accommodation and increasing employer familiarity with the job accommodation process has tremendous potential to improve vocational rehabilitation outcomes in the area of injured worker rehabilitation.

CONCLUSION

The profession of rehabilitation counseling is relatively new, having developed in this century in response to legislative concern regarding the human and financial cost of disability. The rehabilitation of injured workers has always been a major component of the state–federal vocational program because of the incidence of occupational injury in the United States. Since the late 1970s, there has been a movement toward specialization in the area of industrial rehabilitation as employers, workers' compensation insurance carriers, and disability insurance programs have purchased vocational rehabilitation services from private-sector companies to obtain more efficient access and more individualized service.

In the 1990s, there has been a movement away from the use of vocational rehabilitation services in workers' compensation systems in many states. The cost benefit of vocational rehabilitation services and rehabilitation in general is being questioned by employers and insurers. Managed care methods and techniques are hastily being adapted to workers' compensation applications with little in the way of preliminary research or project piloting but with lofty expectations regarding potential cost reduction. Societal barriers to employment and community access that have historically limited individuals with disabilities are being removed by new legal protections at the state and federal levels.

The coming decade will likely see rapid and continued change in the rehabilitation of the injured worker. Given the brief history of vocational rehabilitation in the workers' compensation industry and the dynamic nature of the forces coming to bear on the health care and insurance industries, this is, perhaps, the only prediction that can be made with any degree of certainty.

REFERENCES

Bitter, J. A. (1979). *Introduction to rehabilitation*. St. Louis, MO: Mosby.

Breslin, R. E., & Olsheski, J. A. (1996). The Americans with disabilities act: Implications for the use of ergonomics in rehabilitation. In A. Bhattacharya & J. D. McGlothlin (Eds.), *Occupational ergonomics: Theory and applications* (pp. 669–683). New York: Marcel Dekker.

Chiet, E. F. (1961). *Injury and recovery in the course of employment*. New York: Wiley.

Clifton, D. W. (1995). Managed care and workers' compensation. In S. J. Isernhagen (Ed.), *The comprehensive guide to work injury management* (pp. 698–738). Gaithersburg, MD: Aspen Publishers.

Deneen, L. J., & Hessellund, T. A. (1981). *Vocational rehabilitation of the injured worker*. San Francisco: Rehab Publications.

Diamond, C. R., & Petkas, E. J. (1979). A state agency's view of private-for-profit rehabilitation. *Journal of Rehabilitation*, *45*(3), 30–31.

Gardner, J. (1994). Comments on Weed & Lewis. *Journal of Rehabilitation Administration*, *18*(4), 225–227.

Havranak, J. E. (1993). Historical perspectives on the rehabilitation counseling and the disability management movement: The emergence of a new paradigm. *NARPPS Journal*, *8*(4), 157–167.

Hershenson, D. B. (1990). A theoretical model for rehabilitation counseling. *Rehabilitation Counseling Bulletin*, *33*(4), 268–278.

Jacques, M. E. (1970). *Rehabilitation counseling: Scope and services*. Boston: Houghton-Mifflin.

Kornblau, B. L., & Ellexson, M. T. (1995). Reasonable accommodation and the Americans with Disabilities Act. In S. J. Isernhagen (Ed.), *The comprehensive guide to work injury management* (pp. 781–795). Gaithersburg, MD: Aspen Publications.

Matkin, R. E. (1981). Program evaluation: Searching for accountability in private rehabilitation. *Journal of Rehabilitation*, *47*(1), 65–68.

Matkin, R. E. (1982). Rehabilitation services offered in the private sector: A pilot investigation. *Journal of Rehabilitation*, *48*(4), 31–33.

Matkin, R. E. (1985). *Insurance rehabilitation: Service applications in disability compensation systems*. Austin, TX: ProEd.

Matkin, R. E., & Wallace, W. C. (1985). Disability case management. In R. E. Matkin, *Insurance rehabilitation: Service applications in disability compensation systems* (pp. 91–111). Austin, TX: ProEd.

McCroskey, B. J., Wattenbarger, W., Fields, T., & Sink, J. (1979). *Vocational diagnosis and assessment of residual employability*. Roswell, GA: Vocational Services Bureau.

McMahon, B. T. (1979). Private-sector rehabilitation: Benefits, dangers, and implications for rehabilitation education. *Journal of Rehabilitation*, *45*(3), 56–58.

Miller, L. A. (1980). Everybody's system for interpreting client information like a vocational counselor. In B. S. Bolton & D. W. Cook (Eds.), *Rehabilitation client assessment* (pp. 251–256). Baltimore, MD: University Park Press.

Organist, J. (1979). Private sector rehabilitation practitioners—organize within NRA. *Journal of Rehabilitation*, *45*(3), 52–55.

Shrey, D. E. (1979). The rehabilitation counselor in industry: A new frontier. *Journal of Applied Rehabilitation Counseling*, *9*, 168–172.

United States Department of Labor. (1991). *The revised handbook of analyzing jobs*. Washington, DC: U.S. Government Printing Office.

Weed, R. D., & Lewis, S. H. (1994). Workers' compensation rehabilitation and case management are cost effective. True or false? *Journal of Rehabilitation Administration*, *18*(4), 225–227.

Welch, G. T. (1979). The relationship of rehabilitation with industry. *Journal of Rehabilitation*, *45*(3), 24–25.

Williamson, E. G. (1965). *Vocational counseling: Some historical, philosophical, and theoretical perspectives*. New York: McGraw-Hill.

Worrall, J. D., & Butler, R. J. (1986). Some lessons in workers' compensation. In M. Berkowitz & M. A. Hill (Eds.), *Disability and the labor market: Economic policies and problems* (pp. 111–130). Ithaca, NY: ILR Press.

Wright, G. N. (1980). *Total rehabilitation*. Boston: Little, Brown.

19

Psychosocial Issues

Leonard N. Matheson

OBJECTIVES

The primary objective of this chapter is to address from a client-centered perspective the core psychosocial issues that are encountered in the clinical practice of occupational rehabilitation. In order to focus on the most important psychosocial issues and yet provide a broad scope of applicability, a secondary objective is to describe briefly a new model of occupational development, as well as major psychosocial adjustment problems and intervention strategies that have been found to be useful within the context of occupational rehabilitation.

The occupational competence model of human development will be described as a promising approach to the consideration of issues that link motivation to recovery in occupational rehabilitation. Major theories of personality as they have been applied to persons with disabilities attempting to resume meaningful and valued occupational roles serve as the basis of the model.

URGE TOWARD COMPETENCE

Humans have a psychological need to be competent in the accomplishment of valued roles; that is, we have a need to do what we and others expect of us. This need provides the basic motivation for the development of occupational behavior. In turn, occupational behavior is reinforced by the internal satisfaction that we experience as we perceive our competence, and the approbation provided by society as we demonstrate our competence. The psychosocial nature of this "urge towards competence" was first discussed by Robert W. White (White, 1971), who described it as a primary motivation that directs human behavior. Matheson and Bohr (1997) have described how this motiva-

Leonard N. Matheson • Occupational Therapy Program, Washington University School of Medicine, St. Louis, Missouri 63108-2922.

Sourcebook of Occupational Rehabilitation, edited by Phyllis M. King. Plenum Press, New York, 1998.

tion develops with regard to occupational behavior across the life span. This model provides a framework for this chapter's discussion of psychosocial issues in occupational rehabilitation. Such an approach is useful because these issues are very broad and therefore require a focus that is psychosocial. Additionally, the author believes that psychosocial issues must be approached from a growth-enhancing direction, emphasizing strategies that are likely to be effective when used by rehabilitation professionals working with persons who have a disability. However, before we turn to strategies, we must understand the underlying dynamics of the situation.

Hierarchy of Needs

Goldstein (1963) and Maslow (1971) have described an "actualization motive" as the underlying determinant of behavior that is focused on satisfying the individual's needs across a hierarchy, beginning with survival needs and progressing to needs that provide opportunities for the ultimate expression of the unique, valued characteristics of the person. The expression of these valued characteristics usually occurs in the context of the performance of the person's roles. This context is the basis of the importance of occupational rehabilitation—to assist persons with a disability to "actualize" their experiences, and provide an opportunity for scientists to study the expression of unique human characteristics in the unusual context of impairment and disability. It is thought that this context provides a useful window on the processes of "normal" human development that can be used by scientists to facilitate understanding of these processes.

As the science of rehabilitation has developed, it has become clear that, to the degree that functional limitations impede the expression of role competence, there will be psychological dissonance. This dissonance can motivate the individual to resolve the limitation, overcome the limitation, or accommodate the limitation and minimize its effect on the performance of role tasks. To the degree that the functionally limited person is psychologically healthy, this dissonance may stimulate growth. However, unacceptably high levels of dissonance can also lead to depression and other affective disorders, which can impede growth and the expression of occupational competence. For some people, it appears that such disorders precipitate a decompensation spiral in which diminished competence leads to depression, which leads to diminished self-efficacy, which leads to diminished competence, each exacerbating the other. For many people, however, the urge toward competence presents an ever-present safeguard against decompensation, much in the way that an artesian spring can provide water to continue to slake one's thirst. A rehabilitation professional can assist an impaired person in experiencing occupational competence, so that the cognitive effects of depression can be addressed by an accumulation of objective evidence concerning the impaired person's worth. In this way, the affective or emotional consequences of the disability experience also will be countered by the sense of fulfillment and self-efficacy that is brought on by successful occupational performance, that is, by occupational competence.

Occupational competence is related to the actualization hierarchy described by Maslow (1971). Given that basic needs must be satisfied before higher level needs can be addressed, occupational disability can have a profound effect. It strikes at the survival needs of the individual in his or her valued roles. If disability prevents the individual from working to earn a living, it can threaten income, which in turn threatens shelter and other security needs. This disability will also differentially threaten the individual's family roles, depending on the person's role at the onset of disability. For example, disability that threatens income will have a more profound effect on the person who is in the role of parent as an income provider for the family, than it will have on the person who is a child or who does not have an income responsibility. Mechanisms to meet that responsibility exist in the forms of social support programs and insurance programs. In some cases, such programs can have the unintended effect of creating a "disability trap" for the individual; that is, the mechanism for meeting the role of income provider for the family is dependably met by maintaining the individual's status as a disabled person.

Roles as Opportunities for Societal Value Expression

We mesh with society in the roles we occupy. Society has a stake in our occupational role competence. This is the basic reason for the social support systems that come into play when disability occurs if the individual appears to have the potential to resume an occupational role. Resumption of the occupational role presumes resumption of a contribution to a society that values work.

Roles as Mechanisms for Societal Validation

Occupational roles provide the mechanisms through which society validates the individual and thereby shapes occupational selections. As a member of society, the individual is valued to the degree that he or she is competent in a role that is important to society. It is through the roles that the individual assumes that society rewards the individual. To the degree that the individual is successful in his or her roles, society provides approbation and tangible support. Conversely, to the degree that disability impedes role performance, approbation and support are less available. Society's support for the vocational rehabilitation of persons with disabilities is an inevitable consequence of this situation. Such societal mechanisms have emerged only recently in human history. Thus, the systems are imperfect and much less efficient than they are likely to become. As we understand more about the relationship of the individual to the occupational role and the effects that impairment and disability have on that relationship, we will become more skilled in facilitating the development of that relationship.

Ecology of Person–Role–Environment

It is necessary to take an ecological perspective on the rehabilitation of an occupational disability that is based on work-related impairment. The person, environment, and role must be considered simultaneously as a triad. The person who is experiencing a work-related impairment operates within a role that occurs within an environment. This is true for any impairment one might consider, including those that are described as biomechanical, cardiovascular, metabolic, neurological, or psychological. With regard to the psychosocial issues that are the focus of this chapter, the person, environment, and role can be best understood by considering the person and his or her effectancies, the environment and its affordances, and the role and its challenges (described in Figure 19.1).

Occupational Person

If we begin by considering the person as the first component of the triad, we find that effectancies are those abilities that have developed in response to role demands. Fleishman and Reilly (1992, p. 6) define ability as "a relatively enduring general trait or capacity that is related to performance in a variety of tasks." Abilities can develop

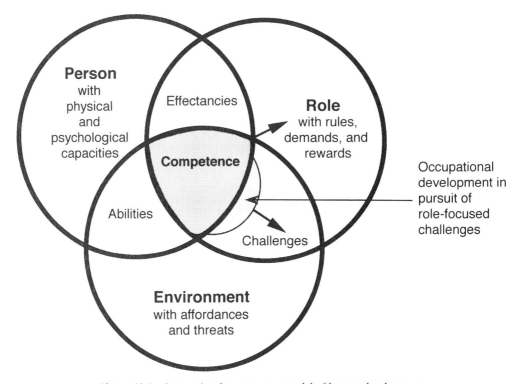

Figure 19.1 Occupational competence model of human development.

independently of role demands and are limited by the capacities of the person. It is not possible for an ability to exceed an individual's capacity. Abilities can be thought of as effectancies that have become quiescent as role demands have shifted or diminished. For example, a child will develop an ability to throw a ball spontaneously and will find that this process is accelerated by the need to meet the role demands of being a member of a baseball team. In this role, throwing the baseball can be thought of as an effectancy because there are specific role demands that stimulate its development. As the individual matures, his or her skill at throwing the ball will develop optimally if he or she continues to be a team member because role demands make a significant contribution to the motivation of the person to practice. The skill will develop up to maturity, though to a lesser extent if the person does not continue to be a team member, simply as a consequence of the general development of the physiologic, psychologic, and other systems that are called on to support this skill. Once the occupational role of team member is no longer maintained by the person, the ability will not develop as rapidly nor will the level of performance that it would have if it continued to be an effectancy, with ongoing challenges by the need to maintain role competence as a team member, be maintained.

The distinction between ability and effectancy is important for three reasons. First, some abilities will not develop at all unless they are effectancies that are stimulated by role demands. Second, there is less of a gradient of development for abilities that naturally develop without a role challenge that there is for those stimulated by a challenge. Third, the ability that is demanded by a role will be better maintained in the face of the deleterious consequences of aging after maturity. The breadth of a person's abilities is much greater than his or her effectancies simply because abilities endure after occupational demands have ceased. Abilities aggregate. Similarly, an ability can become an effectancy once again if an occupational demand is resumed.

We do not yet understand the effect of quiescence on skills and the rapidity with which degradation occurs in the absence of occupational role demand. However, it is clear that the experience of disability imposes types of quiescence that will eventually have a deleterious effect on those abilities. To the degree that the individual who has experienced substantial functional limitations leading to disability can resume the experience of occupational demand in a manner that facilitates expression of the abilities, to that same degree any ability that has been developed as an effectancy will be maintained.

Occupational Environment

If we consider the environment as the second component of the triad, we find that *affordances* are those aspects of the environment that are pertinent to facilitating the person's accomplishment of role tasks (Matheson & Bohr, 1997). It is important to note that affordances must be personally relevant in order to be pertinent. In addition, each affordance must be identified by the person as pertinent. That is, there are many aspects of the environment that are potentially able to support an individual's performance of role tasks so that occupational role responsibilities can be met. However, not all of these will be recognized by the individual, and even fewer will be used. There appears to be a basic cognitive limitation that is affected by the individual's attitudes concerning his or her ability to recognize environmental affordances, which may be a consequence of cognitive ability and self-efficacy with the potential affordance. There also is a limitation imposed on the use of recognized affordances by the creativity that the individual can bring to the invocation of the affordance as a supplement to his or her effectancies so that the role demands can be met.

As people develop, environmental affordances are identified by more experienced members of the community and communicated to those who are less experienced to the degree that the less experienced person is integrated in the community. Affordances also are discovered through the individual's exploratory behavior.

One important consequence of a rapid onset of disability is the magnitude of change that is experienced with regard to environmental affordances. For example, before the onset of disability, a parking lot ramp may not have been recognized by an individual as an affordance because it was not pertinent to him or her, given the ability to walk and the absence of role demands, such as pushing a baby carriage or some other wheeled apparatus. In contrast, the newly disabled individual who uses a wheelchair for mobility finds that the ramp is a pertinent affordance, the utilization of which will depend on development of abilities for wheelchair propulsion that are, in turn, related to the physical characteristics of the ramp, such as its grade, composition, and position in the parking lot. Learning to recognize and use environmental affordances can be facilitated by the transfer of knowledge from more experienced persons, such as rehabilitation professionals, whether they are disabled or nondisabled. It is important to recognize that the use of environmental affordances requires recognition of the affordance and the skill to integrate the affordance into the performance of the role tasks. Affordances that do not contribute to effective task performance of valued roles will not be integrated and will be ignored or discarded.

Occupational Role Challenges

The third component of the occupational triad is the person's valued roles and the demands that those roles place on the person. The importance of challenges presented by role demands cannot be overstated. They are a catalyst to the person's developing and using the effectancies and affordances in his or her environment. To be effective, an occupational challenge must possess the following characteristics:

1. It must be apprehended by the individual. The individual must be aware of the challenge and its pertinence.
2. It must be evaluated by the individual as achievable or, if not, worth the effort and risk to make an attempt.
3. It must be meaningful in that mastery will contribute to competent role performance.

Part of the meaning of an occupational challenge comes from the value of the role that places demands on the person. More valuable roles will have demands that stimulate the development of effectancies to a greater degree than do demands that stem from roles that are less valued. In addition, and this point is not well understood by most rehabilitation professionals, the meaningfulness of a challenge comes from the potential of the person to fail. For many reasons, failure is an important component of accomplishment. Task performance that carries the threat of failure increases the perceived value of success. Additionally, failures help the person to define a temporary performance limit that can become a goal. Goal attainment in the development of an effectancy is meaningful to the degree that the person is at risk of failure.

The meaningfulness of the mastery of an occupational challenge stimulates generalization of the effectancy through the mechanism of self-efficacy. To the degree that the person is successful in meeting meaningful challenges that place her or him at risk, beliefs in the ability to perform will develop and will encourage higher levels of exploration and perseverance. This development, in turn, produces a greater likelihood that the individual will continue to experience success in meeting subsequent occupational challenges.

DISABILITY AS A PSYCHOLOGICAL PROCESS

The experience of disability has many psychological consequences. This experience also has many concomitant psychological effects that can affect the person's functional limitations and make the disability greater or less and are not simply consequences of the impairment. In fact, the psychological concomitants of disability probably exert a more profound effect than any other issue in causing the relationship between impairment and disability to be much less than unitary. Said another way, we cannot predict disability from impairment for many reasons, the most important of which are psychological. To the degree that rehabilitation professionals are able to appreciate the effect of psychological processes in this regard, they will be able to assist the newly impaired person to develop psychological processes that will facilitate resumption of occupational roles and diminution of disability.

Disruption of Roles

Second only to the psychological impact of bodily dysfunction and disfigurement produced by an impairment is the psychological impact of the disruption of roles. Some of the role disruption may be temporary, simply a consequence of the person's need to temporarily inhabit the patient role while receiving medical care and convalescing. However, the person begins to consider longer term effects of the functional limitations on roles within a few hours of the onset of the serious injury or illness. Almost immediately, these considerations produce in the person a fear of loss that usually can be described by that person in graphic terms. Soon after the person experiences the fear of loss, disability may also produce actual loss in terms of income and status. This devaluation of the person occurs at many levels and is psychologically painful, producing anger and resentment. Additionally, unstated fears that are poorly defined can result in anxiety when the individual contemplates difficulties with the future resumption of roles, goals, and his or her lifestyle.

Affective Response

Emotional turmoil, including denial, anger and sadness, is precipitated by the onset of disability. Denial is a self-protective defense mechanism unconsciously employed by the person to avoid the experience of emotions that are unacceptable. It is important and, in the short run, can facilitate psychological adjustment. However, because it prevents the person from experiencing fully his or her new reality, it limits later adaptation. Conversely, anger often disrupts adjustment in the short run but can facilitate it in the long run. Sadness is an important aspect of the disability experience. Although it can provide an opportunity for the individual to deepen an existential awareness, it can also overwhelm and consume some individuals precipitating withdrawal, isolation, and alienation, which, in turn, impede rehabilitation.

Cognitive Interpretation

All of the emotional consequences of disability are filtered cognitively, thus they are magnified or minimized by the person's interpretation. Interpretation that facilitates adjustment can be encouraged by the rehabilitation professional. More specifically, viewing the psychological process of disability in terms of threats to self-confidence and the individual's compensation to those threats in response is most constructive. Although many of the emotional consequences of disability may require professional assistance, most will gradually resolve if the individual is helped to reestablish occupational role competence, the primary focus of work hardening (Matheson, Ogden, Violette, & Schultz, 1985).

REHABILITATION AS A PSYCHOLOGICAL PROCESS

Just as there is a process of rehabilitation that entails the individual's physical domain, there is also a process of rehabilitation that is psychological and psychosocial. Similarly, just as the physical rehabilitation process unfolds and can be tracked, psychological processes are likely to unfold and be tracked. Saying this does not deny that uniqueness of each person's psychological experience. Rather, this is to say that the psychological process of disability is mirrored by the psychological process of rehabilitation. It is involved with the affective response and attendant emotional upset, both of which facilitate the emotional adjustment to disability and are limited by it. Furthermore, it may be that the psychological experience of disability and the attendant psychological process of rehabilitation follow general patterns that can be thought of as stages of psychological rehabilitation.

Identification of Problems in Psychological Adjustment

There are many psychological adjustment problems that are encountered by rehabilitation professionals involved in occupational disability. Some of the most important are presented in sections that follow.

Depression

Depression is a significant problem for Americans in general. Americans who experience chronic disability display an even greater prevalence of depression. Depression may be a preexisting problem that is worsened by the functional consequences of the disability. It may also be a problem that precipitates the injury and impairment, such as in the case of a suicide attempt or other self-destructive behavior. The fourth edition of the *Diagnostic and Statistical Manual of Mental Disorders* (*DSM-IV*) (American Psychiatric Association, 1994) classifies Depressive Disorders as mood disorders because a disturbance in mood is the essential feature. The DSM-IV differentiates Major Depressive Disorder from Dysthymic Disorder in terms of the level of severity, chronicity, and persistence of the mood disorder (p. 320). In the former, a depressed mood must be present for most of the day for a period of at least two weeks. In the latter, a depressed mood must be present for more days than not over a period of at least two years. Features of a Depressive Disorder are reported in the DSM-IV to include the following:

1. Loss of interest or pleasure
2. Reduction in appetite or craving for specific foods
3. Sleep disturbance
4. Agitation or psychomotor retardation, such as slowed speech and thinking
5. Decreased energy, tiredness, and fatigue without physical exertion
6. Sense of worthlessness or guilt with unrealistic negative self-evaluations and ruminations over past failings
7. Impaired ability to think, concentrate, or make decisions, with easy distractibility or memory difficulties
8. Thoughts of death or pending doom, suicidal ideation, or suicide attempts

In addition to the Depressive Disorders and Bipolar Disorders, the *DSM-IV* describes a Mood Disorder Due to a General Medical Condition (p. 366) in which the mood disturbance is the direct physiological consequence of a specific medical condition. In addition to the causation of depression as a "direct physiological consequence" of the impairment, depression also appears to be caused by the disability experience as a consequence of "learned helplessness" (Peterson, Maier, & Seligman, 1993), especially when the environment is viewed by the person as nonresponsive.

Pain Disorder

Pain and the effective and cognitive interference that is a consequence of the pain also produce difficulty with reasoning and with attempts to maintain emotional balance and control the circumstances that produce emotional imbalance. The *DMS-IV* describes Pain Disorder as having that of sufficient severity to warrant clinical attention and cause significant limitation(s) in social or occupational functioning as the predominant clinical characteristic. (Pain Disorder is distinguished from Factitious Disorder or Malingering, which is addressed later in this chapter.) In addition, there are subtypes of Pain Disorder that characterize various etiologies. Consequences and concomitants of a Pain Disorder are reported in the DSM-IV to include the following:

1. Disruption of activities of daily living and normal life involvement
2. Unemployment and family problems
3. Iatrogenic opiod or benzodiazepine dependence or abuse
4. When associated with severe depression or related to a terminal illness, suicide
5. Inactivity and social isolation, leading to a mood disorder
6. Insomnia

Learned Behaviors

Learned behaviors can also be maladaptive responses to rehabilitation. One approach to this phenomenon is described as the symptom magnification syndrome (SMS), which is a "self-destructive, socially reinforced behavioral response pattern consisting of reports or displays of symptoms which function to control the life circumstances of the sufferer" (Matheson, 1991, p. 43). SMS is learned and maintained through social reinforcement and does not constitute a psychiatric diagnosis. SMS has its roots in the "sick role" described by Parsons (1951). Parsons reported that the sick role is conferred on the individual who is ill and is actively involved in treatment. The patient in the sick role is allowed to temporarily escape from other role responsibilities.

Mechanic (1962) introduced the concept of "illness behavior" as a response to symptoms that are idiosyncratically based on personality. Illness behaviors are displayed by persons in the sick role. The purpose of illness behavior was later presented by Mechanic (1975) to be "part of the (patient's) coping repertoire." Pilowsky (1969) introduced the concept of "abnormal illness behavior" to address the problem presented by the patient with physical complaints for which no organic cause could be found. Pilowsky identified abnormal illness behavior as a significant medical issue (1978), defined as "the persistence of an inappropriate or maladaptive mode of experiencing, evaluating and responding to one's own health status" (p. 347).

Behavioral phenomena such as abnormal illness behavior and symptom magnification syndrome are pervasive. Waddell, Bircher, Finlayson, and Main (1984) studied 380 patients with back pain of at least three-months duration and found a strong relationship between inappropriate illness behavior and the amount of treatment. Waddell, Main, Morris, Di Pialo, and Gray (1984) present a model of disability in which physical impairment accounted for approximately 40% of disability, while 23% of the disability was explained by psychological distress factors. An additional 8% of the variance was attributable to "magnified illness behavior."

Symptom magnification syndrome is distinct from Malingering, which is defined in the *DSM-IV* as "the intentional production of false or grossly exaggerated physical or psychological symptoms" (APA, 1994, p. 683). Malingering should be suspected when the client presents in a medicolegal context, and the professional finds a marked discrepancy between the person's claims and the objective findings, and there is a lack of cooperation during the evaluation and treatment, especially in the presence of an Antisocial Personality Disorder.

Malingering differs from Factitious Disorder, which is the intentional production of physical or psychological signs or symptoms in order to assume or maintain the sick role. In Malingering, the symptoms are also intentional, having as their motivation achievement of a goal that is obvious. In Factitious Disorder, there is a psychological need to assume the sick role, which implies psychopathology.

Perhaps the easiest way to distinguish a person who is demonstrating malingering behavior from one who is truly impaired psychologically is to focus on the Antisocial Personality Disorder, which the *DSM-IV* characterizes as a pervasive pattern of disregard for and violation of the rights of others (APA, 1994, p. 645). This pattern begins in childhood or early adolescence and continues in adulthood. On taking a careful history, which may need to be supplemented by school and work records, this person will have indications of a Conduct Disorder during adolescence, demonstrating a pattern of antisocial behavior that continues into adulthood. Some of the most important concomitants of an Antisocial Personality Disorder reported in the *DSM-IV* include the following:

1. A pattern of failure to conform to social norms
2. Disregarding the rights of others
3. Deceitful and manipulative behavior
4. A pattern of impulsivity
5. Irritable and aggressive demeanor
6. Consistent disregard for the safety of themselves or others
7. Consistently and extremely irresponsible with significant periods of unemployment and abandonment of jobs without a plan for getting another
8. Indifference to the consequences of acts

Treatment of Psychological Adjustment Problems

The problems with psychological adjustment described earlier can be approached therapeutically from various perspectives in occupational rehabilitation. One approach favored in rehabilitation in recent years has been called the "biopsychosocial model," a multidisciplinary approach to occupational rehabilitation (Feuerstein, Menz, Zastowny, & Barron, 1994; Waddel, 1987) that addresses the person with a disability in a holistic manner. Actually, it may be that a multidisciplinary team is more likely to be able to assist the injured worker to make a rapid return to the workplace (Feuerstein et al., 1994) and avoid psychological and psychosocial sequelae altogether. This conclusion is especially true if the return to work is undertaken before the patient has "healed" and has returned to preinjury functional capacity. From the patient's perspective, avoidance of "worklessness" (Schulman, 1994) and early resolution and return to work are beneficial, a finding supported across a variety of studies (Banks, 1995; Gervais et al., 1991; Jetté, Smith, Haley, & Davis, 1994; Matheson, Brophy, Vaughan, Nunez, & Saccoman, 1995; Moffroid, Aja, Haugh, & Henry, 1993).

The biopsychosocial clinical model described by Waddell (1987) included recommendations to promote return to work and remediate abnormal illness behavior. Waddell believes that disability based on restriction of the activities of daily living is founded largely on a patient's attitudes and beliefs and is learned. Mayer and his colleagues (Mayer et al., 1985; Mayer et al., 1987) and Hazard and his colleagues (Hazard et al., 1989; Hazard, Haugh, Green, & Jones, 1994) have presented multidisciplinary models of treatment that have developed beyond Waddell's with excellent results. A key aspect of these programs is that they integrate physical challenges to the patient with psychological support for new behaviors, allowing the patient to respond appropriately. A discussion of other strategies that have been advocated follows.

Self-Efficacy Coaching

Self-efficacy is necessary if the individual is to emit exploratory behavior and perseverance in the face of early failures. It may be that self-efficacy blunting occurs as a consequence of therapy. That is, an early dependence on caregivers may rob the individual of opportunities to experience challenges that he or she may be able to meet on an approximate basis with a concomitant level of self-efficacy enhancement. It may be more appropriate to focus on intervention such as that provided by an athletic coach. For example, the therapist's primary strategies are to encourage and support the client to perform tasks that are safe and likely to have therapeutic effects in terms of increasing physical function, skill, or self-confidence. The therapist's emphasis must be on "safety first," with a goal horizon that is equivalent to the therapist's perception of the client's immediate capacity. Conversely, the coach is less concerned with safety and is more concerned with challenge, being certain that the client's immediate capacity lies somewhere beyond her or his current demonstrated ability. Therapist behavior is reinforced by an absence of injury and modest, dependable gains in performance. Coach behavior is reinforced by substantial gains in performance as new "personal records" are set frequently. To some extent, the potential problems created by an emphasis on performance are mitigated through the use of structured and well-planned tasks. The therapist is more likely to employ a creative selection of tasks that are tied to the client's specific interests.

Self-Perception Testing

The individual's functional self-perception is likely to limit performance because people are generally not inclined to attempt to perform beyond their self-perceived levels of ability. Functional self-perception testing is useful in identifying this limit. Testing can be performed on a standardized basis with such devices as the *Loma Linda Activity Sort* (Anzai, 1984) or the *PACT Spinal Function Sort* (Matheson & Matheson, 1989). Serial self-perception testing, which is performed while the client is actually involved in rehabilitation, will mark the client's progress and reinforce attempts to maintain that progress and keep it focused on the tasks that are tied to valued roles.

Progressive Performance Challenge (PPC)

Progressive performance challenge (PPC) is an important and well-recognized strategy of rehabilitation. PPC provides opportunities for the client to experience risk. When success is achieved, the client benefits from the reinforcement that comes with such an experience and the enhancement of self-efficacy occurs. These progressive performance challenges need to be tied to tasks that are involved with the client's valued roles. They also need to be graded so that success occurs often enough to maintain perseverance. The "success-failure ratio" is unique to each client and can only be determined in practice with a particular client. The ratio will tend to be consistent across tasks and may be a characteristic of personality. Some people have much higher tolerance for failure, with a resultant diminution of perseverance, than do others. Other people require almost constant success, requiring challenges that are much more modest to continue to accept the challenges. For individuals involved in occupational rehabilitation, it is important that these challenges maintain a focus on productivity. Productivity is what is valued by the psychosocial environment within which the occupational role is found.

Goaling

A goal is a distinct, complete, and clear communication about one issue that makes life more satisfying. The goaling process helps the client to establish a future orientation, develop a rational basis for planning, and receive positive feedback from his or her community. It also assists the client in communicating clearly those aspects of life that are important. The goaling process has four steps: conducting a structured client interview, developing priorities, conducting a significant other review, and developing and publishing the goal document. The rehabilitation professional may find that the process will feel unnatural to clients. As a consequence, the client may require a considerable degree of encouragement to complete the process. Each of the steps must be completed in this order:

1. *Structured Interview.* The caregiver and client meet in a quiet room. The caregiver asks the client, "What do you want most out of a job?" The caregiver records the client's responses without comment or judgment and works with the client to develop individual goal statements that meet the following criteria:

   a. Each goal is presented as a complete simple sentence.
   b. Each goal is listed in its present or future tense.
   c. Each goal is easily understood and unambiguous.
   d. Each goal is stated in a positive manner.

2. *Developing Priorities.* Each of the goals is listed as it is developed. After from 10 to 15 goals have been identified, the list is presented to the client, who is then asked to select the goal that is least important. After the client does so he or she selects which of the remaining goals is least important. This "negative prioritization" will result in surprises. The client may have difficulty in choosing. The caregiver should encourage the client to make a selection while confirming that all of the goals have importance, but that one is less important than the others.

3. *Significant Other Review.* After the goal list has been organized by priority, a copy is made. The original is provided to the client to take home and review with at least one significant other. The client is encouraged to make any changes that may be appropriate in the goals, including deleting or adding goals. The order of the goals may be changed. Wording may be changed. The client is to return with the goal list after this review.

4. *Developing and Publishing the Goaling Document.* After the client returns with the goal list that has been reviewed, a formal list is prepared. Twenty copies of the goal list are made. The client is instructed to distribute the copies to as many people as he can, but no less than a number selected by the caregiver.

This is a challenging experience for the client. It will involve some level of risk and concern about embarrassment but is potentially very rewarding.

These treatment strategies are most easily implemented in a work-hardening program (Matheson et al., 1985) or a functional restoration program (Hazard et al., 1989; Mayer et al., 1987), although several lend themselves to a work-conditioning program (Darphin, 1995) as well. As occupational rehabilitation develops, additional strategies will be identified that will place the client in the center of the process and focus on improving client safety and productivity in performing valued occupational roles.

TECHNOLOGICAL UNDERPINNINGS

The technological underpinnings to the evaluation and treatment of psychosocial consequences of disability impose real limitations on our abilities as practitioners. Many of the instruments that are in use today have been borrowed from medicine and psychology without adequate appreciation of the unique experience that an individual disability presents. Much of this technology is used in rehabilitation without adequate adjustment being given to those items that are part of the "normal" experience that persons with certain disabilities encounter. The absence of normal values for persons with disabilities produces problems for clinicians and clients in rehabilitation that have not been fully chronicled nor effectively studied.

REHABILITATION SCIENCE'S POSSIBILITIES

One hopeful indicator of the growth of the field of occupational rehabilitation, especially with regard to the identification and treatment of psychosocial issues, is the development of the new field of rehabilitation science. This field has been defined at the Washington University School of Medicine in St. Louis as "the study of basic and applied aspects of biology, medicine, psychology, and engineering as they relate to restoration of an individual's functional capacity and the interaction of that individual with the environment as he or she seeks to fulfill those roles which define the person as an individual" (Baum, personal communication, 1997). This new interdisciplinary science requires collaborative work at the biomedical level, the applied clinical level, and the societal policy level. With regard to psychosocial issues, rehabilitation science seeks to understand how an individual's performance is supported by cognition, communication, physical competence, and psychological well-being, investigates adaptive and compensatory mechanisms, and the ways in which physical, psychological, and social environments can be constructed to minimize disability.

As rehabilitation science evolves and develops, the emphasis on ecological balance among persons, environment, and occupational role is of paramount importance. Rehabilitation scientists who are occupational therapists, psychologists, physical therapists, and physicians will assist the client in addressing the psychosocial issues presented by the disability experience. In fact, the psychosocial aspects that are part of the disability experience can be integrated into the client's evaluation assessment. Situated as it is on the boundaries between medical science and social science, rehabilitation science has the benefit of both. It also has an advantage that is unique to itself in that it is possible for the rehabilitation scientist to study normal human beings caught up in the unique experience of disability. Under these circumstances, the dynamics of human interaction are more easily isolated and understood.

REFERENCES

Anzai, D. (1984). *Loma Linda activity sort*. Ft. Bragg, CA: Work Evaluation Systems Technology.

American Psychiatric Association. (1994). *Diagnostic and statistical manual of mental disorders* (4th ed.). Washington, DC: Author.

Banks, M. (1995). Psychological effects of prolonged unemployment: Relevance to models of work re-entry following injury. *Journal of Occupational Rehabilitation, 5*(1), 37-53.

Darphin, L. (1995). Work-hardening and work-conditioning perspectives. In S. Isernhagen (Ed.), *The comprehensive guide to work injury management* (pp. 443-462). Gaithersburg, MD: Aspen.

Feuerstein, M., Menz, L., Zastowny, T., & Barron, B. (1994). Chronic back pain and work disability: Vocational outcomes following multidisciplinary rehabilitation. *Journal of Occupational Rehabilitation, 4*(4), 229-251.

Fleishman, E., & Reilly, M. (1992). *Handbook of human abilities*. Palo Alto, CA: Consulting Psychologists Press.

Gervais, S., Dupuis, G., Veronneau, F., Bergeron, Y., Millette, D., & Avard, J. (1991). Predictive model to determine cost/benefit of early detection and intervention in occupational low back pain. *Journal of Occupational Medicine, 1*(2), 113-131.

Goldstein, K. (1963). *The organism*. Boston: Beacon Press.

Hazard, R., Fenwick, J., Kalisch, S., Redmond, J., Reeves, V., Reid, S., & Frymoyer, J. (1989). Functional restoration with behavioral support: A one-year prospective study of patients with chronic low-back pain. *Spine, 14*(2), 157-161.

Hazard, R., Haugh, L., Green, P., & Jones, P. (1994). Chronic low back pain: The relationship between patient satisfaction and pain, impairment, and disability outcomes. *Spine, 19*(8), 881-887.

Jetté, A., Smith, K., Haley, S., & Davis, K. (1994). Physical therapy episodes of care for patients with low back pain. *Physical Therapy, 74*(2), 101-115.

Maslow, A. (1971). *The farther reaches of human nature*. New York: Viking.

Matheson, L. (1991). Symptom magnification syndrome structured interview: Rationale and procedure. *Journal of Occupational Rehabilitation, 1*(1), 43-56.

Matheson, L., & Bohr, P. (1997). Occupational competence across the life span: An ecological model of human development. In C. Christiansen & M. Baum (Eds.), *Occupational therapy: Enabling performance and well-being* (2nd ed.) (pp. 428-457). Thorofare, NJ: Slack Publishers.

Matheson, L., Brophy, R., Vaughan, K., Nunez, C., & Saccoman, K. (1995). Workers' compensation managed care: Preliminary findings. *Journal of Occupational Rehabilitation, 5*(1), 27-36.

Matheson, L., & Matheson, M. (1989). *PACT spinal function sort*. Wildwood, MO: Employment Potential Improvement Corporation.

Matheson, L., Ogden, L., Violette, K., & Schultz, K. (1985). Work hardening: Occupational therapy in industrial rehabilitation. *American Journal of Occupational Therapy, 39*(5), 314-321.

Mayer, T., Gatchel, R., Kishino, N., Keeley, J., Capra, P., Mayer, H., Barnett, J., & Mooney, V. (1985). Objective assessment of spine function following industrial injury: A prospective study with comparison group and one-year follow-up. *Spine, 10*(6), 482-493.

Mayer, T., Gatchel, R., Mayer, H., Kishino, N., Keeley, J., & Mooney, V. (1987). A prospective two-year study of functional restoration in industrial low back injury: An objective assessment procedure. *Journal of the American Medical Association, 258*(13), 1763-1767.

Mechanic, D. (1962). The concept of illness behaviour. *Journal of Chronic Diseases, 15*, 189-194.

Mechanic, D. (1975). Response factors in illness: The study of illness behavior. *Social Psychiatry, 1*, 11-20.

Moffroid, M., Aja, D., Haugh, L., & Henry, S. (1993). Efficacy of a part-time work-hardening program for persons with low-back pain. *Work, 3*(3), 14-20.

Parsons, T. (1951). *The social system*. New York: Free Press.

Peterson, C., Maier, S., & Seligman, M. (1993). *Learned helplessness*. New York: Oxford University Press.

Pilowsky, I. (1969). Abnormal illness behavior. *British Journal of Medical Psychology, 42*, 347-351.

Pilowsky, I. (1987). Abnormal illness behaviour. *Psychiatric Medicine, 5*(2), 85-91.

Schulman, B. (1994). Worklessness and disability: Expansion of the biopsychosocial perspective. *Journal of Occupational Rehabilitation, 4*(2), 113-122.

Waddell, G. (1987). A new clinical model for the treatment of low-back pain. *Spine, 2*(7), 632-644.

Waddell, G., Bircher, M., Finlayson, D., & Main, C. (1984). Symptoms and signs: Physical disease or illness behavior? *British Medical Journal, 289*, 739-741.

Waddell, G., Main, C., Morris, E., Di Paola, M., & Gray, I. (1984). Chronic low-back pain, psychologic distress, and illness behavior. *Spine, 9*(2), 209-213.

White, R. (1971). The urge toward competence. *American Journal of Occupational Therapy, 25*, 271-274.

20

Chronic Pain

Joshua C. Klapow, Roger B. Fillingim and Daniel M. Doleys

Of all medical conditions, chronic pain is probably the most challenging and elusive to study, assess, and treat. Unlike a great majority of medical conditions, chronic pain is not a disease process. Pain does not fall into a well-defined organ system, pathophysiological process, or discipline-specific arena. Rather, pain is a symptom, a perception, an experience that afflicts an individual and commonly results in the display of pain behaviors (grimacing, groaning, rubbing), impaired functioning, and associated emotional distress. In fact, although pain is the number one medical condition that drives individuals to seek care, its precise definition has eluded researchers and clinicians for years. Yet, as noted by Boyd (1994), pain is an experience everyone knows regardless of definition. In order to properly evaluate and treat pain, a conceptual base and operational definition must be established. In the case of chronic pain, particularly, failure to conceptualize the condition greatly hinders assessment, diagnostic accuracy, and, ultimately, treatment choice.

Our examination of chronic pain begins with a conceptualization that will serve as a working model. This conceptualization provides a context for the various theories proposed to explain mechanisms of the chronic pain experience. Together, the conceptualization and underlying mechanisms provide a rationale for the various treatment options. Placing treatment approaches within a conceptual model of the pain experience highlights the multidimensionality of chronic pain and emphasizes the need to evaluate and treat pain from a multidimensional perspective.

Joshua C. Klapow and Roger B. Fillingim • Department of Psychology, University of Alabama at Birmingham, Birmingham, Alabama 35294.   **Daniel M. Doleys** • Pain and Rehabilitation Institute, Suite 200, 720 Monteclair Road, Birmingham, Alabama 35209.

Sourcebook of Occupational Rehabilitation, edited by Phyllis M. King. Plenum Press, New York, 1998.

CONCEPTUALIZATION AND DEFINITIONS

Feuerstein (1994) has noted that pain is a concept or construct rather than an entity. As such, definitions vary as a function of individual perceptions and orientations. There are, however, areas of consensus that facilitate our understanding of this concept. It is perhaps easiest to begin with a distinction between the temporal aspects of acute and chronic pain. The International Association for the Study of Pain (IASP) (1986) has defined *chronic* pain as pain that lasts beyond the normal time of healing, using a relatively arbitrary time frame of three months beyond to distinguish acute from chronic pain. As Sullivan, Turner, and Romano (1991) noted, the distinction between acute and chronic pain is often confusing because it does not refer to the quality or severity of the pain experienced but rather temporal factors only. Understanding the temporal component of pain is far less challenging than the definition itself. The IASP definition of pain is the most widely accepted, and it is a useful foundation. Pain is "an unpleasant sensory and emotional experience associated with actual or potential tissue damage, or described in terms of such damage" (Merskey, 1986). As evidenced by this definition, the emphasis when defining pain is not placed upon nociceptive input but on the subjective, sensory, and emotional experience. Therefore, while pain is undoubtedly a "real" medical condition, its understanding goes far beyond the disease process or pathophysiology. Therefore, conceptualization, assessment, and treatment must go beyond nociception.

With any construct of concept comes the need to create a working definition or operationalization. Drawing from the IASP definition, in order to conceptualize chronic pain, we must incorporate several dimensions. The multidimensional nature of pain has been recognized for some time by clinicians and researchers. From a clinical perspective, it is quite common to see patients with the same degree of tissue damage who have varying levels of pain complaints (Klapow et al., 1993). Patients respond to pain with varying coping strategies (Klapow et al., 1995) and react differently to identical therapeutic modalities (Turk & Rudy, 1994). Thus, the clinical presentation of chronic pain varies greatly. Chronic pain patients quite often present with a constellation of related problems, including disability (Fordyce, 1976), depression (Romano & Turner, 1985), addictions (Sternbach, 1974), and disruption of interpersonal relationships (Shealy, 1976). Follick, Aberger, Ahern, and McCartney (1984) have employed the term *chronic pain syndrome* to emphasize (a) the multidimensional nature of chronic pain; (b) the importance of pain as a medical problem in and of itself, regardless of etiology; and (c) the primacy of persistent pain. Marked impairment in daily functioning and emotional distress characterize the most problematic and disabling clinical presentation of a chronic pain condition. Similar conceptualizations have been put forth by others (Merskey, 1986; Poulsen et al., 1987; Turk & Rudy, 1990). Moreover, studies have empirically defined this multidimensional conceptualization of pain in samples of patients with chronic low back pain (Klapow et al., 1993; Klapow et al., 1995), headache (Jamison, Rudy, Penzien, & Mosley, 1994), and temporomandibular disorders (Rudy, Turk, Zaki, & Curtin, 1989). Feuerstein (1994) has proposed a similar conceptualization and operational definition of chronic pain that includes pain sensation, pain behavior, functional status at work, functional status at home, emotional state, and somatic preoccupation.

Although variations in conceptualizations will exist, three broad areas are commonly accepted as essential in the conceptualization of a chronic pain condition. These variations include perceived pain, functional limitations (and pain behaviors), and emotional distress (Follick et al., 1984; Fordyce, 1976; Jamison, 1994; Kerns, Turk, & Rudy, 1985;

Klapow et al., 1993; Sternbach, 1974; Turk & Rudy, 1987). *Perceived pain* can be understood as the experience of pain as reported by the patient. *Functional limitation* is understood as "any restriction or lack of ability to perform an activity in the manner or within the range considered normal for a human being that results from an impairment" (World Health Organization definition of disability, in Feuerstein, 1994). *Pain behaviors* are a set of expressions and observable behaviors that communicate to the world that an individual is experiencing pain. *Emotional distress* is the affective component or suffering that accompanies the pain experience and is most commonly exhibited as anxiety, depression, anger, or irritability. Thus, the clinical presentation of any patient with chronic pain can be seen as the interplay of pain perception, functional limitations, pain behaviors, and emotional distress. (Figure 20.1 graphically describes this interplay.)

Other variables, such as interpersonal support, coping style, personality characteristics, and treatment conditions, can be seen as process dimensions because their primary importance is in how they mediate, moderate, or predict the clinical presentation of the chronic pain experience. The conceptual distinction between process and outcome dimensions is essential for clinical theory development and applied program evaluation research (Cook & Campbell, 1979; Paul, 1969). The assessment of process dimensions is extremely important in understanding the mechanisms of chronic pain. However, given the less than complete understanding of the role of most process variables in chronic pain, it may be particularly important to distinguish, at least conceptually, those variables that serve to define the clinical presentation, and those variables that factor into the mechanisms of the condition (Klapow et al., 1993).

MECHANISMS OF THE CHRONIC PAIN CONDITION

Given the multidimensional conceptualization of pain, it is important to have an understanding of how this presentation may come about. Unfortunately, in the case of chronic pain, underlying mechanisms do not necessarily represent a clear etiology.

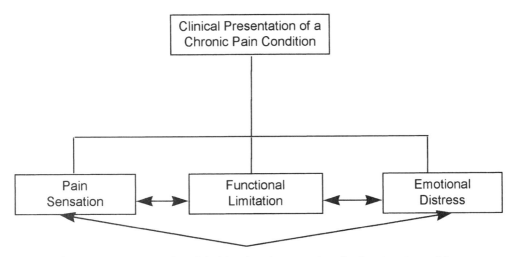

Figure 20.1. Conceptual model of the clinical presentation of a chronic pain condition.

Rather, they serve to present plausible pathways for the clinical presentation. They increase our confidence that what we see clinically is a syndrome rather than an unrelated array of symptoms. Many theories of chronic pain have been put forth. This chapter presents three models of pain, the gate control model, the behavioral model, and the cognitive-behavioral model, that are well known and consistent with the conceptualization presented thus far. These models help to support the clinical conceptualization, suggest areas for evaluation, and have implications for treatment modality.

Gate Control Model

Prior to the publication of the gate control theory in 1965, the prevailing theory of pain was specificity theory, which proposed that injury activates specific pain fibers that transmit impulses via the spinal cord to a pain center in the brain. This theory essentially equated the experience of pain with peripheral injury. The gate control theory represented a very different conceptualization of pain. It proposed that peripheral nociceptive information can be modified at the level of the spinal cord by a gating mechanism located in the dorsal horn (Melzack & Wall, 1965). Specifically, large-fiber input (i.e., a-beta mechanoreceptors) tends to inhibit rostral transmission of nociceptive information, while small-fiber input (i.e., *a*-delta and *c*-fiber nociceptors) tends to facilitate transmission. Thus, the overall pattern of peripheral neural activity determines the experience of pain. The gate control theory was the first theory of pain to propose that neural impulses descending from the brain could modulate the processing of nociceptive information. That is, cognitive–affective processes as well as descending brain activity elicited by peripheral input from specialized large fibers (known as the central control trigger) can influence the spinal gating mechanism.

The gate control model drastically changed the scientific and clinical communities' conceptualizations of pain. No longer was pain considered a basic input–output system in which sensory experience was completely accounted for by peripheral neural activity. Rather, the experience of pain was recognized as a product of the complex integration of multiple peripheral inputs and a descending modulation by activity emanating from higher brain structures. This theory revolutionized pain research, leading to an explosion of scientific activity investigating not only the physiological and neuroanatomical aspects of the theory, but also the efficacy of physical and psychological methods for closing the gate, thereby relieving pain. One example of the therapeutic impact of the theory was the development of transcutaneous electrical nerve stimulation to help close the gate by activating myelinated large-diameter fibers, a treatment that is now widely utilized. Additionally, the application of psychological techniques for treating pain now could be justified and scientifically integrated into mainstream pain research. Thus, the gate control theory of pain set the stage for the multidimensional conceptualization of pain, which is now broadly accepted.

Behavioral Model

Rather than focusing on pain relief, the behavioral model emphasizes the importance of systematically assessing and modifying observable pain behavior. Pain behavior refers to any overt behavior that communicates to observers that the individual is in pain, including verbal complaints, grimacing, guarded movement, and rubbing the affected area. The behavioral model of chronic pain proposes that pain behaviors, like any other form of behavior, can be influenced by its antecedents and consequences through classical and operant conditioning, respectively (Fordyce, 1976). Classical conditioning occurs when a neutral stimulus is paired with a potent stimulus that naturally produces a certain response, and through association the neutral stimulus comes to elicit the same response as the original potent stimulus. For example, a patient who has undergone lumbar surgery naturally exhibits pain behavior when changing positions from sitting to standing because of the potent stimulus of tissue damage. Even after tissue damage has healed, changing position may produce pain behavior because of the previously re-peated association of changing position (the neutral stimulus) with tissue damage (the potent stimulus). Laboratory research suggests that classical conditioning may influence not only overt behavioral responses associated with pain but also the underlying neural processes (Lysle & Fowler, 1988).

In addition to classical conditioning, operant conditioning is believed to exert con-siderable influence on the expression of pain behavior. Operant conditioning suggests that reinforcement of a behavior will increase the likelihood that the behavior will recur, while punishment decreases the frequency of a behavior. Reinforcement for pain behav-iors may come from many sources of chronic pain. For example, financial compensation that is contingent on the demonstration of continued pain (e.g., workers' compensation and/or litigation) may represent a reinforcer. Consistent with this notion are reports that patients receiving workers' compensation payments are less likely to have biomedical findings to explain their pain, and they have less successful outcomes following reha-bilitation or lumbar disc surgery (Aronoff, 1991). Another potential reinforcer for pain behavior is spousal support and attention. For example, one study showed that patients who reported high satisfaction with social support also reported more pain (Gil, Keefe, Crisson, & Van Dalfson, 1987). Although causal interpretations are limited due to the correlational nature of the study, these results are consistent with the interpretation that solicitous spousal behavior may reinforce verbal reports of increased pain. Also, it has been reported that spouse solicitousness is related to increased overt pain behavior in patients with high levels of reported pain (Romano et al., 1995), suggesting that increased rates of reinforcement from spouses are associated with increases in pain behavior. Thus, several lines of evidence support the importance of operant and classical conditioning in chronic pain, and these processes should be integrated into assessment and treatment.

Cognitive–Behavioral Model

Both the gate control model and the behavioral model of pain introduce important factors to the understanding of the chronic pain experience. The gate control model postulates that both ascending and descending mechanisms influence the experience of pain, and thus pain is not simply a sensory experience. The behavioral model introduces the notion of environmental contingencies that can and do influence the perception of pain and the display of pain behaviors. However, it has been argued that both of these models may still have too limited a view of the chronic pain experience (Turk & Rudy, 1994).

The cognitive-behavioral model of chronic pain incorporates an individual's percep-tions and emotions into the environmental contingencies that impact behavior creating a multidimensional model, in which the experience of pain is a product of the multiple interactions between cognition, emotion, and behavior. This model has its origins in the

psychotherapeutic literature as a means to describe the ways in which individuals function, in general. As such, the model is not specific to the understanding of chronic pain. A
cognitive-behavioral conceptualization of function recognizes the role of an individual's
perceptions and the reciprocal interactions between perception, sensory experience,
emotion, and behavior. This reciprocal relationship means that an individual's perceptions impact across sensory, emotional, and behavioral dimensions, and that these dimensions influence the individual's perceptions. Thus, in a cognitive behavioral perspective,
behavior that is reinforced can function to maintain maladaptive perceptions, as much as
distorted perceptions can influence maladaptive behavioral consequences. In this way,
the cognitive-behavioral model is broader than either the behavioral or strictly cognitive
models of function. As applied to chronic pain, this multidimensional perspective is best
recognized and defined by the work of Turk and colleagues (Turk, Meichenbaum, & Genest, 1983; Turk & Rudy, 1994). Drawing from the work of these researchers, the
cognitive-behavioral model of pain defines the condition as an interactive, multidimensional phenomenon in which sensory, affective, behavioral, and cognitive aspects of pain
are all impacted.

Turk and Rudy (1994) described five primary assumptions that characterize the
cognitive-behavioral perspective and guide assessment and treatment. First, individuals
actively process information. That is, individuals make sense of incoming stimuli through
a series of filtering techniques and organizing strategies. An individual's behavior or
covert response to a given stimulus is determined by these information-processing
techniques. Thus, an individual's response is not based on the stimulus itself but rather
the perception or appraisal of that stimulus. These information-processing strategies are
learned over time in reaction to events within the individual's development. Some of
these strategies and techniques may be adaptive, while others are maladaptive. Second,
an individual's thoughts can influence emotional and physiologic arousal, which serve as
a trigger for behavior. This relationship is reciprocal, and thus physiology, emotion, and
behavior will elicit or influence thought processes. The relationship is transactional in
nature and, again, learned over time. Third, and in contrast to a strict behavioral view, an
individual's behavior is not solely determined by the environment. Rather, an individual
interacts with the environment and elicits behaviors (which are cognitively mediated)
that influence the environment around him or her. All interactions between cognition,
behavior, physiological arousal, and emotion, whether adaptive or maladaptive, are assumed to be acquired through the learning process. Therefore, the fourth assumption of
the cognitive-behavioral perspective is that individuals are capable of learning adaptive
ways of thinking, feeling, and behaving. This fourth assumption has direct bearing on
treatment applications, indicating that interventions should address all three dimensions
rather than attempting to modify one dimension with the hope that results will generalize
across the other two. Finally, assumption five is that individuals are capable of playing and
must play an active role in changing maladaptive thoughts, behaviors, and feelings. Just
as individuals have played an active role in learning to function in maladaptive ways,
change will only come about if individuals actively learn adaptive ways of functioning.
In the case of chronic pain, a passive existence will not elicit change in the condition.
Waiting for symptom resolution, as is done in an acute illness episode, will not be effective. Therefore, the individual must seek out ways to think, behave, and feel that promote
relief. The chronic pain patient who has learned over time how to think, behave, and feel
as the result of the impact of a painful condition, must actively pursue a new set of

strategies and behaviors to create interactions that promote relief from the painful experience.

TREATMENT APPROACHES

If the chronic pain condition is conceptually understood as a constellation of sensory, behavioral, and emotional dimensions, treatment must address or impact each of these dimensions. In some cases, a treatment targeted at one dimension may impact the others (i.e., reduction of pain sensation with subsequent improvement in functional abilities). However, treatments that focus solely on either the sensory, affective, or functional dimensions may not be efficacious for patients with more complex chronic conditions. Although each discipline may have an area of concentration and expertise (i.e., occupational therapy and functional limitations, psychology and emotional distress), each discipline must also understand the principles of treatment from other areas that may be applicable for a given patient. Four major treatment approaches for chronic pain conditions will now be described.

Pharmacological Intervention

The use of pharmacotherapy in pain management should be guided by several basic questions. First, what are the target behaviors or symptoms? Second, are medications required? Third, what medication(s) should be used? Fourth, what mechanism of delivery and dosing should be applied? And finally, what are the potential effects and side effects? Unfortunately, the application of pharmacological therapy to the management of pain is often guided by the clinician's predilections. Complaints of pain, accompanying insomnia, and depression, frequently evoke prescription writing. These issues may also be effectively addressed through nonpharmacological means, behavioral and cognitive behavioral therapies being the most effective. Some symptoms reflect a natural response to existing physiological and environmental circumstances. Thus, symptoms should not always be viewed as "chemical deficiencies." The potential need and benefit of medications in the management of pain is, therefore, best determined in an interdisciplinary setting. In such an environment, various approaches to a single problem can be evaluated, and those best suited for the patient selected. Attempts to isolate and treat individual complaints or symptoms pharmacologically can lead to polypharmacy, which may be confusing and detrimental to the patient. The patient's complaints and behaviors must be put in the proper context. Often times, medication dependence, misuse, or overuse is blamed on the patient, when in fact it may be iatrogenic.

Clearly, some patients will benefit from the use of medications. The particular symptoms must be identified. Symptoms may include muscle spasms, mood disorders, inflammation, sleep disorder, "pain," and nociception. It is important to discriminate between medicating the patient's "verbal reports" versus documented symptoms. All too often, we assume a one-to-one correlation between the patient's reports and the actual behavior or complaint. A careful clinical interview and ongoing assessment can be very useful in clarifying the symptom (Doleys, Murray, Klapow, & Coleton, 1997b). Not all symptoms are of equal importance or accessibility. For example, a patient's experience of pain may be altered by providing antidepressant medication for sleep and mood disturbance. It may be easier to treat the sleep and mood disturbance than to attempt to alter the overall elusive experience of "pain." Common agreement should be reached by the patient and treatment team as to what symptoms are to be targeted for pharmacological intervention, what types of preparations will be used over what period of time, and how the outcome will be evaluated.

Once the target symptoms are determined, one must choose among the various agents available. There is, for example, a wide range of antidepressants, including selective serotonin reuptake inhibitors (SSRI's) that can serve various purposes. Nonsteroidal anti-inflammatory drugs, opiates, muscle relaxers, tranquilizers, and anticonvulsants have each found their way into the treatment of the pain patient (cf. Fields & Liebeskind, 1994). Although the preparations within each given category share certain pharmacological properties, there are differences in the pharmacokinetics. Many of these preparations cannot and should not be casually applied. Certain antidepressants, for example, are more sedating than others (Gilman, Rall, Nies, & Taylor, 1990). Anticonvulsants have been found to be beneficial in treating neuropathic pain, though not with equal efficacy.

There are many options regarding the mode of delivery and dosing. Medication can be provided orally, intravenously, intramuscularly, epidurally, intra-articularly, and intrathecally. Preparations come in the form of liquid, pills, transdermal patches, and injectable solutions. They can be provided in divided doses or in a single dose. There are slow-acting and sustained-release preparations. It is generally agreed that medications given on a chronic basis, such as opiates for pain control, are best used on a fixed time rather than an as needed (i.e., prn) schedule. Most facilities prescribing pain medications, particularly opiates, have developed an individualized therapeutic "contract" signed by the patient and facility. This contract outlines the responsibility of both parties. Although the use of chronic opiate therapy in the case of noncancer pain has become more acceptable and wide spread, this therapy is not without its potential problems and should be applied by a trained and knowledgeable clinician (Portenoy, 1994).

The utilization of implantable drug administration systems (DAS) is increasing in popularity. These systems provide for a programmed release of suitable substances to the epidural or intrathecal space. It is believed that administration in these areas can be more effective and efficient. Although potentially very beneficial, this application of pharmacological intervention should be applied within the strictest of guidelines so as to minimize potential side effects and complications (Krames & Schuchard, 1995).

Pharmacological therapy is not without its effects and side effects. All too often, casual reports by the patient are used as the sole source of data for altering medications. Observations by the staff, family members, and the use of self-report diaries should supplement verbal reports. With many of the pain medicines, such as narcotics, there is the potential for the patient's developing dependence and tolerance, however true "addiction" is an overstated concern (Portenoy, 1994). Proper application of medications to the patient with a past or active history of addiction requires a good deal of experience and sophistication. Addicts are susceptible to suffering from pain, much like any other patient, and should not be denied analgesics merely on the basis of addiction.

One must be concerned about the physiological effects of chronic medication management. Liver function enzymes must be monitored in an effort to detect potential damage. There is growing evidence that opiates can affect hormonal activity. Reduced testosterone levels have been identified (Doleys et al., 1997a). This side effect may predispose the patient to osteoporosis and thus add another complicating factor.

The use of pharmacotherapy for pain management has expanded to exploring "preemptive analgesia." in this instance, medications are utilized preoperatively in an effort to prevent or minimize the development of chronic pain conditions, such as hyperalgesia. Postop and acute pain pharmacological management may be very beneficial in aiding rehabilitation therapy by reducing the likelihood of the development of pain behaviors that are inadvertently reinforced by the environment. Finally, there are those preparations that may be considered for long-term utilization. Clearly, medication management can be a very effective and useful adjunct in the treatment of many chronic pain conditions when applied properly.

Behavioral Intervention

Treatments based on the behavioral model emphasize reducing pain behaviors and increasing "well" behaviors (e.g., increased activity and verbal reports of decreased pain). From a classical conditioning perspective, inducing this behavior requires breaking the connection between certain antecedent events and subsequent pain behaviors. For example, a patient who underwent back surgery and experienced considerable pain when ambulating due to postsurgical inflammation and tissue damage may develop an association between ambulation and limping. This association may continue even after healing of the tissue damage has occurred; therefore, a goal of treatment would be to break the connection between walking and the pain behavior of limping, using gait training combined with desensitization. From an operant conditioning perspective, treatment should emphasize removing reinforcers for pain behaviors and applying reinforcement following well behaviors. For instance, a patient whose spouse provides extra attention when the patient complains of pain would be instructed to give the attention following more functional, well behavior and to extinguish the pain complaints by acknowledging the patient in a neutral, matter-of-fact manner.

Before behavioral treatment can be implemented, a thorough behavioral assessment must be conducted. This assessment involves a functional behavioral analysis that identifies relevant pain behaviors and well behaviors, the antecedents and consequences of these behaviors, and some indication of the patient's and family's willingness to cooperate in treatment. Important behaviors to assess include activity level, medication consumption, and the specific overt pain behaviors exhibited by the patient (e.g., limping, verbal complaints, grimacing), as well as functional behaviors that are to be maintained. Many of these variables can be assessed by having the patient keep a daily diary in which she or he records activities, pain reports, and medication. Overt pain behavior can be quantitatively assessed by videotaping patients and using specific rating systems or by using automated devices; however, these methods can be quite costly and time intensive. Alternatively, a variety of pain behavior checklists that allow clinicians and/or family members to more easily assess overt pain behaviors through direct observation have been developed (Richards, Nepomuceno, Riles, & Suer, 1982; Turk, Wack, & Kerns, 1985). Following a thorough behavioral assessment, realistic goals for treatment must be determined, taking into account the patient's physical pathology and other potential limiting factors. Patient involvement in goal setting is one important method of increasing the patient's sense of control and enhancing cooperation with treatment. Finally, behavior change must be monitored throughout treatment in order to track patient progress and to guide treatment modifications.

Overt pain behaviors are generally reduced by removing their reinforcers, a process known as extinction. In turn, well behaviors are increased by using reinforcement. For example, in treatment, patients should be attended to and praised when exhibiting well behavior, such as exercise, and social reinforcement should be withdrawn when pain behaviors are exhibited. This extinction of pain behaviors and reinforcement of well behaviors should be continued by the patient's family members outside of the treatment setting. Additionally, response prevention or substitution may be needed if subjects are to decrease or discontinue certain types of pain behavior and replace them with well behavior. Instructing a patient to bear weight equally on both legs rather than walking with an assistive device would be an example of response prevention and substitution. Gait training may also require the behavioral technique known as shaping, which involves reinforcing the patient for successive approximations of the desired behavior. That is, rather than waiting until the patient demonstrates a completely normal gait, he or she is reinforced for incremental progress that takes them closer to the goal of a normal gait. Another important component of behavioral treatment is observational learning. Patients must have the opportunity to observe others engaging in the appropriate behaviors. In order to teach patients proper body mechanics, it is important that therapists and treatment staff "practice what they preach." Also, in group treatment settings, if a patient observes another patient being reinforced for engaging in well behaviors, this experience can be an even more effective method of observational learning.

These techniques generally involve applying a positive reinforcer following a healthy behavior; however, another important aspect of behavioral treatment is reducing the negative reinforcement of pain behaviors. Negative reinforcement occurs when a behavior is followed by the removal of an unpleasant stimulus. For example, a patient may experience increased pain from activity, and then lay down, reducing the pain. In this scenario, the patient is being reinforced for "downtime," or inactivity, because this behavior results in the reward of pain relief. Thus, to prevent activity avoidance, activity should not be pain contingent. Rather, activity increases should be based on predetermined quotas. That is, patients should not be instructed to exercise until their pain increases to a certain level; they should be given realistic objective goals for exercise (e.g., stationary cycling for 10 minutes) that are increased in a systematic fashion (Doleys et al., 1982). A previous case study of a chronic pain patient (Dolce, Crocker, Moletteire, & Doleys, 1986) demonstrated that exercise quotas of this type not only increased exercise levels but also increased perceived ability to exercise and decreased anxiety related to exercise. Similarly, many patients take pain medication only when they are experiencing increased pain, which is called pain-contingent medication use. This leads to pain relief that is a negative reinforcer; patients are reinforcing themselves for medication consumption. Medication intake should be switched from a pain-contingent basis to a time-contingent basis to ensure that patients are no longer negatively reinforced for medication use. It has been demonstrated that, compared to pain-contingent medication intake, time-contingent medication provided better pain relief and enhanced mood among chronic pain patients (Berntzen & Gotestam, 1987; White & Sanders, 1985).

Several important considerations must be recognized when applying behavioral methods in the treatment of chronic pain (Sanders, 1996). First, the patient and family must be willing to cooperate with treatment and apply these methods both inside and outside the treatment setting. Also, behavioral methods take time to work, and the process of extinction typically involves an initial increase in the pain behaviors before they start decreasing. Therefore, the patient and the treatment team must be committed to applying these methods and giving them time to produce the desired effects. Another important point is that behavioral methods can be effective for patients with acute as well as chronic pain. For example, Fordyce and colleagues (1986) demonstrated that a behavioral treatment program, including time-contingent medication usage and a quota-based program for incrementing activity, was more effective than traditional medical treatment for acute back pain. A final issue regarding behavioral treatment is that these methods should not be used in isolation; rather, they should be integrated into an interdisciplinary treatment approach, including other psychological as well as physical and medical interventions.

Cognitive-Behavioral Intervention

Treatment from a cognitive-behavioral perspective is drawn directly from the conceptualization of the pain experience as well as the assumptions of the cognitive behavioral model. Because pain is viewed as a multidimensional experience in which sensory, affective, cognitive, and behavioral components are constantly interacting, treatment approaches must proceed accordingly. Thus, the cognitive-behavioral treatment approach is one that encompasses several specific interventions from within each of these dimensions. It is impossible and unnecessary to exhaustively cover all of these treatment modalities, given the wealth of literature that provides these specifics (e.g., Karoly & Kanfer, 1982; Turk et al., 1983). It should be noted that the cognitive-behavioral treatment model has been utilized in a wide variety of pain conditions, including headache (Holroyd, Nash, Pingel, Cordingley, & Jerome, 1991), arthritis (Bradley et al., 1987), and temporomandibular pain (Olson & Malow, 1988). As noted by the NIH Technology Assessment Panel (1996), cognitive-behavioral interventions have been shown to be superior to placebo and routine care for low back pain, rheumatoid arthritis, and osteoarthritis. The primary premise of a cognitive-behavioral approach to chronic pain management is that an individual's experience is comprised of the collective interaction of perception, cognition, emotion, and behavior. As such, treatment then should target the perceptive, cognitive, affective, and behavioral components of the pain experience. Thus, from a cognitive-behavioral perspective, the use cognitive and behavioral techniques to help the individual make changes "across the board" is indicated.

Chronic pain management from a cognitive-behavioral perspective focuses on changes in the patient's perceptions, cognitive style, and behavior that function to keep the patient feeling overwhelmed and controlled by their pain problem. The emphasis of the interventions is not on "removing" the sensory experience of pain, but rather on helping patients reconceptualize the experience and empower themselves to function in a more "healthy" and normal manner. Alleviation of the sensory experience is not the sole focus of treatment because the experience of pain is a complex and multidimensional one. Attempts to alleviate the sensory experience alone are not likely to be efficacious.

Prior to treatment, a thorough assessment must be conducted. Because the cognitive-behavioral perspective of pain postulates that perceptual, affective, and functional variables all define the pain condition, assessment must be multidimensional. Assessment of chronic pain from a cognitive-behavioral perspective closely resembles the biopsychosocial ideal put forth by Engle (1977), taking into consideration the physical, behavioral, and psychological factors that define the pain experience. Turk and Rudy (1994) have broken down the assessment process into three major dimensions, which have been incorporated into the Multiaxial Assessment of Pain model (Turk & Rudy, 1987). Evaluation of these dimensions may require the integration of information from laboratory, psychometric, and functional assessment instruments.

1. Medical/Physical. A determination should be made of the patient's injury, disease status, and physical impairment. This information can be obtained through physical exam, laboratory procedures, and/or functional measures of strength, mobility, and flexibility.
2. Psychosocial. An assessment should be made of the patient's pain perceptions, level of distress, and social and role-functioning limitations due to pain.
3. Behavioral. Responses to pain, including pain behaviors and their antecedents and consequences; activity levels; use of the health care system; and medication usage should be observed and evaluated.

Helping patients change the long-standing belief that they are helpless against their chronic pain problems and reconceptualize that belief as one that they can exert control over (Turk & Rudy, 1994), is essential to cognitive-behavioral treatment. Reconceptualization includes effective skills that patients can learn to use to respond more successfully to the chronic pain problem. Furthermore, patients learn that exerting control over the pain problem means that their roles in treatment and management will be active rather than passive or reactive. Reconceptualization begins with the patient's understanding that thoughts, emotions, perceptions, and behaviors are interactive, and that these interactions can often be maladaptive. With this foundation, patients then learn a variety of skills, both cognitive and behavioral, to deal with problems associated with the pain experience (i.e., pain exacerbations, thoughts of failure, feelings of hopelessness, physical deconditioning). These skills must be well learned so that patients are able to concentrate efforts on identifying when and in what situations the skills should be applied. To foster generalizability and maintenance of these skills, patients learn how to attribute changes and treatment benefits to the work they have done rather than to chance or external forces. Encouraging patients to attribute success directly to efforts they have exerted helps to increase their perception of control over the pain problem. Finally, with foundation of skills in place and the patient's having experienced a series of successful changes, problem-solving and relapse prevention plans can then be addressed to ensure maintenance of treatment effects and skills acquisition over time.

These overarching objectives create avenues for a variety of specific treatment components. Treatment components typically cover *education*, *skills development*, *practice*, and *relapse prevention*. These components can be implemented by providers with a wide range of expertise and varied backgrounds; thus, they are not limited solely to mental health professionals or pain psychologists. Each discipline involved in the patient's care (e.g., occupational therapy, physical therapy, vocational rehabilitation, psychology) can contribute specifics within these components; however, it is essential that the patient develop a general understanding of how these treatment components fit together as a single approach to pain management. Each treatment component lays out objectives that are necessary for control over the chronic pain problem. Very often these objectives are achieved through ongoing interaction with a psychologist skilled in cognitive-behavioral interventions. The psychologist can facilitate the integration by teaching the patient how each of the treatment components fit into the interactive process among thoughts, feelings, perceptions and behaviors, and how each component serves as a part of the treatment plan.

Education is often misconceptualized as "telling" the patient what he or she needs to do or must do. From a cognitive-behavioral perspective, information alone is not effective if the patient has no rationale for or understanding of its usefulness. Thus, the educational component begins with the rationale that education itself is an effective tool for managing the pain problem, and that education is the first step towards mastering it. Education begins to set the tone for further intervention. Several specific topics are typically conveyed to the patient. First, the notion that treatment, by definition, is a collaborative effort, and that treatment will not involve doing something *to* the patient but rather working *with* the patient. Second, education involves dispelling several myths and misconceptions. Patients should be provided with information about the stability of their condition, and an understanding that exercise will not produce further injury, that they are not limited in activity because of their physical condition. Education also focuses on why the patient continues to have pain, and why behavioral, cognitive, and emotional factors are contributing components to the pain experience. Tailoring this information to the individual characteristics of the patient by utilizing behavioral and psychosocial assessment data serves to make the educational component more meaningful and salient.

Skills building is an essential component of the cognitive-behavioral intervention. The chronic patient learns specific skills to make changes in his or her life. These skills include relaxation training, cognitive restructuring, quota-based physical activity, distraction and imagery, stress management, communication skills, and active problem solving. The specific use of these techniques has been described in a number of studies (Turk et al., 1983; Turk, Holzman, & Kerns, 1985). Again, the primary emphasis of these specific techniques is to enable the chronic pain patient to impact the cognitive, emotional, perceptual, and behavioral interactions that drive the experience of pain. Mastery of these skills facilitates this process and gives a sense of control over the pain problem.

In order to ensure maintenance of the new skills, cognitive and behavioral practice or rehearsal is a central part of the overall intervention. Practice involves the use of mental imagery, the patient visualizes himself or herself employing the newly acquired skills in the face of problems or difficult situations. Role playing with the provider enables the patient to run through specific situations and interactions in which the new skills are applicable. Homework is a critical portion of the cognitive and behavioral practice. It serves not only as an assessment of the patient's newly acquired abilities, but also as a mechanism for reinforcement and behavior change. Completion of graduated tasks allows the patient and provider to empirically document progress outside of the treatment setting. Each homework assignment is set at a level that the patient is capable of completing and gradually increases in difficulty. As Turk and colleagues (1983) noted, completing tasks outside of the treatment setting serves several important functions. Information can be obtained regarding typical responses of the patient and significant others to pain and pain behaviors. Factors that either exacerbate, cerebrate, or reduce pain and pain behavior can be identified. Adaptive and maladaptive responses to pain and pain behavior also can be identified. Coping skills and exercise strategies learned in the treatment setting can be applied in a real-world setting. Treatment progress can be demonstrated to the patient and significant others, which reinforces the notion that the patient can live functionally despite the existence of pain. This reinforcement serves to promote perceptions of control self-efficacy. Finally, homework is a means for providing "data" to evaluate progress and identify areas that need modification.

Education, practice, and rehearsal enable the chronic pain patient to acquire a repertoire of new behaviors, thinking styles, and conceptualizations of the pain problem. However, crucial to the maintenance of treatment effects is the provision for generalization and relapse prevention. Relapse prevention strategies help the patient to anticipate problems and proactively set strategies to address them. By reviewing situations that are likely to propose challenges for the pain patient (i.e., a family outing, situations of pro-longed exercise or exertion, or stressful situations) and laying out the previously learned coping skills (i.e., reframing of the situation, pacing of activity, etc.), the patient not only sets a plan for dealing with these problems, but continues to practice the newly acquired skills. This process reinforces the patient's learning and continues to promote self-efficacy. Central to relapse prevention and generalization of treatment effects is the patient's understanding that the changes that have occurred during treatment need to be adopted as part of a lifestyle. Thus, maintaining treatment effects means using the cognitive and behavior skills on a daily basis.

The cognitive-behavioral approach to chronic pain is by definition a multidimen-sional one and is drawn directly from a conceptualization of the pain experience, which is complex and interactive. As such, cognitive behavioral treatment often entails several specific treatment components (education, skills building, practice, and relapse preven-tion), delivered in a number of different manners (didactics, role playing, imagery, and homework), across a variety of settings (treatment program, at home, in rehabilitation, and at work). Despite the variety and complexity of this approach, the basic objectives of treatment remain the same. Therefore, although implementation of a cognitive-behavioral treatment program should include a trained pain psychologist, covering the sensory, functional, and emotional components of the chronic pain condition often requires a team of providers. Regardless of subspecialty (e.g., physical therapy, occupa-tional therapy, vocational rehabilitation, or psychology), each provider can contribute to the overall approach to chronic pain management. Essential to this treatment approach, however, is an understanding of the cognitive-behavioral model of pain by members of each discipline involved in the treatment program.

Interdisciplinary Intervention

Each of the treatment approaches described here highlights the physical, behavioral, and psychosocial complexities that can and do present in a chronic pain condition. Unlike acute injuries, such as splinting for a broken limb, demobilization for a muscle strain, or medication to reduce edema and pain, which often resolve with time and proper unidimensional treatment, chronic pain conditions have not resolved with time and frequently are resistant to unidimensional treatment approaches. Referring back to the conceptualization of the clinical presentation of a chronic pain condition (see Figure 20.1, p. 371), we are reminded that the chronic pain experience is one that impacts an individual across physical, functional, and emotional domains. As such, interventions must either directly or indirectly address each of these dimensions in order to be efficacious. Although it is possible for some patients to experience generalization of treatment effects from unidimensional treatment, it is not the case for all patients. For patients who do not see treatment carry over, the integration of treatment components from several disciplines may be necessary.

An interdisciplinary pain management team is typically comprised of members representing the disciplines of medicine, psychology, nursing, occupational therapy, physical therapy, and vocational rehabilitation. In this way, the pain management team is similar to rehabilitation teams that treat spinal cord or brain injuries. As Chapman (1994) noted, not all patients with a chronic pain condition need this type of program. Many patients with chronic pain conditions are able to manage the problem with minimal to moderate levels of intervention. The interdisciplinary treatment program is often reserved for those patients who's constellation of symptoms is so severe that they are simply unable to manage effectively from day-to-day. It has been proposed that these patients represent a unique subgroup that can be described as suffering from a chronic pain syndrome (Follick et al., 1984; Klapow et al., 1993). Therefore, the interdisciplinary pain program should be saved for the most complex, treatment-refractory patients.

As Turk and Rudy (1994) have noted, a distinction should be made between multi-disciplinary programs in the comprehensive treatment of a pain condition. Multidisci-plinary treatment typically refers to the use of several providers with a range of specialties to provide treatment for a given patient. In contrast, interdisciplinary treatment refers to the integration of specialties in an overall treatment approach. This difference is notable because multidisciplinary treatment often translates into a large amount of outside consultation with little integration or continuity of care. Again, if we refer back to the conceptualization of the chronic pain condition, we see that the condition itself is a well-integrated syndrome not a group of unrelated symptoms. Interdisciplinary treatment, that is treatment provided in an integrated team approach, is more likely to be efficacious than that of a large number of providers working independently with the patient.

Essential to the interdisciplinary team approach is a uniformed front of care. This care requires close communication among team members, a common approach to treat-ment, reinforcement of each others efforts and special abilities, and a constant awareness and understanding of what each member of the team is doing with the patient. Treatment goals must be clear and carefully laid out to the patient. Because the patient will be seen by a great number of providers (occupational therapy, physical therapy, psychology, and vocational rehabilitation) and asked to make several changes in her or his life, clear, definable short- and long-term goals must be specified. One fundamental advantage of the interdisciplinary treatment approach is the opportunity of the patient to learn and apply skills from each discipline across a variety of treatment settings, thus promoting skill generalization. For example, relaxation strategies for self-control of pain can and should be implemented during occupational or physical therapy sessions. The patient should be encouraged by the occupational therapist to implement these skills to facilitate comple-tion of the therapy session. In this manner, the occupational therapist must have an understanding of the patient's skill level and the basic skills involved in relaxation. Furthermore, the therapist will need to reinforce the patient's implementing these skills in order to foster generalization.

Treatment Format: Inpatient versus Outpatient

The University of Washington's inpatient pain management program has been the prototype for most current inpatient pain treatment programs. Such comprehensive programs last up to six weeks and address all aspects of the chronic pain condition. The model of care is rehabilitative, focusing on physical, behavioral, psychological, social, and vocational dimensions. Imbedded in this format is the application of strict operant principles for the modification of pain behavior (Fordyce, 1976). Pain relief is not a primary goal of the program, although many patients experience modest pain relief. Patient education, quota-based physical activity, medication tapering, nonreinforcement of pain behavior with reinforcement of healthy behavior, and vocational retraining are all central to the program.

The inpatient setting offers a number of advantages for this type of program. Treatment intensity, control, and continuity are all enhanced in the inpatient setting.

Reinforcement schedules for activity, health behavior, and medication can all be maintained virtually around-the-clock. Assessment and supervision by the treatment team is intensified, allowing for immediate revisions and modifications in the treatment regimen when needed. The self-report strategies can be less emphasized, using direct observation as a substitute. For medication-tapering purposes, the inpatient setting provides the necessary safety and medical facilities. Finally, by removing the patient from his or her familiar surroundings, reinforcement contingencies for pain behavior and disability are not kept in place. The new setting enables the patient to more easily learn the new set of skills without the competing reinforcement for old, maladaptive behaviors. Inpatient treatment programs have demonstrated efficacy across the dimensions of pain intensity, functional disability, and emotional distress (Chapman, Brena, & Bradford, 1981). Furthermore, they have demonstrated significant cost savings (Stieg, Williams, & Timmermans-Williams, 1985).

The classic inpatient model of treatment has given rise to a number of variations and related programs. Given the substantial costs of inpatient care, outpatient programs have become a viable and growing alternative. Within the outpatient program realm exists two models of care. The outpatient residential program in which individuals stay in a hotel or nonhospital setting during the treatment program, and the outpatient program in which patients reside at home and commute to the program on a daily basis. Although the setting differs, outpatient treatment programs generally employ the same treatment philosophy as inpatient models.

Several basic factors of the outpatient treatment setting are appealing. First, costs associated with outpatient programs are substantially less. Second, the outpatient setting decreases the number of disruption and logistical difficulties patients face in the inpatient setting. Patients may return home, and in some cases continue to work, while participating in the treatment program. Difficulties that arise at home or work and are related to the pain condition (i.e., pacing of activities, spousal solicitousness, or work-related stress) may be dealt with directly and integrated into the treatment program. Furthermore, behavior change strategies can be implemented outside of the treatment setting and then evaluated and modified if needed. Scheduling of activities, therapies, and education can be more easily tailored to the needs of the patient. Moreover, family members may have easier access to the patient and the program, which facilitates their participation in treatment. Termination may also be facilitated in an outpatient setting, as treatment session fading can occur. Patients can be faded from a daily to weekly schedule, and then to a monthly schedule. Fading may enhance generalizability of the treatment effects.

The disadvantages of the outpatient setting are relatively clear. First, intensity levels of the treatment may not compare with the inpatient setting. Second, if the individual resides at home rather than at a separate nonhospital setting during the treatment program, changes in existing behavior patterns will be difficult to achieve. When residing at home, the individual's old behavior patterns and reinforcement contingencies compete directly with the newly acquired skills and contingencies. This competition can hinder behavior change.

Few studies have examined the relative efficacy of inpatient versus outpatient interdisciplinary programs. Those that have, have not found a clear difference in efficacy between the two options, with both producing significant improvements across a variety of physical, psychological, and behavioral outcome variables (Chapman et al., 1981; Peters & Large, 1990). As Chapman (1994) noted, the choice of program is more reliant on the treatment components and level of treatment intensity than on inpatient or out-patient status.

The choice of an interdisciplinary versus less comprehensive approach and an in-patient versus outpatient program should be made on a case-by-case basis. As mentioned previously, not all patients will require the intensity and comprehensiveness of an interdisciplinary treatment program. Furthermore, those who are candidates for an interdisciplinary program may not be suitable for an inpatient program. Suitability for an inpatient program will be influenced by factors ranging from the severity of clinical presentation to insurance coverage to ability to pay.

CONCLUSION

This chapter has presented a conceptual model of chronic pain that highlights its multidimensional nature and describes the underlying mechanisms that drive the often complex clinical presentation. Given the complexity of chronic conditions, it is essential that care providers not be lulled into a discipline-specific, unidimensional understanding of the condition. The occupational therapist involved in care for the chronic pain patient may be part of an integrated team, may function as one of many independent care providers, or may be solely responsible for providing intervention. In any of these sce-narios, it is crucial that the therapist understand that the sensory, behavioral, and emo-tional components of the chronic pain condition can and will impact the intervention effects. Every encounter with the patient should be approached from a broad perspec-tive, examining how the interplay of these dimensions affect treatment response. The patient who has difficulties completing tasks may not be intentionally noncompliant but under a contingency of reinforcement that competes with the treatment regimen. Finan-cial incentives, reinforcement for "sick" behaviors from family and friends, release from household, work, and social responsibilities are likely to influence patient performance in therapy. Often the patient is not aware of these factors and their affect on performance. Other factors influencing performance include clinical depression, medication side-effects, and anticipatory anxiety. Although it is not the primary role of the occupational therapist to provide comprehensive treatment, it is necessary to understand and assess factors across the behavioral, psychological, and functional domains that may be affecting treatment. Proper use of outside consultation (e.g., physical medicine, psychology, voca-tional rehabilitation, and physical therapy) can be facilitated. In the end, the management of a chronic pain condition will be challenging and complex, but the proper understand-ing of the condition, its mediating and moderating factors, and the multidimensional avenues for treatment will make management easier.

REFERENCES

Arnoff, G. (1991). Chronic pain and the disability epidemic. *Clinical Journal of Pain, 7,* 330.

Ashburn, M. A., & Rice, L. J. (Eds.). (1997). *The management of pain.* New York: Churchill & Livingston.

Berntzen, D., & Gotestam, K. G. (1987). Effects of on-demand or fixed-interval schedules in the treatment of chronic pain with analgesic compounds: An experimental comparison. *Journal of Consulting and Clini-cal Psychology, 55,* 213–218.

Boyd, D. B. (1994). Taxonomy and classification of pain. In C. D. Tollison, J. R. Satterthwaite, & J. W. Tollision (Eds.), *Handbook of pain management* (2nd ed., pp. 7–10). Baltimore, MD: Williams & Wilkins.

Campbell, D. T., & Stanley, J. C. (1963). *Experimental and quasi-experimental designs for research.* Chicago: Rand McNally.

Chapman, S. L. (1994). Outpatient chronic pain management programs. In C. D. Tollison, J. R. Satterthwaite, & J. W. Tollison (Eds.), *Handbook of pain management* (2nd edition, pp. 677–686). Baltimore, MD: Williams & Wilkins.

Chapman, S. L., Brena, S. F., & Bradford, L. A. (1981). Treatment outcome in a chronic pain rehabilitation program. *Pain, 11,* 255–268.

Cook, T. D., & Campbell, D. T. (1979). *Quasi-experimentation.* Boston: Houghton-Mifflin.

Dolce, J. J., Crocker, M. F., Moletteire, C., & Doleys, D. M. (1986). Exercise quotas, anticipatory concern, and self-efficacy expectancies in chronic pain: A preliminary report. *Pain, 24,* 365–372.

Doleys, D. M., Crocker, M. F., & Patton, D. (1986). Response of patients with pain to exercise quotas. *Physical Therapy, 62,* 1111–1114.

Doleys, D. M., Dinoff, B. L, Page, L., Tutak, U., Willis, K. D., & Coleton, M. I. (1997a). *Sexual dysfunction and other "side effects" associated with intraspinal opiate management of chronic non-cancer pain.* Unpublished manuscript, Pain and Rehabilitation Institute, Birmingham, AL.

Doleys, D. M., Murray, J. B., Klapow, J. C., & Coleton, M. I. (1997b). Behavioral medicine/psychological assessment of the pain patient. In M. A. Ashburn & L. J. Rice (Eds.), *The management of pain.* New York: Churchill Livingston.

Engel, G. L. (1977). The need for a new medical model: A challenge for biomedicine. *Science, 196,* 129–136.

Feuerstein, M. (1994). Definitions of pain. In C. D. Tollison, J. R. Satterthwaite, & J. W. Tollision (Eds.), *Handbook of pain management* (2nd ed., pp. 3–6). Baltimore, MD: Williams & Wilkins.

Fields, N. H. L., & Liebeskind, J. C. (Eds.). (1994). *Pharmacological approaches to the treatment of chronic pain: New concepts in critical issues.* New York: Pergamon Press.

Flor, H., Fydrich, T., & Turk, D. C. (1992). Efficacy of multidisciplinary pain treatment centers: A meta-analytic review. *Pain, 49,* 221–230.

Follick, M. J., Aberger, E. W., Ahern, D. K., & McCartney, J. R. (1984). The chronic low back pain syndrome: Identification and management. *Rhode Island Medical Journal, 67,* 219–224.

Fordyce, W. E. (1976). *Behavioral methods for chronic pain and illness.* St. Louis, MO: Mosby.

Fordyce, W. E., Brockway, J. A., Bergman, J. A., & Spengler, D. (1986). Acute back pain: A control-group comparison of behavioral versus traditional management methods. *Journal of Behavioral Medicine, 9,* 127–140.

Gil, K. M., Keefe, F. J., Crisson, J. E., & Van Dalfson, P. J. (1987). Social support and pain behavior. *Pain, 29,* 209–217.

Gilman, A. G., Rall, T. W., Nies, A. S., & Taylor, P. (Eds.). (1990). *Goodman and Gilman's The pharmacological basis of therapeutics.* New York: Pergamon Press.

Holzman, A. D., Turk, D. C., & Kerns, R. D. (1986). The cognitive-behavioral approach in the management of chronic pain. In A. D. Holzman & D. C. Turk (Eds.), *Pain Management: A handbook of psychological treatment approaches* (p. 40). Elmsford, NY: Pergamon Press.

International Association for the Study of Pain. (1986). Classification of chronic pain: Descriptions of chronic pain syndromes and definitions of pain terms. *Pain Supplement, 3,* 1–225.

Jamison, R. N., Rudy, T. E., Penzien, D. B., & Mosley, T. H. (1994). Cognitive-behavioral classifications of chronic pain: Replication and extension of empirically derived patient profiles. *Pain, 57,* 277–292.

Judd, C. M., & Kenny, D. A. (1981). *Estimating the effects of social interventions.* Cambridge: Cambridge University Press.

Kaplan, R. M., & Anderson, J. P. (1988). A general health policy model: Update and application. *Health Services Research, 23,* 203–234.

Karoly, P., & Kanfer, F. M. (Eds.). (1982). *Self management and behavior change.* Elmsford, NY: Pergamon Press.

Keefe, F. J., & Block, A. R. (1982). Development of an observation method for assessing pain behavior in chronic low back pain patients. *Behavior Therapy, 13,* 363–375.

Keefe, F. J., Bradley, L. A., & Crisson, J. E. (1990). Behavior assessment of low back pain: Identification of pain behavior subgroups. *Pain, 40,* 153–160.

Kerns, R. D., Turk, D. C., Holzman, A. D., & Rudy, T. E. (1986). Efficacy of a cognitive-behavioral approach for the treatment of chronic pain. *Clinical Journal of Pain, 1,* 195–203.

Kerns, R. D., Turk, D. C., & Rudy, T. E. (1985). The West Haven-Yale multidimensional pain inventory (WHYMPI). *Pain, 23,* 345–356.

Klapow, J. C., Slater, M. A., Patterson, T., Atkinson, J. H., Doctor, J. N., & Garfin, S. (1993). An empirical evaluation of multidimensional clinical outcome in chronic low back pain patients. *Pain, 55,* 107–118.

Klapow, J. C., Slater, M. A., Patterson, T. L., Atkinson, H. J., Weichgenant, A. L., Grant, I., & Garfin, S. R. (1995). Psychosocial factors differentiate multidimensional clinical groups of chronic low back pain patients. *Pain, 62,* 349-355.

Krames, E. S., & Schuchard, M. (1995). Implantable intraspinal infusion analgesia: Management guidelines. *Pain Reviews, 2,* 243-267.

Lysle, D. T., & Fowler, H. (1988). Changes in pain reactivity induced by unconditioned and conditioned excitatory and inhibitory stimuli. *Journal of Experimental Psychology: Animal Behavior, 14,* 376-389.

Meichenbaum, D., & Turk, D. C. (1987). *Facilitating treatment adherence: A practitioner's guidebook.* New York: Plenum Press.

Melzack, R., & Wall, P. D. (1965). Pain mechanisms: A new theory. *Science, 150,* 971-979.

Merskey, H. (1986). Classification of chronic pain: Descriptions of chronic pain syndromes and definitions. *Pain, 3,* S1-S225.

Morse, R. H. (1983). Pain and emotions. In S. F. Brena & S. L. Chapman (Eds.), *Management of patients with chronic pain* (pp. 36-53). New York: SP Medical and Scientific Books.

NIH Technology Assessment Panel. (1996). Integration of behavioral and relaxation approaches into the treatment of chronic pain and insomnia. *Journal of the American Medical Association, 276,* 313-318.

Olson, R. E., & Matow, R. M. (1988). Effects of biofeedback and psychotherapy on patients with myofascial pain dysfunction who are not responsive to conventional treatments. *Rehabilitation Psychology, 7,* 527-544.

Peters, J. L., & Large, R. G. (1990). A randomized control trial evaluating in and outpatient pain management programs. *Pain, 41,* 283-293.

Portenoy, R. K. (1994). Opiod therapy for chronic nonmalignant pain: Current status. In H. L. Fields & J. C. Liebeskind (Eds.), *Progress in pain research and management,* Vol. 1. Seattle, WA: IASP Press.

Poulsen, D. L., Hansen, H. J., Langemark, M., Olesen, J., & Beck, P. (1987). Discomfort or disability in patients with chronic pain syndrome: Psychotherapy. *Psychosomatics, 48,* 60-62.

Richards, J. S., Nepomuceno, C., Riles, M., & Suer, Z. (1982). Assessing pain behavior: The UAB pain behavior scale. *Pain, 14,* 193-198.

Romano, J. M., & Turner, J. A. (1985). Chronic pain and depression: Does the evidence support a relationship? *Psychological Bulletin, 97,* 18-34.

Romano, J. M., Turner, J. A., Jensen, M. P., Friedman, L. S., Bulcroft, R. A., Hops, H., & Wright, S. F. (1995). Chronic pain patient-spouse behavioral interactions predict patient disability. *Pain, 63,* 353-360.

Rudy, T. E., Turk, D. C., Zaki, H. S., & Curtin, H. D. (1989). An empirical taxometric alternative to traditional classification of temporomandibular disorders. *Pain, 36,* 311-320.

Sanders, S. H. (1996). Operant conditioning with chronic pain: Back to basics. In R. J. Gatchel & D. C. Turk (Eds.), *Psychological approaches to pain management: A practitioner's handbook* (pp. 112-130). New York: Guilford Press.

Seals, H. L., & Liebeskind, J. C. (Eds.). (1994). *Pharmacological approaches to the treatment of chronic pain: New concepts in critical issues.* Seattle, WA: IASP Press.

Shealy, C. N. (1976). *The pain game.* Millbrae, CA: Celestial Arts.

Steig, R. L., Williams, R. C., & Timmermans-Williams, G. (1985). Cost benefits of interdisciplinary chronic pain treatment. *Clinical Journal of Pain, 1,* 189-195.

Sternbach, R. A. (1974). *Pain patients: Traits and treatments.* New York: Academic Press.

Sternbach, R. A. (1984). Behavior therapy. In P. D. Wall & R. Melzack (Eds.), *Textbook of pain* (pp. 57-71). London: Churchill Livingstone.

Sullivan, M. D. Turner, J. A., & Romano, J. (1991). Chronic pain in primary care: Identification and management of psychosocial factors. *Journal of Family Practice, 32*(2), 193-199.

Turk, D. C., Holzman, A. D., & Kerns, R. D. (1985). Chronic pain. In K. A. Holroyd & T. L. Creer (Eds.), *Chronic disease: A handbook of self-management approaches* (pp. 88-103). New York: Academic Press.

Turk, D. C., Meichenbaum, D., & Genest, M. (1983). *Pain and behavioral medicine: A cognitive behavior perspective.* New York: Guilford Press.

Turk, D. C., Wack, J. T., & Kerns, R. D. (1985). An empirical examination of the "pain behavior" construct. *Journal of Behavioral Medicine, 8,* 119-130.

Turk, D. C., & Rudy, T. E. (1986). The assessment of cognitive factors in chronic pain: A worthwhile enterprise? *Journal of Consulting & Clinical Psychology, 54,* 760-768.

Turk, D. C., & Rudy, T. E. (1987). Toward the comprehensive assessment of chronic pain patients: A multiaxial approach. *Behavior Research Therapy, 25,* 237-249.

Turk, D. C., & Rudy, T. E. (1988). Toward an empirically derived taxonomy of chronic pain patients: Integration of psychological assessment data. *Journal of Consulting & Clinical Psychology, 56,* 233-258.

Turk, D. C., & Rudy, T. E. (1990). The robustness of an empirically derived taxonomy of chronic pain patients. *Pain, 43,* 27–35.

Turk, D. C., & Rudy, T. E. (1994). A cognitive-behavioral perspective on chronic pain: Beyond the scalpel and syringe. In C. D. Tollison, J. R. Satterthwaite, & J. W. Tollision (Eds.), *Handbook of pain management* (2nd ed., pp. 136–151). Baltimore, MD: Williams & Wilkins.

Turner, J. A., & Chapman, C. R. (1982). Psychological interventions for chronic pain: A critical review: II. Operant conditioning, hypnosis, and cognitive-behavior therapy. *Pain, 12,* 23–46.

White, B., & Sanders, S. H. (1985). Differential effects on pain and mood in chronic pain patients with time versus pain-contingent medication delivery. *Behavior Therapy, 16,* 28–38.

21

Effective Worksite-Based Disability Management Programs

Donald E. Shrey

This chapter provides a comprehensive overview of effective worksite-based disability management programs. The basic principles of disability management are reviewed, emphasizing the direct involvement of the employer, the disabled worker, and other worksite representatives. The importance of "early intervention" as a key to effective disability management outcome is emphasized. The merits of the "therapeutic" worksite are discussed and contrasted with traditional clinical interventions and rehabilitation programs. Disability management is conceptualized at the clinical, organizational, and statutory levels. Each of these three levels is reviewed in terms of its relative importance to the injured worker, the employer, and the community.

This chapter features a case study that illustrates the forces that have an impact on an injured worker in the absence of an effective disability management system. Worker and employer benefits of disability management programs are reviewed, as are some of the "commonsense" perspectives on disability management. Another case study illustrates the importance of disability management "controls" within a changing corporate environment. The steps in the work-injury management process are delineated, and key controls for building a worksite-based disability management infrastructure are reviewed. Disability management program outcomes that are based on survey research are summarized in this chapter, including special features of worksite-based disability management programs among U.S. and Canadian employers.

Donald E. Shrey • Department of Physical Medicine and Rehabilitation, University of Cincinnati Medical Center, Cincinnati, Ohio 45244.

Sourcebook of Occupational Rehabilitation, edited by Phyllis M. King. Plenum Press, New York, 1998.

BASIC PRINCIPLES OF WORKSITE-BASED DISABILITY MANAGEMENT

Disability management is a proactive process that minimizes the impact of an impairment (resulting from injury, illness, or disease) on the individual's capacity to participate competitively in the work environment (Shrey, 1995b). The ultimate goals of worksite-based disability management are to control unnecessary workers' compensation and disability costs and to promote the sustained employment of workers with injuries and disabilities. Disability management strategies and interventions are focused on three basic objectives: (1) reducing the number and magnitude of injuries and illnesses, (2) minimizing the impact of disabilities on work performance, and (3) decreasing lost time associated with injuries, illnesses, and resulting disabilities.

Employer Involvement

Trends show that employers are taking a more active role in disability management. The employer is the central decision-maker, planner, and coordinator of interventions and services in the worksite-based disability management process (Akabas, Gates, & Galvin, 1992). Worksite representatives (i.e., supervisors, managers, union representatives, and co-workers) are directly involved in rehabilitation interventions that emphasize job retention, positive work adjustment, and accommodation. These are the primary methods of promoting sustained employment among workers with disabilities, while reducing the financial liabilities of the employer.

Worksite-based disability management interventions capitalize on the therapeutic value of working while the worker is recovering from an injury or illness. Workers are treated as valued employees regardless of their impairments, and accommodations are made to facilitate continued meaningful employment. Disability management interventions introduced by the employer, within the ecological context of the workplace, strengthens the bond between the worker with functional restrictions and the worksite (Shrey & Olsheski, 1992).

In business and industry, controlling the cost of disability and its ultimate impact on employee productivity is a complex process. It involves an intricate interplay of employer goals, resources, and expectations; the needs and self-interests of workers, health care providers, labor unions, and attorneys; and external community resources. The ability of the employer to effectively manage resources and to participate in an interdisciplinary fashion will contribute to the control of costs and the maintenance of the disabled worker's sustained employment.

Early Intervention

Historically, "early intervention" has been universally accepted as necessary for a successful rehabilitation outcome. Any unnecessary delays in providing treatment and rehabilitation interventions results in a greater likelihood of prolonged lost time and an increased potential for the development of psychosocial and secondary health problems (Boschen, 1989; Galvin, 1985; Linveh, 1986; Seligman, 1991; Shrey, 1995b; Walker, 1992). Although early intervention is necessary for maximizing positive rehabilitation results, it is insufficient in achieving ultimate success in disability management. To control costs and maintain the worker's productive employment, effective disability management requires both early intervention and early return to work. By illustration, many clinical treatment programs for injured workers promote an early intervention philosophy. However, the early intervention may be followed by several weeks of clinical treatment and conditioning services. Extensive involvement in such clinical programs often results in extended lost time, during which the injured employee loses his or her identity as a worker (Shrey, 1995a).

The Therapeutic Worksite

Workers with disabilities may experience significant rehabilitation gains while involved in active therapies and conditioning programs. However, a safe and timely return to work will not be realized unless the worksite has a strong infrastructure that supports the worker's transition back to work. Effective return-to-work programs need to be strongly supported by labor and management, and written policies are needed to guide return-to-work activities and to support disability management interventions. Likewise, worksite procedures and protocols that address jobsite accommodations, transitional work options, worker evaluation, job analysis, and other important "controls" are required to ensure successful outcomes. Effective disability management is focused on bringing the clinical interventions to the worksite rather than taking the worker to the clinic. The focus is on enabling the worker to get well while working rather than waiting for the worker to get well in order to return to work.

The Three Levels of Disability Management

Level 1 is the *micro* or "clinical" level, which is focused specifically on the individual with an injury or disability. Worksites that effectively address the multidisciplinary needs of their workers with disabilities achieve much success in reducing unnecessary lost time and associated costs. Much of what happens at the micro level depends on the relationship between workers with disabilities, their supervisors, co-workers, case managers, and others who intervene to support each worker's safe and timely return to work.

Level 2 is the *macro* or "organizational" level of disability management. At this level, the worksite's policies and resources are organized and coordinated in support of the clinical activities that take place at Level 1. Return-to-work success for the injured worker is remote without a strong organizational infrastructure. Important "controls" to support disability management activities at Level 2 consist of accommodations, creative return-to-work options, flexible policies, responsible labor and management representatives, accountability among supervisors, and strong labor–management support. Supportive community-based rehabilitation services are also a necessary component of the macro level.

Level 3 is the *mega* or "statutory" level of disability management, which is characterized by workers' compensation statutes, disability insurance policies, and legislative mandates (e.g., Americans with Disabilities Act). The laws and regulations that govern disability benefits and health care services are a significant force in shaping the "organizational" response to worker injury and disability, which occurs at Level 2, the macro level. Likewise, clinical interventions with injured workers at the micro level (Level 1) are directly linked to rehabilitation services that are legislated, approved, or authorized at the mega level.

RESOLVING DISABILITY PROBLEMS: CASE STUDY

Injury and disability in the workplace are commonly treated as medical–legal problems. However, negative labor relations can be the most pervasive barrier to resolving a worker's disability claim. Workers who dislike their jobs, their supervisors, and their co-workers are more likely to exaggerate medical problems and symptoms associated with an injury. Likewise, the supervisor who dislikes a particular worker may actively prevent that employee from returning to work after a lost-time injury. In either case, the results are similar: more lost time, extensive medical involvement and associated costs, and uncontrolled disability claims. Consider the following case study, which was illustrated by Shrey (1995a) in *Principles and Practices of Disability Management in Industry*. This study illustrates the significance of the three levels of disability management, especially when proper "controls" are not established.

> Bill is a 35-year-old machinist who sustained a low back injury when he fell on a slippery floor at work. He had back surgery six months ago and has been involved in physical therapy for the past four months. He attends therapy sessions three times per week. There is no indication that his condition has improved as a result of therapy. Bill complains that his treating physician gives him no indication of his prognosis for recovery.
>
> After the accident, Bill was hospitalized for several days, during which time he was not contacted by his employer. He received three or four telephone calls from an insurance claims adjuster representing his employer. The adjuster seemed to be more interested in investigating the details of his accident than in Bill's injury and treatment. Bill did not receive his first workers' compensation check until three months after his injury, due to a lengthy claims investigation process and administrative delays. Bill now receives about 70% of his average weekly wages as well as supplemental benefits from his employer.
>
> Bill was a good, productive worker. However, it seemed that he could never please his supervisor, who was excessively demanding and unrealistic about production goals. Work was plentiful prior to Bill's accident, but Bill's employer recently lost a major production contract to a competitor, and there were rumors of anticipated lay-offs at the plant. Bill was concerned about his job security, lack of contact from his employer, unclear medical prognosis, and economic uncertainty. He recently retained the services of an aggressive workers' compensation attorney.
>
> Bill's workers' compensation case is currently in litigation, and his attorney is seeking a significantly high settlement for permanent and total disability. Bill does not understand the legal process, but he has put total trust in his attorney, who has assured Bill of a major financial award. No one has suggested vocational rehabilitation to Bill, particularly in light of the poor prognosis cited in the most recent medical report from Dr. Jones, a physician recommended to Bill by his attorney.
>
> Things look very bleak to Bill. He has lost all contact with his employer. Everything is in the hands of his attorney, the physicians, and the workers' compensation board. Bill's future depends on the outcome of the litigation process. Anger, frustration, uncertainty, and stress continue to mount. Things have also deteriorated at home. Bill's relationship with his wife seems to be one continuous argument—mostly about Bill's excessive drinking and complaining. Even the kids have lost respect for Bill because all he does is sit around all day "feeling sorry for himself."

Case Study Analysis

On examining this case study, it becomes clear that several negative forces are having an impact on return-to-work goals for the injured worker. Ineffective or prolonged therapy and poor communication with the treating physician (at the micro level) result in this worker's diminished hope for recovery. As the period of work disruption increases, the worker becomes dependent on treatment providers. Concurrently, communication between the worker and his employer has terminated, and the worker-employer relationship has deteriorated. Lengthy claims investigation processes and delays in receiving benefits (at the mega level) created a deeper adversarial climate between the worker and his employer. Many workers, after having reached this point, choose to punish their employers by becoming uncooperative and continuing to draw weekly compensation benefits at the employer's expense.

Disabled worker-employer relationships typically deteriorate during the claims investigation process when the worker experiences delays in claims processing and fails to receive his or her due benefits. Claims adjusters who lack empathy, understanding, and sensitivity often create additional stress for the worker. Conflicts arise when the worker's interest in economic self-sufficiency is challenged by the insurance carrier's (or third-party administrator's, or managed care organization's) self-interested goals of controlling medical costs and challenging questionable disability claims. The result is often extended work disruption, litigation, and greater personal and economic costs for the employer and the worker.

In the case study, labor relations (at the macro level) appear to have played a major role in this employee's potential for returning to work. The marginal relationship with his supervisor, the threat of a reduction in the workforce, and the risk of losing economic security have a significant impact on the worker's loyalty to the employer. The worker's self-interest in controlling the negative impact of the work environment conflicted with the employer's self-interest in reduced lost time and increased productivity.

Litigation activity then becomes the battleground in which worker-employer adversity is played out. Independent medical examiners become mercenaries, while attorneys draw up the battle plans. Once the war has ended, the generals claim their victories, which are measured in legal fees, while injured workers are counted among the casualties.

Corporate attorneys may try to gather and present evidence that minimizes the disabled worker's functional impairment and work disability. If the extent and consequences of disability are reduced, then the cash settlement is also reduced, and the short-term self-interest of the employer is satisfied. However, the attorney's failure to recognize the subjective nature of the worker's disability often competes with the injured worker's need to secure financial independence because of a significantly disabling condition. Litigation, by its adversarial nature, causes further animosity. Labor relations between the employer and the worker (including some sympathetic co-workers) is often irreversibly damaged.

The injured worker's attorney uses a different strategy, hoping to offer evidence that maximizes the client's impairments and disabilities. More extensive impairments translate into larger settlements (and larger attorney's fees). The self-interest of the attorney is often financial in nature rather than rehabilitative in spirit. The disabled worker may be discouraged from participating in vocational rehabilitation and return-to-work activities during the litigation process. As time passes, the injured worker's general health often deteriorates, the family structure is frequently disrupted, and psychological, social, and stress problems begin to dominate.

Battles involving injured-worker issues are fought in the home as well as the courtroom. As the previous case study revealed, secondary psychosocial problems typically emerge as lost work time increases. Relationships with family members often deteriorate rapidly under the strain of self-abusive behaviors and learned helplessness. Maladaptive behaviors resulting from work disruption are common. When other family members are affected by the "fall out" of a litigated disability claim, pathological relationships within the family emerge. The disabled worker undergoes "role changes." Family members experience "role-change reactions." The once independent, self-supporting worker now takes on a role of passive dependency. Resentment abounds when the family is disrupted by the presence of an ever-demanding, sometimes angry, and often depressed individual. This is a typical outcome of unresolved labor relations problems, fueled by stress, and ignited by litigation activity and intense adversarial proceedings. Although the relationship among these forces is not always understood, the damage is usually profound.

Disability Management Benefits to Employers and Workers

Problems reflected in the earlier case study can be avoided through the development of effective disability management programs at worksites. Such programs enable the employer to do the following:

- Gain control of the adverse consequences of disabilities
- Improve corporate competitiveness
- Reduce work disruptions and unacceptable lost time
- Decrease the incidence of accidents and magnitude of disability
- Reduce illness and disability duration (and costs)
- Promote early involvement and preventive interventions
- Maximize the use of internal (worksite) resources
- Strengthen the accountability of external community service providers

The worker with an injury or disability benefits when the disability management program accomplishes the following:

- Reduces the human cost of disability
- Enhances morale by valuing employee physical and cultural diversity
- Protects the employability of the worker
- Insures compliance with ADA and other legislation
- Reduces the adversarial nature of disability and litigation
- Improves labor relations
- Promotes joint labor–management collaboration
- Facilitates direct worker involvement in work-return planning
- Increases worksite accommodation options to maintain productive work activity

COMMONSENSE PERSPECTIVES ON DISABILITY MANAGEMENT

Implementing disability management programs at worksites is a complex process that is often impeded by adverse labor relations, competing self-interests, lack of accountability, negative attitudes toward persons with disabilities, and lack of knowledge or skills among worksite personnel. However, much of disability management practice is rooted in "commonsense" principles. The following sections illustrate a few of these principles on which effective disability management programs can be designed and implemented (Shrey, 1997).

Paying Disabled Workers

Many worksites continue to embrace the policy of not returning injured workers to work until they are 100% fit for duty. It is unfair that injured workers are required to be 100% productive on returning to work, while many workers without disabilities continue working at less than 100% efficiency. Nevertheless, many injured workers unnecessarily face barriers imposed by such archaic attitudes and illogical expectations. However, many advanced engineering and ergonomic technologies and endless accommodations have enabled the most severely disabled persons to become productive employees.

Impairment and Occupational Disability

An impairment becomes an occupational disability only when accommodations are unavailable to permit the worker to perform the essential job functions. Impairments with no disabilities are present in blind secretaries, deaf engineers, one-armed mechanics, and computer operators who are quadraplegics.

Physicians' Familiarity with Physical Job Demands

The vast majority of physicians know little about occupational disability, and they spend little or no time at worksites (Scheer, 1995). Therefore, they have little knowledge of work environments, job tasks, working conditions, work processes, and labor relations. Aside from having little or no training in performing functional assessments, most physicians do not have access to the requisite testing equipment, nor do they schedule their patients for the lengthy appointments required to undergo functional capacity assessments. However, return-to-work decisions are often left to physicians who are unable to make valid determinations. Physicians need to be educated about the nature of work environments so that their opinions on work restrictions are valid. Also, they must be accountable for producing objective evidence to support their opinions regarding functional limitations and work disability.

Failure of Light-Duty Programs

Light duty is often perceived negatively by labor and management, particularly because traditional light-duty programs have met with only limited success. The reasons for light-duty failure are often simple and obvious. Perhaps the most common problem associated with the traditional light-duty model is that the period of light-duty work is typically open-ended. Many workers remain in light-duty assignments for indefinite periods of time, sometimes resulting (unnecessarily) in permanent placements. This situation is usually the result of a lack of therapeutic supervision and monitoring of the injured worker. Other problems of light duty arise out of conflicts caused by collective bargaining agreements that make it possible for a more senior employee to bump an injured worker out of a light-duty job. A situation such as this stems from ineffective coordination with the union and the lack of a formal policy responsive to such issues.

It is important to distinguish *transitional work* from traditional light-duty programs. The transitional work program model is preferable to the limited light-duty model. Transitional work is focused on real-work activities at the worksite as an interim step in the return-to-work process. It includes a transitional period of adjustment and adaptation, along with temporary accommodations, physical reconditioning, and safe work practices education for the injured worker. One major advantage of transitional work over traditional light-duty assignments is the ongoing monitoring and progressive upgrading of real-work activities, which gradually result in safely returning the worker to full duty (i.e., the original job). Light-duty programs typically rely on inexperienced work supervisors in attempting to accomplish this objective. However, this approach is risky unless supervisors have the experience and clinical skills to achieve the worker's safe and successful transition. Time spent in a light-duty program is sometimes insufficient to enable a worker to return to full duty. Transitional work concepts make it possible to use work activities as therapeutic modalities and progressively condition the worker to resume her or his usual job duties.

Return-to-Work Outcomes

Strong research evidence in disability management suggests that return-to-work outcomes are greater among worksites that assume internal responsibility and accountability for their workers with disabilities (Habeck, 1993). Regardless of the worker's physical recovery process, an effective return to work will not occur without a facilitative and receptive work environment. It is important for employers to develop an infrastructure that creates opportunities for temporary accommodations and alternative, productive work options while the worker is completing the physical recovery process. Together, labor and management representatives are intimately familiar with labor relations issues, the corporate culture, and co-worker/supervisor receptivity to reintegrating workers with disabilities. Conversely, outside third parties often lack an intimate knowledge of internal worksite resources and the potential "points of resistance" in a return-to-work effort. Therefore, it is important for worksite representatives to assume control over the return-to-work process, which may include delegating responsibility to external third parties, holding them accountable for what they offer to the return-to-work plan.

Worker Motivation to Return to Work

All injured workers are motivated. Some are motivated to return to work. Others are motivated to avoid returning to work. Worker disability is often more closely associated with labor relations problems than with medical problems. Workers who derive high levels of satisfaction from their work feel a sense of loss when they experience a major work disruption. They are often motivated to recover their losses by returning to work as quickly as possible. However, dissatisfied workers often feel that nothing has been lost when they are separated from the work environment. In fact, avoiding work can be quite rewarding; such workers may be eluding adverse relationships with co-workers or supervisors, or they may be escaping job tasks and responsibilities that contribute to job dissatisfaction. Conflicts at the worker-supervisor level can be a major factor contributing to unnecessary lost time. Common sense would dictate that many worker disability and lost-time problems could be resolved by avoiding such conflicts or by applying appropriate conflict resolution strategies. Labor and management representatives can benefit greatly from an awareness of disability management concepts, many of which address labor relations issues and interpersonal relationships between injured workers and others.

Worksite Disability Management Coordinator Training

At many worksites, disability management roles and functions are often delegated to individuals who lack the essential knowledge and skills to perform these important responsibilities. This situation can lead to management frustration and inadequate service coordination among injured workers. There is a growing need for disability management coordinators to carry out the day-to-day activities involved in assisting workers with disabilities. These coordinators work with safety committee members, human resources and benefits officers, health service and rehabilitation providers, and insurance and benefit program staff to manage a process that includes steps taken prior to injury, at injury, during recovery, and after the employee's return to work.

THE DISABILITY MANAGEMENT PROGRAM WITHIN THE CORPORATE ENVIRONMENT

Increasing workers' compensation and health care costs are threatening the survival of business and draining resources otherwise allocated for future economic development. Despite the rapidly escalating costs of injury and disability, rehabilitation technologies and disability management resources are available to facilitate immediate and recurrent savings for business and industry. Disability management policies, procedures, and strategies properly integrated into the worksite provide the infrastructure that enables employers to effectively manage disability and continue to compete in a global environment (Mital & Shrey, 1996).

Consider the following case study, in light of essential disability management controls and the employer's capacity to effectively manage injury and disability problems.

Disability Management Program Development: Case Study Analysis

The Alpha Corporation is a unionized worksite with 900 employees. Work was plentiful at Alpha Corporation during past years. However, because of worldwide competition, Alpha has recently lost its bids for several major production contracts. Alpha has undergone the first stage of organizational restructuring, which has resulted in the consolidation of several management positions and the elimination of 150 jobs. There have been rumors of additional lay-offs at the plant, and workers are concerned about the loss of job security. In order to remain competitive, Alpha has initiated discussions with a close competitor, Beta Corporation, regarding the advantages of merging the two companies to gain strength in the marketplace.

Historically, labor relations and the corporate culture at Alpha reflected feelings of labor–management conflict, mistrust, and resistance to disability management principles. Management has viewed injured workers as opportunists who prefer lost-time benefits to working. Labor sees management as being manipulative and inconsistent in its response to workers with disabilities. Adversarial relationships between workers with disabilities and management are expected when disability claims are filed. Recently, however, labor and management have indicated an interest in developing a disability management program. There has been some degree of tolerance between labor and management, but considerable changes in attitudes are required on both sides if an effective disability management program is to emerge. Labor wants to protect its injured or disabled members' jobs. Management wants to reduce unnecessary costs.

The average number of workers' lost-time days has nearly doubled over the past three years. Management recognizes the need to reduce rapidly escalating workers' compensation and disability insurance costs. Beta Corporation has expressed some reservations regarding a possible merger with Alpha due to the liabilities associated with these uncontrolled disability costs.

Alpha Corporation is seriously inadequate in internal and external communications related to effective disability management. Generally, no one establishes direct contact with treating physicians. Work return activities are often initiated by the injured worker or an external rehabilitation provider; there is little worksite representative involvement. There is considerable confusion at this worksite as to where the responsibility lies for return-to-work coordination. There is a safety manager at the worksite who has been trying to coordinate return-to-work activities, working without sufficient support, direction, or resources. This individual is seriously deficient in knowledge and skills and ineffective in coordinating work-return activities for workers with disabilities. Lacking a full commitment to transitional work, Alpha often operates an "informal" return-to-work process. Coordination is typically left to chance, with no one specifically accountable for reducing unnecessary lost time or for accommodating workers with disabilities.

Overall, Alpha tends to be "reactive" to occupational injury and disability. There is no evidence of coordination between the administration of worker's compensation claims and other disability insurance claims (i.e., short-term and long-term disability). Interventions are often late rather than early, and they tend to be responsive only in crises. Monitoring of injured workers by Alpha's occupational health nurse is sporadic, and it is often perceived by workers as being intrusive rather than facilitative. All case management activities have been relinquished to an external rehabilitation specialist with very limited involvement at the worksite. Case management is generally limited to the telephonic monitoring of medical treatments during the injury recovery process.

KEY CONTROLS FOR EFFECTIVE DISABILITY MANAGEMENT

The Alpha Corporation is strongly characterized as a worksite with weak controls with respect to disability management. Generally, many employers are viewed as having a combination of strengths and weaknesses related to disability management strategies, interventions, and necessary controls. The ultimate goal in disability management strategic planning is to introduce proper controls where absent while strengthening existing controls. An effective disability management program at the worksite should reflect a "seamless" process of rehabilitation and return-to-work activities, beginning with the initial illness or injury experience and ending with the worker safely accommodated in meaningful productive work activity.

Steps in the Work-Injury Management Process

Initial Reporting

Once an accident occurs, all steps in the work-return process, beginning with the initial report of injury, must be properly managed. Typically, it is the supervisor who first becomes aware of the initial illness or injury because most employers expect their workers to promptly report injuries and illnesses to their immediate supervisors. Internal communication of illnesses and injuries often involve accident reports being sent to the human resources department, and OSHA-recordable injuries being filed with the employer's safety representative. External communications involve reporting to insurance carriers, workers' compensation boards, managed care organizations, and third-party claims administrators.

Emergency Treatment

Following an accident, the injured worker is typically transported to a local treatment facility. Doing this opens up an opportunity to establish the initial point of communication between the treatment physician, the injured worker, and the employer. The direct involvement of the supervisor during the initial injury experience assures the worker that the employer cares about the worker's recovery and values responsive medical treatment. This early involvement of the supervisor also enables the employer to provide the physician with accurate information regarding the worker's job, including the kinds of accommodations that the employer will offer to influence a safe and timely return to work.

Early Response to Expected Lost Time

When lost time is anticipated as a result of an injury or illness, it is important to initiate immediate contact with the worker's treating physician. This is the critical time to communicate to the physician the physical demands of the worker's job and to ascertain from the physician the worker's restrictions and functional abilities. When expected periods of work disruption are relatively short (7 days or less), the worksite's disability manager or case manager meets with the worker's supervisor to review the employee's work restrictions and to identify accommodations needed to facilitate an effective return to work. Options are communicated to the physician to influence the worker's timely release to return to the original job or to a temporary, modified job. More lengthy work disruptions may require multiple interventions and more extensive case management, especially when few return-to-work options exist, or when the multidisciplinary needs of the worker become more complex.

Individualized Transitional Work Plans

The return-to-work plan is developed concurrently with an assessment of the worker's functional abilities as related to the physical demands of the job. Workers who require more than basic accommodations may benefit from involvement in a transitional work program. The worker's transitional work plan is a written document, designed with the worker's active involvement to identify specific tasks to be performed for designated time periods. Worker participation in conditioning activities may be combined with work activities for optimal strengthening and safe work performance. Job-site modifications and accommodations are also important components of a transitional work plan, ensuring greater compatibility between physical job demands and the worker's functional capacities.

The success of the transitional work program is only limited by the flexibility and creativity of those involved in developing transitional work options for the injured worker. Transitional work is defined as *any combination of tasks, functions, or jobs that a worker who has functional restrictions can perform safely, for pay, and without the risk of injury to self or other workers* (Shrey & Lacerte, 1995). Transitional work programs are typically 8–12 weeks in duration rather than permanent job placements. They require ongoing evaluation of the worker's job performance, with gradual upgrading of job tasks as the worker gains strength and endurance through proper exercise, therapy, and conditioning activities.

Transitional work programs are often strengthened by developing a *job bank*, a reservoir of temporary, meaningful, and productive jobs or job tasks (sedentary to light-work activity) that can be performed while the worker is making a recovery from injury or illness. Work tasks and jobs from the job bank can be flexibly assigned to workers on a day-to-day basis to facilitate a return to the worker's regular job or to a permanent, modified job. For example, if the worker is unable to perform the essential functions of his or her regular job, the worker is enabled to perform only those original jobs tasks that are compatible with his or her functional capacities. The job bank is an effective resource thàt helps to reduce or eliminate lost time, which relates directly to reducing workers' compensation and other disability costs.

Worker Monitoring

After the worker begins the transitional work program, ongoing monitoring of her or his progress is performed by the supervisor or another designated worksite representative. In some worksites, physical or occupational therapists perform periodic monitoring of workers to document progress. As the worker progresses through conditioning and work readjustment, the job tasks are upgraded to be more physically challenging, and more of the worker's original job tasks are reintroduced. The worker's time involvement in transitional work activity may also be gradually increased (work hours or work days) as he or she achieves higher levels of performance. Worker monitoring, when done in a caring fashion, gives assurance that labor and management value the injured worker as a contributing member of the work group.

DISABILITY MANAGEMENT CONTROLS: BUILDING THE WORKSITE INFRASTRUCTURE

This section summarizes the key controls necessary for establishing a strong workplace disability management infrastructure that will support disability management and return-to-work-objectives. Increasing evidence suggests that the ability to control workers' compensation and disability costs are, for the most part, within the employer's grasp (Shrey, 1995b). Habeck (1993) reported that the results of a survey of 124 Michigan firms supported the assumption that many factors causing unacceptable workers' compensation costs are internal to companies and within the employer's power to control. The study identified two distinct and equally weighted processes involved in disability management: those involving injury prevention, and those involving disability management after injury occurrence. Management philosophy, policies, and practices were found to be strongly related to successful claims outcome. Factors related to favorable claims experiences included an open management style, a human resource orientation, a more rigorous adoption of safety and prevention interventions, and specific procedures to prevent and manage disabilities.

According to Shrey (1995a), the following disability management strategies have been demonstrated to control the adverse effects of workplace injury:

1. Analyze management's capacity to respond to injury and disability.
2. Know your organization's strengths and weaknesses as well as the resources available to properly manage the injured worker's safe and timely return to work.
3. Understand the corporate culture, including the attitudes, motivations, and self-interests of labor and management regarding injury prevention, worksite accommodation, and injured-worker rehabilitation.
4. Recognize the unique patterns of injury and disability in the workforce, including types of impairments, ages of workers, lost-time statistics, accident data, and costs associated with disability claims.
5. Promote early interventions and the systematic monitoring of injured workers.
6. Design benefit plans to reward disabled workers for returning to work and remaining healthy and productive.
7. Develop flexible and creative work-return transition options and reasonable accommodations for disabled workers.
8. Support positive labor relations that promote job satisfaction and worker involvement in decision making.
9. Be sensitive to the psychological and social consequences of injury and disability and the overall impact of work disruption on the worker's family.
10. Actively promote accident prevention and risk reduction programs by encouraging employee input.
11. Do not relinquish all company control and responsibility to "outside" third parties, such as insurance carriers, claims administrators, and attorneys. Rather, develop functional alliances between quality resources and the employer-based disability management system.
12. Understand the value of securing vocational rehabilitation and effective case management services for workers with restrictions.
13. Create expectations among employees regarding the policies and procedures to follow from the point of injury to the safe return to work.
14. Provide treating physicians with information regarding the physical demands of the injured worker's job, and invite them to visit production sites and work areas.
15. Get directly involved by identifying, utilizing, and evaluating effective medical and rehabilitation services in the community. "Internalize" these external resources, making them part of the worksite's disability management infrastructure. Then, guide injured workers to responsible service providers.
16. Seek independent medical and physical capacity evaluations when evaluating questionable claims or when reviewing medical reports that fail to objectively substantiate the worker's alleged impairments and medical restrictions.
17. Create labor–management agreements that protect the employability of the worker by identifying alternatives to costly work disruptions and chronic absenteeism.
18. Analyze jobs that cause injuries, and develop effective ergonomic modifications that prevent future work disabilities.

The key controls for effective disability management are organized within three major categories: (1) disability management policy and worksite resources, (2) disability prevention, and (3) early intervention and timely return-to-work process.

Disability Management Policy and Worksite Resources

Joint Labor–Management Support and Empowerment

The foundation of worksite disability management is joint labor–management support and empowerment. Both unions and managers are key contributors in the disability management process when they participate cooperatively as decision-makers, planners, and coordinators of interventions and services. Joint labor–management support occurs when senior labor and management representatives exercise their leadership influence to facilitate a spirit of cooperation among all workplace stakeholders. Together, labor and management create expectations for success, jointly developing disability management policies and practices.

Responsibility and Accountability

Effective worksite disability management programs require high levels of communication and coordination within the workplace and between the worksite and the community. The strength and effectiveness of a worksite disability management program often depends upon the extent to which *responsibility*, *accountability*, and *authority* are vested in the designated disability management coordinator.

Corporate Culture—Worker and Supervisor Expectations

Effective worksite disability management programs require that the intentions of employers and the expectations of workers be consistent with one another. When formal return-to-work processes are not in place, workers often expect that the only consequence of a lost-time injury is paid compensation. Concurrently, managers and supervisors often expect that workers' compensation costs are merely the "costs of doing business." In reality, disability costs are frequently the cost of "not taking care of business." It is important that workers and supervisors receive a proper orientation regarding the importance of worksite disability management, the benefits to workers with disabilities, and the value of disability management practices to the employing organization.

Internal and External Communications

At the worksite, the operational aspects of the worksite disability management program require consistent and accurate internal communications between employees, managers, supervisors, and labor representatives. External communications enhance the employer's relationship with treating physicians, claims managers, rehabilitation service providers, and workers' compensation administrators.

Knowledge and Skills of the Disability Management Coordinator

Highly effective worksites typically have a designated disability management coordinator who has demonstrated a broad range of knowledge and skills in the development of disability management policies and procedures and the coordination of return-to-work activities for workers with disabilities.

Disability Prevention

Accident Prevention and Safety Programs

When no accidents occur, there are no adverse consequences for the worker or the employer. Therefore, to a great extent, the success of a worksite's disability management program depends on the strength of accident prevention and safety initiatives. Optimal worksites have formal safety departments or joint labor–management safety committees that are responsible for administering the safety program and investigating accidents and injuries. There is close monitoring of all potential risks and hazards at the worksite, and workers who become ill or injured receive prompt and proper medical care.

Occupational Ergonomics

Ergonomics aims at fitting the task to individuals and represents a proactive approach to injury control. It ensures that the tasks are designed so that the demands imposed on individuals are within their capabilities. When this goal is accomplished, the risk of injury is greatly reduced. It should also be realized that even when workplaces, equipment, and tools are ergonomically designed, some injuries will occur. The injured workers then need to be accommodated in the workplace. The role of ergonomics is not simply making job accommodations to integrate injured workers. Rather, it involves determining the residual work capacities of injured workers, developing ergonomically designed physical training programs to enhance workers' capabilities, designing work and schedules during the transition from being occupationally disabled to a full return-to-work status, and making changes in the workplace, if needed, to accommodate the individual (Mital, 1995; Mital & Shrey, 1996).

Health Promotion and Wellness

Those workplaces that demonstrate a caring attitude for the health and wellness of their workers are likely to have greater success in controlling workers' compensation and disability costs. Health promotion and wellness programs at the worksite have experienced great popularity and growth over the past decade. They may include weight-loss programs, smoking cessation clinics, aerobic exercising, stress management, intramural sports, jogging groups, and a multitude of activities performed at corporate fitness centers.

Injury, Disability, and Lost-Time Patterns

Data establishing the unique disability patterns within any worksite are necessary when designing a disability management program that is responsive to types of injuries among workers in various age groups employed in different work categories. The interventions and services that characterize a worksite's disability management system should be based on carefully diagnosed problems and factors specific to the workforce. Otherwise, the interventions used may fail to resolve the problems at hand.

Disability Cost Data

An employer's total cost of injury can be elusive because the hidden costs of disability have been calculated to exceed those costs that are more easily ascertained. For example, hidden costs often include all the costs of replacing a nonproductive injured worker. The analysis of disability patterns and their associated costs are essential to building the worksite's foundation for disability management. The financial success of a disability management program is measured in reduced expenditures. Therefore, it is important to achieve a baseline measure of a worksite's cost patterns from the beginning. Cost patterns associated with community treatment providers and service outcomes also allow an employer to survey the market and compare for cost-effectiveness.

Early Intervention and Timely Return-to-Work Process

Early Intervention and Worker Monitoring Protocol

Early intervention and worker monitoring is critical to the return-to-work process, and it begins with the initial injury that is expected to result in work restrictions or lost time. Monitoring should be "worker-centered," focusing on the physical, psychosocial, economic, occupational, and family needs of the worker with a disability. Monitoring should be supportive of the worker, ensuring that he or she has access to information related to medical treatment, job-site accommodations, and resources to facilitate the return-to-work process. In optimal disability management programs, the worksite disability management coordinator maintains direct continuous contact with the injured worker, monitoring medical treatments, outcomes, and all objectives of the return-to-work plan. Monitoring, when done in a caring fashion, gives assurance that labor and management value the injured worker as a contributing member of the work group.

Case Management Procedures

Case management services are necessary to facilitate the development and implementation of disability management strategies and return-to-work plans for workers with disabilities. The case manager serves as a central disability management team member by functioning as a liaison between employers, labor representatives, injured workers, community health care providers, and others. Case managers coordinate the worksite's response to injury and disability through the development and implementation of rehabilitation plans and work-return/work transition programs.

Return-to-Work Coordination

Effective return-to-work programs require a high level of internal (worksite) coordination and communication, as well as the coordination of activities among external (community) medical services, rehabilitation providers, and others. Return-to-work coordination requires an understanding of the worker with a disability and the work environment. Among optimal disability management programs, the steps from injury to work return are clearly delineated and understood by workers and employers. Essential coordination roles of the disability management coordinator are to (a) establish communication lines, (b) explain the program's objectives to the injured worker, (c) develop and implement the return-to-work plan with the injured worker and others, and (d) monitor the worker's progress and coordinate additional services or interventions, as required.

Transitional Work Options

Transitional work, as described earlier in this chapter, represents a proactive disability management strategy that formalizes the work-return process by providing organization, structure, and accountability. The transitional work assignments must be meaningful and productive; these assignments must contribute to the company's operations and provide a returning worker with a worthwhile job. Creating senseless jobs for the sole purpose of getting the person back to work insults the worker's integrity and undermines the therapeutic value of transitional work. Effective transitional work programs at worksites are often managed by a joint labor–management committee, the members of which represent key worksite departments and labor unions (Shrey & Lacerte, 1995).

Worksite Accommodations

Worksite accommodations include modifications or adjustments to the job, job site, or the way that a job is performed that allow a person with an injury or disability to perform work tasks safely and with increased independence. Many managers, labor representatives, and workers have been implementing job modifications and accommodations informally for many years. Increasingly, worksite accommodations are being recognized as effective tools in disability management planning.

Program Coordination and Ongoing Maintenance

Established return-to-work programs must be efficiently coordinated. They must also be continuously evaluated, improved, and maintained. Accomplishing this requires a high level of internal (worksite) coordination and communication and the coordination of activities between external (community) medical services, rehabilitation providers, and others. Return-to-work coordination requires an understanding of the worker with a disability and the work environment. Among optimal disability management programs, the steps from injury to work return are clearly delineated and understood by workers and employers. The disability management coordinator's essential roles are to (a) establish communication lines, (b) explain the program's objectives to the injured worker, (c) develop and implement the return-to-work plan with the injured worker and others, and (d) monitor the worker's progress and coordinate additional services or interventions, as required.

OUTCOMES OF MODEL DISABILITY MANAGEMENT/TRANSITIONAL WORK PROGRAMS

In recent years, U.S. business and industry have consistently reported significant outcomes as a result of having developed and implemented disability management programs. Consumer Power Company's program resulted in a 48% decrease in the number of work days lost due to recordable lost-time injuries. Safeway Stores saved eight dollars for each dollar spent and reduced back injuries and related costs by 50%. Marriott, with 20,000 employees in 50 states, reduced the number of workers' compensation cases by from 30 to 50%, saved four dollars for every dollar spent, and reduced litigated workers' compensation cases by 50%. Lockheed Missile and Space Company reduced worker visits for physical therapy and associated costs by 50% during the first year of its operation (Shrey, 1995a).

This author has developed several disability management programs in the United States and Canada, many of which have shown reductions of 30% or more in workers' compensation and disability costs. One model program at TS Trim Industries, a U.S.-based company in Ohio, reported exceptionally strong outcomes for its worksite-based disability management program. A consulting physical therapist at the worksite has been a key factor in successful return-to-work results. Prior to establishing the program in fiscal year 1994–1995, TS Trim had 17 lost-time workers' compensation claims, resulting in 508 total lost days. Medical costs totaled $240,282; wage replacement costs were $144,083. Outcomes reported from June 1996 to May 1997 were 23 lost-time claims, totaling 311 lost days. Wage replacement costs were reduced to $41,460.

A customized transitional work program was developed for all workers with restrictions for the city of Oregon, Ohio. This program featured a joint labor–management committee on disability management that included representatives from management and five major unions. The program reduced lost time and associated costs by offering a systematic return-to-work program for employees, including firefighters, police, wastewater treatment workers, street workers, and other municipal employees. A similar program, which will feature a joint labor–management committee, transitional work options, and established job banks for all city divisions, is currently being developed for the city of Cincinnati's disability retirement and workers' compensation benefits program.

This author has worked with management of the Hubert Company in Cincinnati to establish an internal disability management committee. Together we designed a customized disability management system, which included a formal policy and procedure manual for work-injury management, an early intervention system, accident and incident reporting forms, a charge-back system to ensure accountability for work return among all departments, a job bank with over 40 temporary alternative duty options for injured workers, and a customized transitional work program. This program achieved immediate success in reducing lost time by introducing return-to-work options for workers with chronic disabling conditions who had accumulated extensive lost time. This program is currently controlling Hubert's workers' compensation and short-term disability costs.

Effective Disability Management in Canadian Business and Industry

The author of this chapter has assisted in developing Canada's National Institute for Disability Management and Research, an organization that actively promotes joint labor–management training in disability management. The institute has actively promoted disability management concepts in Canada through a number of research and training initiatives (Shrey, 1997). The following outcomes have been reported among Canadian worksites that have adopted variations of disability management and transitional work models.

At the Alberni Specialties Division of MacMillan Bloedel, Port Alberni, British Columbia, the worksite's long-term disability (LTD) and short-term disability (STD) costs were found to be three times the industrial average. A disability management program was developed in 1995, which showed a total return of 38 workers as of February 1997. The average lost time among these workers was 16 months, which is significant in that one year or more lost time typically results in a minimal probability of return to work. LTD premium costs were reduced by 25%; STD premium costs were reduced by 20%. A savings of $1.25 million was realized in one year.

At the Somass Division of MacMillan Bloedel, a formal disability management program was initiated in 1994 as a pilot program to demonstrate the impact of joint labor–management collaboration. Of 120 workers who participated in the program, 112 had returned to work as of July 1996. Length of lost time ranged from 4 weeks to 13 years. Fourteen workers on LTD returned to work; six of these workers had a total of 148 years of benefits payments remaining, at a net present value of $2.486 million. Workers' compensation costs were reduced by 50%, and the number of workers involved in lost-time accidents was reduced from 48 to 8. The number of workers on workers' compensation was reduced from 37 in 1991 to 5 in 1996.

Two internal disability management coordinators jointly manage the return-to-work program of British Columbia Hydro and Power Authority, a provincial Crown corporation and the third-largest electrical utility in Canada, employing approximately 5,000 workers. Lost time at BF Hydro has decreased by 65%, which resulted in a reduction of workers' compensation premiums of $700,000 in 1996. Projected savings are estimated at over $1 million over the next four years. Lost-time cases of 10 days or more have been reduced from 82 in 1995 to 51 in 1996. BC Hydro's original return-to-work pilot program realized a savings of $449,862 over a six-month period.

Recent research conducted reflects similar outcomes among worksites that have embraced a disability management philosophy. For example, Fletcher Challenge Canada in Campbell River, British Columbia, reported a decrease in lost-time days from 1,250 in 1994 to 850 in 1996. Total cost savings were conservatively estimated at $792,000 from 1994 to 1996.

The city of Lethbridge, Alberta, adopted a modified work program model, with time lines of 2 weeks to 3 months for injured workers who are participating. Employees are paid 100% of wages while participating in the program. Costs for lost-time disability payments are being charged back to the budgets of the workers' original departments, which creates incentives for supervisor accountability in the work-return process. Lethridge boasts results that include a reduction of claims from 40 in 1990 to 14 in 1995, and only 7 lost-time claims reported for the first half of 1996.

Similar outcomes were reported by the city of Vancouver, with its workforce of 8,000 employees. The city uses two in-house disability management coordinators to track employees with lost time, provide case management services, resolve supervisor-employee conflicts, and coordinate services and referrals. In 1993–1994, the city experienced a reduction of 2,020 hours of lost time. It was again reduced by 1,200 hours in 1994–1995, and by 800 hours in 1995–1996. Reductions in wage losses for these three years were estimated at $650,000, $300,000, and $210,000 respectively. Also, workers' compensation assessments were reduced by $150,000 in 1995, $200,000 in 1996, and an estimated $800,000 for 1997.

Interlink Freight Systems in Willowdale, Ontario, is moving toward a formal disability management system for its 2,400 unionized employees (Transportation Communications Union). Compensation costs were high and Interlink was in a penalty workers' compensation rating. The company was purchased by its own employees and initiated a joint labor–management program to manage workers' compensation, LTD, and STD claims. Current outcome statistics reported 419 lost-time injuries resulting in 16,117 total lost days in 1994. In 1995, lost-time injuries were reduced to 313, for a total of 7,061 lost days. In 1996, further reductions to 256 lost-time injuries were reported, with a total of 5,559 lost days.

Highland Valley Copper in Logan Lake, British Columbia, in collaboration with United Steelworkers of America Local 7619, initiated a work transition center for their mining operation's 1,100 employees. The return-to-work goal is established by the treating doctor, who identifies guidelines for levels of physical activities and work restrictions. The injured worker's department is canvassed for suitable temporary work, based on these guidelines. When options are unavailable, the Modified Work Centre is accessed, which makes supervised opportunities available to the worker from 8 A.M. to 4 P.M. 5 days per week. The center's main volume of work opportunities is focused on the recycling of mine supplies, reuse of items, and reduction of waste. Total work days saved by accommodations at regular job sites totaled 1,656; 694 work days were saved by accommodating workers at the center. Bottom-line workers' compensation savings in 1996 were calculated at $86,512, with weekly indemnity savings of $123,510 (based on days not charged to these accounts). Additionally, goods produced at the center, along with services provided to other mining operations departments, amounted to an added value of $640,000, with operational costs of $419,123.

Westmin Resources-Gibralter Mines, at Mileesa Lake, British Columbia, a smaller mining operation with 275 unionized workers (Canadian Auto Workers Local 3018), was faced with high workers' compensation premiums, high insurance carrier premiums, and 666 days of lost time for 24 accidents in 1991. In 1996, this worksite's disability management program reported only two lost-time accidents for nine days of total lost time. Short-term disability costs were reduced from $58,000 in 1993 to $12,000 in 1995. Among workers accommodated at this worksite were three with injuries that included a broken foot, a broken ankle, and a fractured arm. None experienced more than five days lost time.

CONCLUSIONS

Overall, worksite-based disability management programs have produced important benefits for workers with disabilities and their employers. Research results reflect recurrent savings among worksites that adopt caring attitudes and formal return-to-work programs. More important are the outcomes for workers with disabilities who are enabled to maintain meaningful, productive employment and provide for their families. Building a strong disability management infrastructure at a worksite requires a strong commitment and careful planning by labor and management.

Clearly, the worksite holds great potential for being a responsive, proactive, therapeutic environment for workers with disabilities. We are on the threshold of a new paradigm in work-injury management. The focus is shifting from community-based medical treatment programs to accommodating worksites with transitional work options. Vocational rehabilitation expertise, which has been traditionally in the domain of external service providers, is giving way to rapidly evolving disability management models and return-to-work programs that are coordinated by worksite-based representatives.

REFERENCES

Akabas, S., Gates, L., & Galvin, D. (1992). *Disability management*. New York: Amacom.

Boschen, K. A. (1989). Early intervention in vocational rehabilitation. *Rehabilitation Counseling Bulletin, 32,* 34-45.

Galvin, D. (1985). Employer-based disability management and rehabilitation programs. *Annual Review of Rehabilitation,* 5.

Habeck, R. (1993). Achieving quality and value in service to the workplace, *Work Injury Management, 2*(3), 1, 3-5.

Linveh, H. (1986). A unified approach to existing models of adaptation to disability: Part I. A model adaptation. *Journal of Applied Rehabilitation Counseling, 17*(1), 5-16, 56.

Mital, A. (1995). Ergonomics, injury prevention, and disability management. In D. Shrey & M. Lacerte (Eds.), *Principles & Practices of Disability Management in Industry* (pp. 157-171). Winter Park, FL: GR Press.

Mital, A., & Shrey, D. (1996). Back problems in health professionals: Extent of the problem and an integrated approach for its management. *Critical Reviews in Physical and Rehabilitation Management, 8*(3), 201-219.

Seligman, M. (1991).*Learned optimism*. New York: Alfred A. Knopf.

Scheer, S. J. (1995). The role of the physician in disability management. pp. 175-205.

Shrey, D. (1995a). Disability management practice at the work site: Developing, implementing and evaluating transitional work programs. In D. Shrey & M. Lacerte (Eds.), *Principles & Practices of Disability Management in Industry* (pp. 55-105). Winter Park, FL: GR Press.

Shrey, D. (1995b). Worksite disability management and Industrial Rehabilitation. In D. Shrey & M. Lacerte (Eds.), *Principles & Practices of Disability Management in Industry* (pp. 3-53). Winter Park, FL: GR Press.

Shrey, D. (1997, July 4). *Disability case management: The "Hot Issues."* Keynote address at the Association of Workers' Compensation Boards of Canada, Halifax, Nova Scotia, Canada.

Shrey, D., & Lacerte, M. (Eds.). (1995).

Principles and practices of disability management in industry. Winter Park, FL: GR Press.

Shrey, D., & Olsheski, J. (1992). Disability management and industry-based work return: Transition programs. In C. Gordon & P. E. Caplan (Eds.), *Physical Medicine & Rehabilitation: State of the Art Review* (pp. 303-314). Philadelphia: Hanley & Belfus.

Walker, J. M. (1992). Injured worker helplessness: Critical relationships and systems level approach for intervention. *Journal of Occupational Rehabilitation, 2*(4), 201-209.

Index

ISBN 0-306-45842-X

90000

9 780306 458422